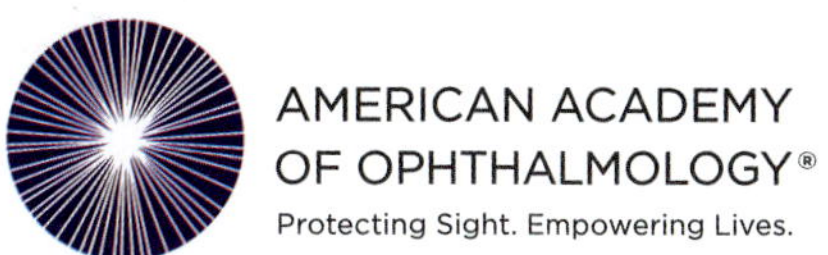

10 | Glaucoma

Major Revision Edition

2024–2025

BCSC

Basic and Clinical Science Course™

EB

Published after collaborative review with the European Board of Ophthalmology subcommittee

The American Academy of Ophthalmology is accredited by the Accreditation Council for Continuing Medical Education (ACCME) to provide continuing medical education for physicians.

The American Academy of Ophthalmology designates this enduring material for a maximum of 10 *AMA PRA Category 1 Credits*™. Physicians should claim only the credit commensurate with the extent of their participation in the activity.

CME expiration date: June 1, 2027. *AMA PRA Category 1 Credits*™ may be claimed only once between June 1, 2024, and the expiration date.

To claim *AMA PRA Category 1 Credits*™ upon completion of this activity, learners must demonstrate appropriate knowledge and participation in the activity by taking the posttest for Section 10 and achieving a score of 80% or higher. For further details, please see the instructions for requesting CME credit at the back of the book.

The Academy provides this material for educational purposes only. It is not intended to represent the only or best method or procedure in every case, nor to replace a physician's own judgment or give specific advice for case management. Including all indications, contraindications, side effects, and alternative agents for each drug or treatment is beyond the scope of this material. All information and recommendations should be verified, prior to use, with current information included in the manufacturers' package inserts or other independent sources, and considered in light of the patient's condition and history. Reference to certain drugs, instruments, and other products in this course is made for illustrative purposes only and is not intended to constitute an endorsement of such. Some material may include information on applications that are not considered community standard, that reflect indications not included in approved FDA labeling, or that are approved for use only in restricted research settings. **The FDA has stated that it is the responsibility of the physician to determine the FDA status of each drug or device he or she wishes to use, and to use them with appropriate, informed patient consent in compliance with applicable law.** The Academy specifically disclaims any and all liability for injury or other damages of any kind, from negligence or otherwise, for any and all claims that may arise from the use of any recommendations or other information contained herein.

Cover image: From BCSC Section 4, *Ophthalmic Pathology and Intraocular Tumors.* Photomicrograph of focal posttraumatic choroidal granulomatous inflammation. *(Courtesy of Vivian Lee, MD.)*

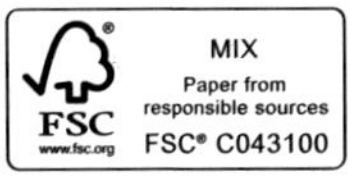

Printed in India.

Basic and Clinical Science Course

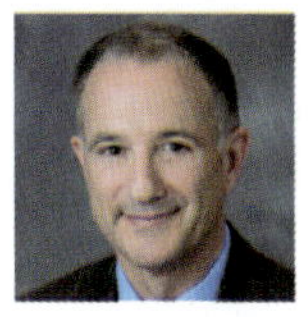

Christopher J. Rapuano, MD, Philadelphia, Pennsylvania
Senior Secretary for Clinical Education

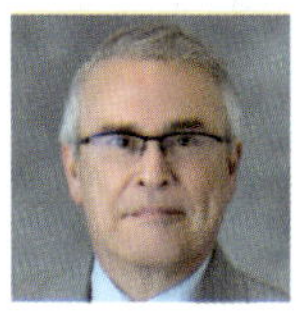

J. Timothy Stout, MD, PhD, MBA, Houston, Texas
Secretary for Lifelong Learning and Assessment

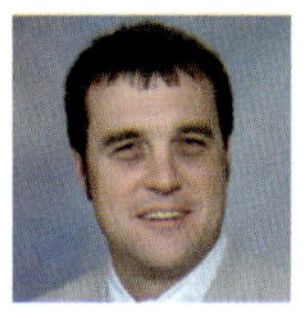

Colin A. McCannel, MD, Los Angeles, California
BCSC Course Chair

Section 10

Faculty for the Major Revision

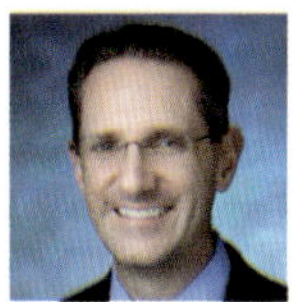

Michael V. Boland, MD, PhD
Chair
Boston, Massachusetts

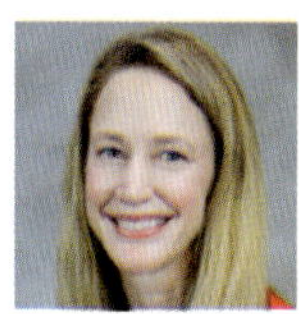

Kelly Walton Muir, MD, MHSc
Durham, North Carolina

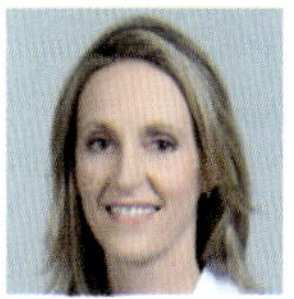

JoAnn A. Giaconi, MD
Los Angeles, California

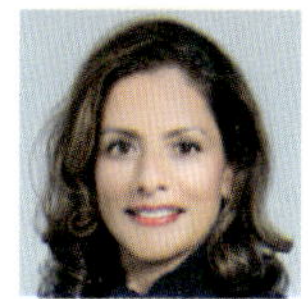

Shalini Sood, MD
Cleveland, Ohio

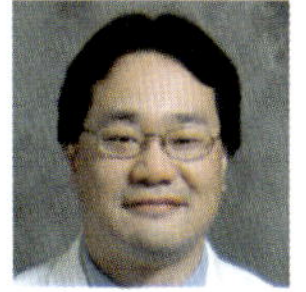

Richard K. Lee, MD, PhD
Miami, Florida

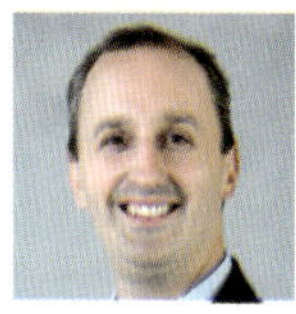

Derek S. Welsbie, MD, PhD
La Jolla, California

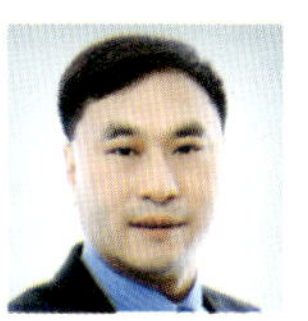

Shan C. Lin, MD
San Francisco, California

The Academy acknowledges the *American Glaucoma Society* for recommending faculty members to the BCSC Section 10 committee.

The Academy acknowledges the following committees for review of this edition:

Committee on Aging: Jonathan Young, MD, PhD, Portland, Oregon

Vision Rehabilitation Committee: Mona A. Kaleem, MD, Bethesda, Maryland

BCSC Resident/Fellow Reviewers: Sharon L. Jick, MD, *Chair,* St Louis, Missouri; Judy L. Chen, MD; Enny Omolara Oyeniran, MD; Kristi Y. Wu, MD

Practicing Ophthalmologists Advisory Committee for Education: Troy M. Tanji, MD, *Primary Reviewer,* Waipahu, Hawaii; Bradley D. Fouraker, MD, *Chair,* Tampa, Florida; George S. Ellis Jr, MD, New Orleans, Louisiana; Kevin E. Lai, MD, Carmel, Indiana; Philip R. Rizzuto, MD, Providence, Rhode Island; J. James Rowsey, MD, Largo, Florida; Gaurav K. Shah, MD, San Francisco, California; Scott X. Stevens, MD, Bend, Oregon

The Academy also acknowledges the following committee for assistance in developing Study Questions and Answers for this BCSC Section:

Resident Self-Assessment Committee: Amanda D. Henderson, MD, *Chair,* Baltimore, Maryland; Misha Syed, MD, Galveston, Texas

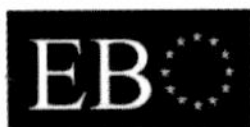

European Board of Ophthalmology: Anna P. Maino, MBBS, PGCert, *Liaison,* Manchester, England; Ian Rodrigues, PGCert, FEBOS-Glaucoma, *Chair,* London, England; Hana Abou Zeid, MD, FEBO, Geneva, Switzerland; Pouya Alaghband, MD(res), PGCert, York, England; Theodoros Filippopoulos, MD, Athens, Greece; Panayiota Founti, MD, PhD, FEBO, London, England; Dimitrios Giannoulis, MD, FEBO, Thessaloniki, Greece; Stylianos A. Kandarakis, MD, Athens, Greece; Antonio Moreno Valladares, MD, PhD, Albacete, Spain; Chiara Posarelli, MD, Lucca, Italy; Francesco Stringa, MBChB, FEBO, Southampton, England; Marc Toeteberg-Harms, MD, FEBO, Augusta, Georgia

Recent Past Faculty

Chandrasekharan Krishnan, MD
Felipe A. Medeiros, MD, PhD
Sayoko E. Moroi, MD, PhD
Arthur J. Sit, MD
Angelo P. Tanna, MD

The Academy also gratefully acknowledges the contributions of numerous past faculty and advisory committee members who have played an important role in the development of previous editions of the Basic and Clinical Science Course.

American Academy of Ophthalmology Staff

Dale E. Fajardo, EdD, MBA, *Vice President, Education*
Beth Wilson, *Director, Continuing Professional Development*

Denise Evenson, *Director, Brand & Creative*
Susan Malloy, *Acquisitions and Development Manager*
Stephanie Tanaka, *Publications Manager*
Jasmine Chen, *Manager, E-Learning*
Sarah Page, *Online Education and Licensing Manager*
Rayna Ungersma, *Manager, Curriculum Development*
Lana Ip, *Senior Designer*
Amanda Fernandez, *Publications Editor*
Beth Collins, *Medical Editor*
Kenny Guay, *Program Manager, Publications*
Debra Marchi, *Online Education Specialist*

Financial Disclosures

Academy staff members who contributed to the development of this product state that within the 24 months prior to their contributions to this CME activity and for the duration of development, they have had no financial interest in or other relationship with any entity whose primary business is producing, marketing, selling, reselling, or distributing health care products used by or in patients.

The authors and reviewers state that within the 24 months prior to their contributions to this CME activity and for the duration of development, they have had the following financial relationships:*

Dr Abou Zeid: Entre Vues Opticiens SA (O)

Dr Alaghband: Santen Pharmaceutical Co, Ltd (C), Théa Pharmaceuticals (L)

Dr Boland: Allergan (C), Carl Zeiss Meditec AG (C, L), Janssen Pharmaceuticals (C), Topcon Medical Systems, Inc (C)

Dr Founti: Théa Pharmaceuticals (L)

Dr Fouraker: AJL Ophthalmic, SA (C, L), Alcon Laboratories (C, L), OASIS Medical, Inc (C, L)

Dr Giaconi: Allergan (C, L), LightTouch (C), MediPrint Ophthalmics (C, SO)

Dr Giannoulis: AbbVie Inc (L)

Dr Lai: Twenty/Twenty Therapeutics LLC (C)

Dr Lee: Johnson & Johnson Vision (US), Mitsubishi Tanabe Pharma Development America, Inc (S), Pfizer Inc (US)

Dr Lin: Aerie Pharmaceuticals, Inc (C, L), Allergan (C), Bausch + Lomb Corporation (C, L), Eyenovia, Inc (C), IRIDEX Corporation (C), Santen Pharmaceutical Co, Ltd (C), Tomey Corporation (C)

Dr Posarelli: FB Vision (L), Johnson & Johnson (C), Santen Pharmaceutical Co, Ltd (L)

Dr Rodrigues: Altacor Ltd (C), iSTAR Medical (C), Santen Pharmaceutical Co, Ltd (L)

Dr Rowsey: HEO3 (C, P)

*C = consultant fee, paid advisory boards, or fees for attending a meeting; EE = hired to work in an executive role for compensation or received a W-2 from a company; L = lecture fees or honoraria, travel fees or reimbursements when speaking at the invitation of a commercial company; O = equity ownership/stock options in publicly or privately traded firms, excluding mutual funds; P = beneficiary of patents and/or royalties for intellectual property; S = grant support or other financial support from all sources, including research support from government agencies, foundations, device manufacturers, and/or pharmaceutical companies; SO = stock options in a public or private company; US = equity ownership or stock in publicly traded firms, excluding mutual funds (listed on the stock exchange)

Dr Shah: Allergan (C, L, S), DORC International BV (S), Focus Vision Supplements (SO), Regeneron Pharmaceuticals, Inc (C, L, S)

Dr Sood: Carl Zeiss Meditec AG (C), Ivantis, Inc (C), Ocular Therapeutix, Inc (C), Sight Sciences, Inc (C)

Dr Stringa: Santen Pharmaceutical Co, Ltd (L)

Dr Toeteberg-Harms: Alcon, Inc (L), Allergan (L), ELT Sight (C), EyeLight, Inc (C), Glaukos Corporation (L), Heidelberg Engineering GmbH (L), IRIDEX Corporation (C, L, S), MLase AG (C), Novartis AG (L), Santen Pharmaceutical Co, Ltd (C, L, S), Théa Pharmaceuticals (L)

Dr Welsbie: Medivation, Inc (P), Perceive Biotherapeutics, Inc (C, EE, O, SO)

All relevant financial relationships have been mitigated.

The other authors and reviewers state that within the 24 months prior to their contributions to this CME activity and for the duration of development, they have had no financial interest in or other relationship with any entity whose primary business is producing, marketing, selling, reselling, or distributing health care products used by or in patients.

American Academy of Ophthalmology
655 Beach Street
Box 7424
San Francisco, CA 94120-7424

Contents

Introduction to the BCSC

The Basic and Clinical Science Course (BCSC) is designed to meet the needs of residents and practitioners for a comprehensive yet concise curriculum of the field of ophthalmology. The BCSC has developed from its original brief outline format, which relied heavily on outside readings, to a more convenient and educationally useful self-contained text. The Academy updates and revises the course annually, with the goals of integrating the basic science and clinical practice of ophthalmology and of keeping ophthalmologists current with new developments in the various subspecialties.

The BCSC incorporates the effort and expertise of more than 100 ophthalmologists, organized into 13 Section faculties, working with Academy editorial staff. In addition, the course continues to benefit from many lasting contributions made by the faculties of previous editions. Members of the Academy Practicing Ophthalmologists Advisory Committee for Education, Committee on Aging, and Vision Rehabilitation Committee review every volume before major revisions, as does a group of select residents and fellows. Members of the European Board of Ophthalmology, organized into Section faculties, also review volumes before major revisions, focusing primarily on differences between American and European ophthalmology practice.

Organization of the Course

The Basic and Clinical Science Course comprises 13 volumes, incorporating fundamental ophthalmic knowledge, subspecialty areas, and special topics:

1 Update on General Medicine
2 Fundamentals and Principles of Ophthalmology
3 Clinical Optics and Vision Rehabilitation
4 Ophthalmic Pathology and Intraocular Tumors
5 Neuro-Ophthalmology
6 Pediatric Ophthalmology and Strabismus
7 Oculofacial Plastic and Orbital Surgery
8 External Disease and Cornea
9 Uveitis and Ocular Inflammation
10 Glaucoma
11 Lens and Cataract
12 Retina and Vitreous
13 Refractive Surgery

References

Readers who wish to explore specific topics in greater detail may consult the references cited within each chapter and listed in the Additional Materials and Resources section at the back of the book. These references are intended to be selective rather than exhaustive, chosen by the BCSC faculty as being important, current, and readily available to residents and practitioners.

Multimedia

This edition of Section 10, *Glaucoma,* includes videos and online case studies related to topics covered in the book. The videos and case studies are available to readers of the print and electronic versions of Section 10 (aao.org/bcscvideo_section10 and aao.org/bcsccasestudy_section10). Mobile-device users can scan the QR codes below (a QR-code reader may need to be installed on the device) to access this content.

Videos

Case Studies

Self-Assessment and CME Credit

Each volume of the BCSC is designed as an independent study activity for ophthalmology residents and practitioners. The learning objectives for this volume are given on page 1. The text, illustrations, and references provide the information necessary to achieve the objectives; the study questions allow readers to test their understanding of the material and their mastery of the objectives. Physicians who wish to claim CME credit for this educational activity may do so by following the instructions given at the end of the book.*

Conclusion

The Basic and Clinical Science Course has expanded greatly over the years, with the addition of much new text, numerous illustrations, and video content. Recent editions have sought to place greater emphasis on clinical applicability while maintaining a solid foundation in basic science. As with any educational program, it reflects the experience of its authors. As its faculties change and medicine progresses, new viewpoints emerge on controversial subjects and techniques. Not all alternate approaches can be included in this series; as with any educational endeavor, the learner should seek additional sources, including Academy Preferred Practice Pattern Guidelines.

The BCSC faculty and staff continually strive to improve the educational usefulness of the course; you, the reader, can contribute to this ongoing process. If you have any suggestions or questions about the series, please do not hesitate to contact the faculty or the editors.

The authors, editors, and reviewers hope that your study of the BCSC will be of lasting value and that each Section will serve as a practical resource for quality patient care.

*There is no formal American Board of Ophthalmology (ABO) approval process for self-assessment activities. Any CME activity that qualifies for ABO Continuing Certification credit may also be counted as "self-assessment" as long as it provides a mechanism for individual learners to review their own performance, knowledge base, or skill set in a defined area of practice. For instance, grand rounds, medical conferences, or journal activities for CME credit that involve a form of individualized self-assessment may count as a self-assessment activity.

Objectives

Upon completion of BCSC Section 10, *Glaucoma,* the reader should be able to

- state the epidemiologic features of glaucoma, including the social impacts of the disease
- describe hereditary and genetic factors in glaucoma
- describe the physiology of aqueous humor dynamics and the control of intraocular pressure (IOP)
- describe the clinical evaluation of patients with glaucoma, including history and general examination, gonioscopy, optic nerve examination, and visual field testing
- list the clinical features of the patient considered a glaucoma suspect
- describe the clinical features, evaluation, and treatment of primary open-angle glaucoma and normal-tension glaucoma
- list the various clinical features of and therapeutic approaches for the secondary open-angle glaucomas
- state the underlying causes of the increased IOP in various forms of secondary open-angle glaucoma and the impact that these underlying causes have on disease management
- describe the pathophysiology of primary angle-closure glaucoma
- describe the pathophysiology of secondary angle-closure glaucoma, both with and without pupillary block
- describe the pathophysiology of and therapy for primary congenital and juvenile-onset glaucomas

- describe the various classes of medical therapy for glaucoma, including efficacy, mechanism of action, and safety
- state the indications and techniques for laser and incisional surgical procedures for glaucoma, as well as complications of these treatments

CHAPTER 1

Introduction to Glaucoma

Highlights

- Glaucomas are classified by etiology (primary vs secondary), gonioscopic assessment of the iridocorneal angle (open vs closed), and age at onset (childhood vs adult).
- Elevated intraocular pressure (IOP) is a major risk factor for primary open-angle glaucoma (POAG); however, a large proportion of patients with POAG have IOP in the statistically normal range.
- Glaucoma is a major public health problem and a leading cause of irreversible blindness worldwide.
- Glaucoma linked to a single gene is not common, but many genomic regions have been found to be associated with various types of glaucoma.

Optic Nerve Anatomy

The term *glaucoma* refers to a group of optic neuropathies characterized by optic nerve head (ONH) excavation, or *cupping,* and corresponding patterns of retinal ganglion cell (RGC) loss. An understanding of the normal and pathologic appearances of the optic nerve enables the clinician to detect and monitor glaucoma. The entire visual pathway is described and illustrated in BCSC Section 5, *Neuro-Ophthalmology.* For further discussion of retinal involvement in the visual process, see Section 12, *Retina and Vitreous.* The following discussion is intended to provide a concise review of optic nerve anatomy.

The optic nerve is composed of RGC axons, glial tissue, extracellular matrix, and blood vessels. The human optic nerve consists of approximately 1.2–1.5 million RGC axons, although considerable individual variability exists. The cell bodies of the RGCs lie in the ganglion cell layer of the retina, and their axons synapse primarily in the lateral geniculate nucleus of the thalamus.

The average diameter of the ONH, or *optic disc* (both terms are used interchangeably in the literature) is approximately 1.5–1.7 mm as measured with planimetry but varies widely among individuals and ethnic groups. On exiting the globe, the optic nerve expands to approximately 3–4 mm in diameter. This increase in size is due to axonal myelination, the presence of glial tissue, and the beginning of the leptomeninges (optic nerve sheath). The axons are separated into fascicles within the optic nerve, with the intervening spaces occupied by astrocytes.

Figure 1-1 shows the distribution of retinal nerve fibers as they enter the ONH. The arcuate nerve fibers entering the superior and inferior poles of the ONH are more susceptible to glaucomatous damage, possibly because of the larger size of the pores of the lamina cribrosa in these regions. This susceptibility may explain the frequent occurrence of arcuate visual field defects in eyes with glaucoma. The arrangement of axons in the ONH and their differing susceptibility to damage determine the patterns of visual field loss in glaucoma, which are described and illustrated in Chapter 6.

The intraocular portion of the optic nerve is divided into 2 regions, anterior and posterior, by the lamina cribrosa. The lamina cribrosa is a fenestrated connective tissue layer that is continuous with the sclera and allows passage of axons through the scleral coat. Anterior to the lamina, axons of the optic nerve are unmyelinated, while posterior to the lamina, they are myelinated. Most anteriorly, the superficial nerve fiber layer is continuous with the nerve fiber layer (NFL) of the retina and is composed primarily of RGC axons in transition from superficial retina to the neuronal component of the optic nerve.

The lamina cribrosa provides the primary structural support of the optic nerve as it exits the eye. This layer is a reticulated network of connective tissue beams composed primarily of collagen (Fig 1-2) and extracellular matrix components (ie, elastin, laminin, and fibronectin). The laminar beams contain the capillaries that supply nourishment for

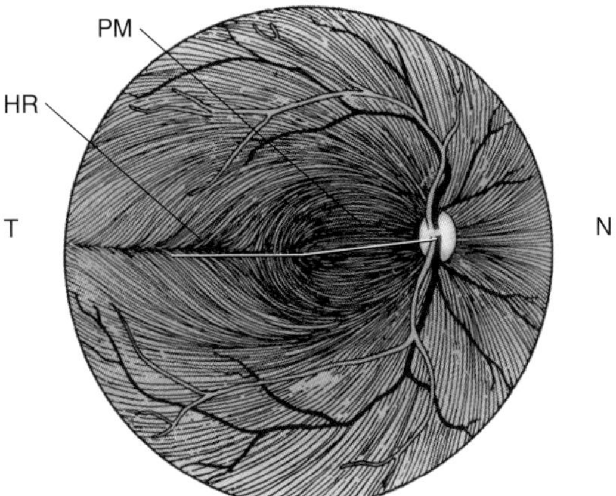

Figure 1-1 The pattern of the nerve fiber layer of axons from retinal ganglion cells to the optic nerve head (ONH). Temporal axons originate above and below the horizontal raphe (HR) and take an arching course to the ONH. Axons arising from ganglion cells in the nasal macula project directly to the ONH. Axons from ganglion cells supplying the fovea approach the ONH as the papillomacular bundle (PM). Peripheral fibers run closer to the choroid and exit in the periphery of the optic nerve, whereas fibers originating from ganglion cells closer to the ONH run closer to the vitreous and occupy a more central portion of the nerve. In most eyes, the fovea is located inferior to the horizontal meridian (see red line from ONH to fovea). Among individuals, there is variability in the relationship between the ONH and the fovea, and this is now recognized to be important for retinal nerve fiber layer imaging that extends into the macula. N = nasal; T = temporal. *(Reproduced from Kline LB, Foroozan R, eds.* Optic Nerve Disorders. *2nd ed. Ophthalmology Monographs 10. Oxford University Press, in cooperation with the American Academy of Ophthalmology; 2007:5.)*

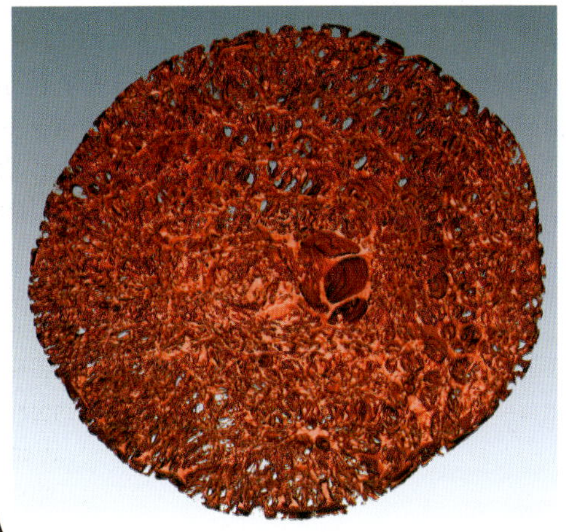

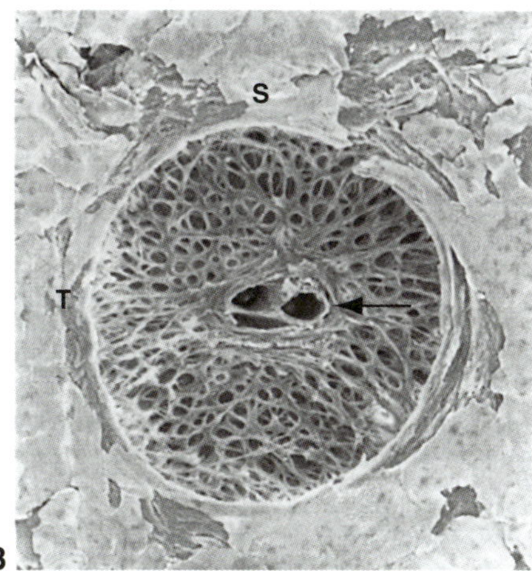

Figure 1-2 Imaging of the lamina cribrosa, a reticulated network of connective tissue beams. **A,** Anterior view of the human lamina cribrosa from a healthy donor, obtained from a 3-dimensional episcopic autofluorescent reconstruction illustrating the fenestrated network of supportive connective tissue. **B,** Scanning electron micrograph of a nonglaucomatous human lamina cribrosa after trypsin digestion viewed *en face*. The openings for the central retinal vessels are shown *(arrow)*. The density of the connective tissue and the size of the laminar pores vary by region. The lamina cribrosa is believed to be more structurally vulnerable to damage at the inferior and superior poles of the optic nerve head because of the larger pores in these locations. S = superior region; T = temporal region. *(Part A courtesy of Crawford Downs, PhD, and Christopher Girkin, MD; part B courtesy of Harry A. Quigley, MD.)*

this critical region. Neural components of the optic nerve pass through these connective tissue beams. In addition, relatively large central fenestrations allow passage of the central retinal artery and central retinal vein. Scanning electron microscopy of the healthy lamina cribrosa reveals a lower density of connective tissue and extracellular matrix material at its inferior and superior poles, where the laminar pores are larger compared with those in the nasal and temporal regions. This difference may explain the increased susceptibility to damage of the inferior and superior regions of the optic nerve. The laminar pores are often seen by ophthalmoscopy at the base of the *optic cup*, a central depression within the ONH. Between the optic nerve and the adjacent choroidal and scleral tissue lies a rim of connective tissue called the *ring of Elschnig*.

Downs JC. Optic nerve head biomechanics in aging and disease. *Exp Eye Res.* 2015;133: 19–29.

Blood Supply to the Optic Nerve

The anterior optic nerve vasculature can be divided into 4 regions (Fig 1-3):

- superficial nerve fiber layer
- prelaminar
- laminar
- retrolaminar

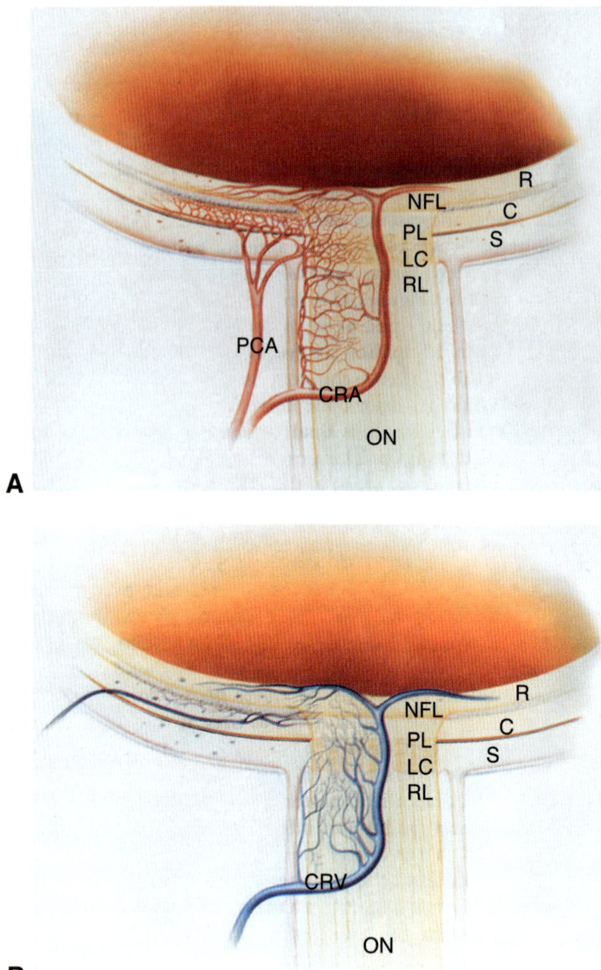

Figure 1-3 Anterior optic nerve vasculature. **A,** Arterial supply to the anterior optic nerve and peripapillary choroid. **B,** Venous drainage of the anterior optic nerve and peripapillary choroid. C = choroid; CRA = central retinal artery; CRV = central retinal vein; LC = lamina cribrosa; NFL = nerve fiber layer; ON = optic nerve; PCA = posterior ciliary artery; PL = prelamina; R = retina; RL = retrolamina; S = sclera. *(Reproduced from Cioffi GA. In Ritch R, Shields MB, Krupin T, eds.* The Glaucomas. *2nd ed. Mosby; 1996:178, 183, Figs 8-2, 8-12.)*

The arterial supply of the anterior optic nerve is derived entirely from branches of the ophthalmic artery via 1–5 posterior ciliary arteries. Typically, between 2 and 4 posterior ciliary arteries course anteriorly before dividing into approximately 10–20 short posterior ciliary arteries, which occurs before their entry into the posterior globe. These arteries penetrate the perineural sclera of the posterior globe to supply the peripapillary choroid and most of the anterior optic nerve. A discontinuous arterial circle, the *circle of Zinn-Haller,* is often present within the perineural sclera. The central retinal artery, also a posterior orbital branch of the ophthalmic artery, penetrates the optic nerve approximately 10–15 mm posterior to the globe. The central retinal artery has few, if any, intraneural branches; the exception is an occasional small branch within the retrolaminar region, which may anastomose with the pial system. The central retinal artery courses adjacent to the central retinal vein within the central portion of the optic nerve.

The superficial NFL is supplied principally by recurrent retinal arterioles branching from the central retinal artery. The prelaminar region is principally supplied by direct branches of the short posterior ciliary arteries and by branches of the circle of Zinn-Haller (when present). Similar to the prelaminar region, the laminar region receives its blood supply from branches of the short posterior ciliary arteries or from branches of the circle of Zinn-Haller. These precapillary branches perforate the outer aspects of the lamina cribrosa before branching into an intraseptal capillary network. The retrolaminar region is supplied by branches of the short posterior ciliary arteries and by branches of the pial arteries coursing adjacent to this region. The pial arteries originate both from the central retinal artery, before it pierces the retrobulbar optic nerve, and from branches of the short posterior ciliary arteries more anteriorly. The central retinal artery may supply several small intraneural branches in the retrolaminar region.

The rich capillary beds of each of the 4 regions of the anterior optic nerve are anatomically confluent. Venous drainage of the anterior optic nerve occurs almost exclusively via the central retinal vein. In the NFL, blood drains directly into the retinal veins, which then join to form the central retinal vein. In the prelaminar, laminar, and retrolaminar regions, venous drainage also occurs via the central retinal vein or axial tributaries to the central retinal vein.

Pathophysiology

Characteristic ONH changes are among the defining features of glaucoma (Fig 1-4). Histologic examination reveals that early glaucomatous cupping begins with structural damage to the lamina cribrosa. Subsequently, there is loss of RGCs and their axons, blood vessels, and glial cells. RGC axonal damage begins at the level of the lamina cribrosa and is most pronounced at the superior and inferior poles of the ONH. In many cases, structural optic nerve changes may precede detectable functional loss, as measured by standard perimetry.

As previously mentioned, the lamina cribrosa is the fenestrated portion of the posterior sclera through which RGC axons exit the eye to become the optic nerve. It represents a weak point in the eye wall, susceptible to physical forces. In patients with glaucoma, a variety of factors, including intraocular pressure (IOP) and retrolaminar cerebrospinal fluid pressure, interact to create stress on the lamina cribrosa. Depending on the eye's structural features (eg, elasticity, axial length, ONH size) and an individual's genetic predisposition, these stresses can lead to strain on and remodeling of the lamina cribrosa (Fig 1-5A). This remodeling in turn leads to damage of the intervening axons through mechanisms that remain unclear, although mechanical compression, energy supply/demand mismatch, mitochondrial dysfunction, and neuroinflammation may all play a role. Axonal injury impairs the transport of pro-survival factors, such as brain-derived neurotrophic factor (BDNF), and leads to the generation and/or activation of pro-degenerative factors, such as dual leucine zipper kinase/mitogen-activated kinase kinase kinases 12 (DLK/MAP3K12) and sterile alpha and TIR motif containing 1. This triggers axonal degeneration, which is

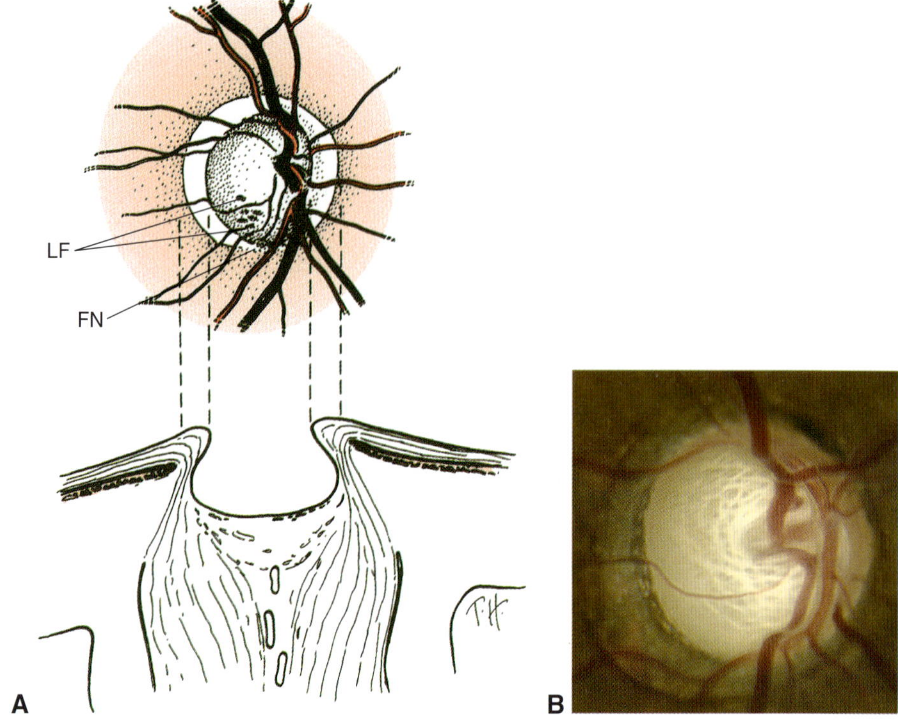

Figure 1-4 Two views of glaucomatous optic nerves. **A,** Anterior optic nerve head and transverse view, right eye. Note thinning, undermining, and focal notching (FN) of the inferior neuroretinal rim; enlarged central cup with visible laminar fenestrations (LF); nasal shift of retinal vessels; and peripapillary atrophy. **B,** Clinical view of a glaucomatous optic nerve head demonstrating extensive loss of the neuroretinal rim. *(Part A reproduced with permission from Wright KW, ed.* Textbook of Ophthalmology. *Williams & Wilkins; 1997. Part B courtesy of Ronald L. Gross, MD.)*

later followed by cell death via apoptosis. As RGCs are responsible for preprocessing and transmitting visual information to the thalamus and midbrain, RGC death causes loss of the visual field. The long-term impact on higher-order visual centers and thus the potential for vision restoration remains unknown. Of note, although RGCs are lost in other progressive optic neuropathies, the characteristic cupping and optic nerve excavation seen in glaucoma (Fig 1-5B) are not prominent. The central role of laminar deformation in glaucoma leads to these features.

IOP at any level within the range observed in the general population is a continuous risk factor for the development of glaucoma. Moreover, IOP is not elevated above the statistically normal range (10–21 mm Hg) in a substantial proportion of patients with primary open-angle glaucoma (POAG), and elevated IOP and is not a defining characteristic of the disease. More than one-third of patients with POAG in North America have IOP levels within statistically normal limits. And for reasons that are unclear, an even larger proportion of patients with POAG in certain Asian populations,

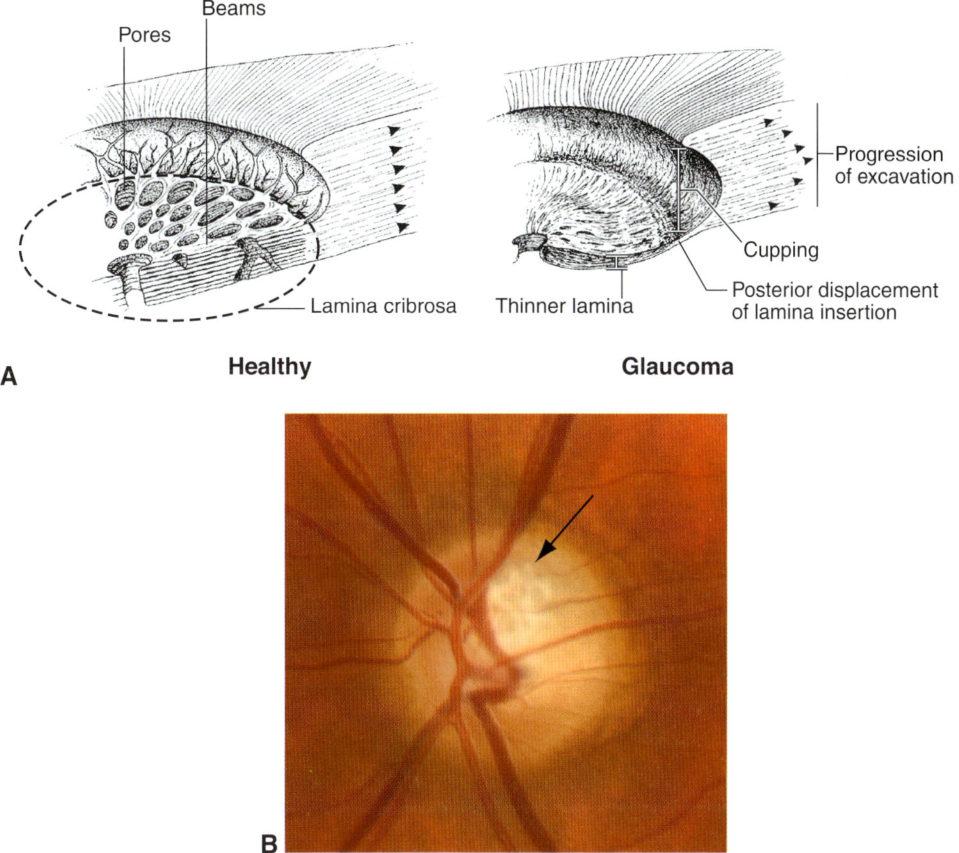

Figure 1-5 Lamina cribrosa and optic nerve head. **A,** The illustration depicts a healthy lamina cribrosa *(left)* and the deformation and remodeling that occur in glaucoma *(right)*. **B,** The photograph shows optic nerve head excavation, or "cupping." Note the focal neural rim loss *(arrow)* and exposed laminar pores superiorly. *(Part A illustration modified with permission from Burgoyne CF, Downs JC, Bellezza AJ, Suh JK, Hart RT. The optic nerve head as a biomechanical structure: a new paradigm for understanding the role of IOP-related stress and strain in the pathophysiology of glaucomatous optic nerve head damage.* Prog Retin Eye Res. *2005;24(1):39–73. Fig 7, p 49. Part B courtesy of Angelo P. Tanna, MD.)*

such as Japanese and Korean, have statistically normal IOP (eg, 90% of Japanese POAG patients).

While IOP at any level is a risk factor for glaucoma, mildly elevated IOP is neither necessary nor sufficient for the development of glaucoma. A large proportion of patients with *ocular hypertension,* defined as the presence of statistically elevated IOP in the absence of visual field or ONH damage, do not go on to develop glaucoma. Clinicians often imprecisely use the word *glaucoma* to describe conditions in which the IOP is elevated in the absence of known glaucomatous neuropathy. Although this is common parlance, it should be avoided.

Whether there are any pathophysiologic differences between glaucoma at low and high IOP is unknown (see Chapter 7). In patients with glaucoma, the baseline IOP—even when "normal"—is too high for RGC function and survival. It has been shown that in most patients with glaucoma, lowering the IOP stops or slows visual field loss. However, in some eyes, optic nerve damage may progress despite treatment to lower the IOP.

Quigley HA. Glaucoma. *Lancet.* 2011;377(9774):1367–1377.

Weinreb RN, Aung T, Medeiros FA. The pathophysiology and treatment of glaucoma: a review. *JAMA.* 2014;311(18):1901–1911.

Classification

Adult forms of glaucoma are classified as open angle or angle closure and as primary or secondary (Table 1-1). Pediatric forms of glaucoma are discussed in Chapter 11. Distinguishing open-angle glaucoma from angle-closure disease is essential from a therapeutic standpoint.

Table 1-1 Classification of Glaucoma and Related Conditions[a]

I. Open Angle

- A. Primary
  1. Primary open-angle glaucoma
  2. Normal-tension glaucoma
  3. Juvenile open-angle glaucoma
- B. Secondary
  1. Pseudoexfoliation syndrome
  2. Pigmentary glaucoma
  3. Traumatic glaucoma (in patients with angle recession, traumatic hyphema, or other evidence of trauma)
  4. Corticosteroid-induced glaucoma
  5. Glaucoma associated with intraocular inflammation
  6. Hemolytic glaucoma (hemoglobin-laden macrophages obstruct TM)
  7. Ghost cell glaucoma (degenerated RBCs obstruct TM)
  8. Glaucoma associated with intraocular tumors (neoplastic cells, cellular material, debris, or RBCs obstruct outflow)
  9. Glaucomatocyclitic crisis (Posner-Schlossman syndrome)
  10. Fuchs uveitis syndrome
  11. Uveitis-glaucoma-hyphema syndrome
  12. Lens associated
      - a. Phacolytic glaucoma (leaked lens proteins obstruct TM)
      - b. Lens particle glaucoma (retained lens material after surgery or trauma)
      - c. Phacoantigenic glaucoma (inflammatory response after surgical or accidental lens trauma)
  13. Glaucoma associated with elevated episcleral venous pressure
  14. Glaucoma associated with siderosis, chalcosis
  15. Schwartz-Matsuo syndrome (IOP elevation caused by photoreceptor outer segment release in association with rhegmatogenous retinal detachment)
  16. Glaucoma due to IOP elevation associated with repeated anti-VEGF intravitreous injection

(Continued)

Table 1-1 *(continued)*

II. Angle Closure

- A. Primary[b]
    1. Primary angle-closure suspect (≥180° iridotrabecular contact without IOP elevation, PAS, or glaucomatous optic neuropathy)
    2. Primary angle closure (≥180° iridotrabecular contact with statistically elevated IOP and/or PAS in the absence of glaucomatous optic neuropathy)
    3. Primary angle-closure glaucoma (≥180° iridotrabecular contact with statistically elevated IOP and/or PAS and evidence of glaucomatous optic neuropathy)
    4. Acute primary angle closure, also called acute angle-closure crisis (closed angle with symptomatic IOP elevation)
    5. Plateau iris configuration (persistent iridotrabecular contact after a patent laser peripheral iridotomy without IOP elevation after pupil dilation)
    6. Plateau iris syndrome (persistent iridotrabecular contact after a patent laser peripheral iridotomy with IOP elevation after pupil dilation)
- B. Secondary
    1. With pupillary block
        - a. Lens-induced
            - i. Phacomorphic[c]
            - ii. Ectopia lentis
            - iii. Pseudophakic pupillary block (especially with ACIOL)
            - iv. Microspherophakia
        - b. Aphakic pupillary block
        - c. Posterior synechiae
    2. Without pupillary block
        - a. Anterior pulling mechanism
            - i. Neovascular glaucoma
            - ii. Iridocorneal endothelial syndrome
            - iii. Posterior polymorphous corneal dystrophy
            - iv. Consolidation of inflammatory material
            - v. Anterior synechiae due to trauma
        - b. Posterior pushing mechanism
            - i. Malignant glaucoma
            - ii. Uveal effusion
            - iii. Anterior rotation of ciliary body (eg, due to CRVO, scleral buckle, PRP)
            - iv. Phacomorphic[c]
            - v. Cysts of iris or ciliary body
            - vi. Persistent fetal vasculature
            - vii. Retinopathy of prematurity

III. Combined-Mechanism Glaucoma (Mixed-Mechanism Glaucoma)

Ongoing glaucomatous damage in an eye that had successful treatment for angle closure with laser peripheral iridotomy or removal of the crystalline lens.

ACIOL = anterior chamber intraocular lens; CRVO = central retinal vein occlusion; IOP = intraocular pressure; PAS = peripheral anterior synechiae; PRP = panretinal photocoagulation; RBCs = red blood cells; TM = trabecular meshwork; VEGF = vascular endothelial growth factor.

[a] For childhood glaucomas, see Chapter 11.

[b] The mechanism of primary angle closure usually involves pupillary block. Plateau iris configuration and syndrome are also usually accompanied by some degree of pupillary block. Those conditions can be reliably diagnosed only after an iridotomy is performed (see Chapter 9).

[c] Phacomorphic glaucoma can be caused by pupillary block and non–pupillary block mechanisms.

Open Angle

In *open-angle glaucoma (OAG),* there is evidence of glaucomatous injury to the ONH, but no obstruction of the trabecular meshwork by the iris is visible on gonioscopic examination of the anterior chamber angle. The condition is further classified as *primary* OAG (POAG) when no macroscopic abnormality is seen that could disrupt outflow of aqueous humor. OAG is classified as *secondary* when an abnormality that can decrease outflow (excluding iris malposition, in which case the condition would be classified as angle closure) is identified. Differentiating between primary and secondary OAG may be important for determining target pressures, because optic nerve injury is more likely to occur at lower pressures in POAG than in secondary OAG.

In POAG with elevated IOP, the etiology of the outflow obstruction is believed to be an abnormality in the extracellular matrix of the trabecular meshwork and in trabecular meshwork cells in the juxtacanalicular region, or an abnormality in the function of the endothelial cells lining the inner wall of the Schlemm canal (see Chapter 2). The term *normal-tension glaucoma* is often used for POAG with IOP that is within the statistically normal range. The conceptual basis for this distinction and for the term itself is controversial and is discussed in Chapter 7.

Angle Closure

Angle closure refers to an anatomical configuration in which there is mechanical blockage of the trabecular meshwork by the peripheral iris. This form may be classified as *primary,* in which no underlying pathologic condition can be identified to explain the angle narrowing; or *secondary,* in which the angle closure can be attributed to certain disease processes (see Table 1-1). Primary angle-closure disease is further classified as follows:

- *Primary angle-closure suspect.* The patient has narrowing of the anterior chamber angle (when it is visualized by gonioscopy) with ≥180° iridotrabecular contact but without elevated IOP, peripheral anterior synechiae, or signs of glaucomatous optic neuropathy. The angle narrowing may be an anatomical variant with little clinical consequence for many patients.
- *Primary angle closure.* The narrow angle has led to statistically elevated IOP (>21 mm Hg) and/or adhesions between the peripheral iris and the cornea/trabecular meshwork, referred to as *peripheral anterior synechiae (PAS).*
- *Primary angle-closure glaucoma.* The narrow angle has led to glaucomatous optic neuropathy.

Normal aqueous humor flow in the anterior segment is illustrated in Figure 1-6A. In primary angle closure (and in some forms of secondary angle closure), the flow of aqueous humor from the posterior to the anterior chamber is obstructed at the pupil (Fig 1-6B). The resulting pressure increase in the posterior chamber causes the peripheral iris to bow forward into the anterior chamber angle. The iris bowing increases the resistance to outflow and raises eye pressure; this is referred to as *pupillary block.* In some forms of angle closure and in plateau iris, the peripheral iris or the entire lens–iris interface is mechanically *pushed* forward, again narrowing the iridocorneal angle (see Chapter 9). This can

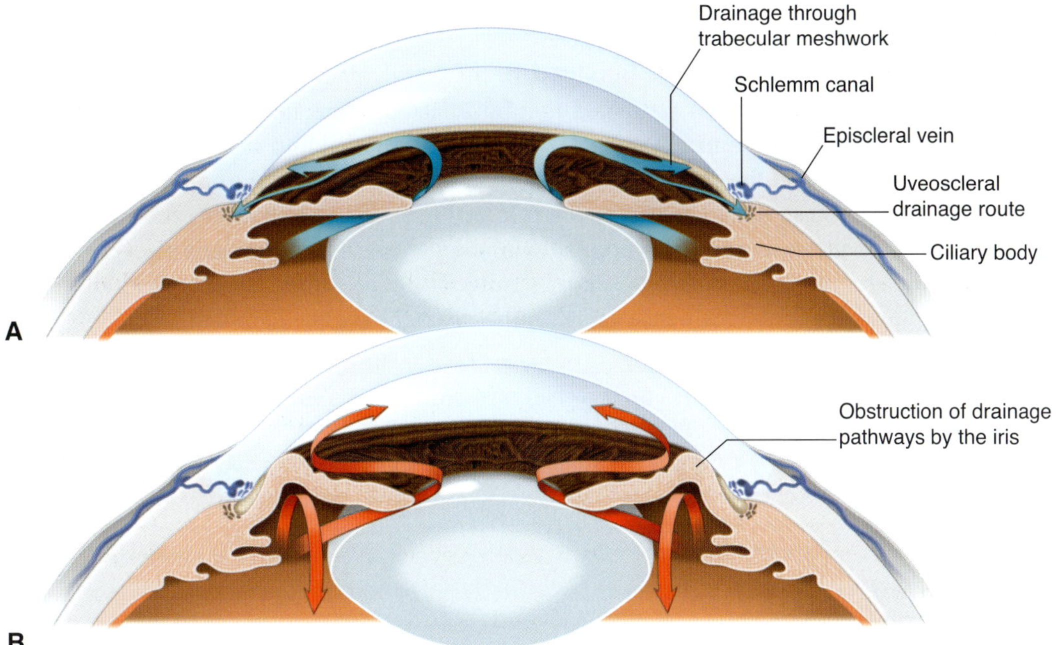

Figure 1-6 Aqueous humor flow. **A,** Normal flow of aqueous humor from the posterior chamber, through the pupil, and into the anterior chamber. Aqueous humor exits the eye through 2 pathways: conventional flow through the trabecular meshwork and the uveoscleral pathway. **B,** In primary angle closure due to pupillary block, the flow of aqueous through the pupil is obstructed, resulting in a positive pressure gradient between the posterior and anterior chambers, anterior displacement of the peripheral iris, and closure of the anterior chamber angle. *(Illustration by Mark Miller.)*

result from a ciliary body abnormality, posterior segment tumor, hemorrhage, or other causes (see Chapter 10). Patients with angle closure can have angle narrowing because of a combination of pupillary block and an abnormal ciliary body position. In other forms of secondary angle closure, the peripheral iris is *pulled* forward, typically by contraction of a cellular, fibrovascular, or inflammatory membrane. These conditions are called *non–pupillary block angle closure.*

Combined Mechanism

Combined-mechanism glaucoma (or *mixed-mechanism glaucoma*) refers to the condition in which an eye with glaucomatous optic neuropathy that has undergone successful treatment for angle closure with either laser peripheral iridotomy or removal of the crystalline lens continues to demonstrate reduced outflow facility and elevated IOP in the absence of PAS. Given that other combinations of mechanisms can occur and lead to elevated IOP or glaucoma—such as neovascular glaucoma after a vein occlusion in a patient with POAG, or IOP elevation due to inflammation and corticosteroid use in a patient with uveitis—this term should be used judiciously so as to avoid confusion.

Epidemiology

As a leading cause of irreversible blindness in the world, glaucoma poses a significant public health problem. It was estimated that by 2020, approximately 80 million people worldwide would have glaucoma, with 11.2 million bilaterally blind as a result. A meta-analysis estimated that the global prevalence of this disease is 3.5% in the population aged 40–80 years. Because older age is a major risk factor for glaucoma and because life expectancies are increasing in most populations, the prevalence of glaucoma is expected to increase sharply in the coming decades. (Note: The confidence intervals around the estimated prevalence and incidence values in this chapter have been omitted.)

Bourne RR, Taylor HR, Flaxman SR, et al. Number of people blind or visually impaired by glaucoma worldwide and in world regions 1990–2010: a meta-analysis. *PLoS One.* 2016;11(10):e0162229. doi:10.1371/journal.pone.0162229

Tham YC, Li S, Wong TY, Quigley HA, Aung T, Cheng CY. Global prevalence of glaucoma and projections of glaucoma burden through 2040: a systematic review and meta-analysis. *Ophthalmology.* 2014;121(11):2081–2090.

Primary Open-Angle Glaucoma

Prevalence and incidence

The prevalence (total number of individuals with a disease at a specific time) and incidence (number of new cases that develop during a specific period) of POAG vary widely across population-based samples owing to differences in ethnic and racial representation (Fig 1-7). In the Baltimore Eye Survey, the prevalence of POAG among White individuals ranged from 0.9% in those aged 40–49 years to 2.2% in those aged ≥80 years, whereas the prevalence among Black individuals ranged from 1.2% to 11.3%, respectively. The overall population-based prevalence was 4–5 times higher among Black individuals than White individuals.

In the Rotterdam Study, a longitudinal population-based study of northern Europeans, the observed prevalence was 1.1% among participants aged ≥55 years. In the same study cohort, the incident risk of developing glaucoma at 10 years was 2.8%. In both the Baltimore Eye Survey and the Rotterdam Study, half of the participants with glaucoma were unaware of their diagnosis.

The prevalence of glaucoma in the Barbados Eye Study (a predominantly African Caribbean population) was 7% in individuals aged ≥40 years, and the 4-year incidence of glaucoma was 2.2%. Again, older age was found to be a major risk factor for the prevalence and incidence of glaucoma.

The observed prevalence of OAG in the Los Angeles Latino Eye Survey (LALES), a longitudinal population-based study of Latino individuals (mostly Mexican ancestry) aged ≥40 years, was 4.7%, with 75% unaware of their diagnosis at baseline. The prevalence among those aged ≥80 years was nearly 22%. The 4-year incidence rate of OAG was 2.3%.

In the Tajimi Study (Japan), the prevalence of POAG among participants aged ≥40 years was 3.9%. The IOP was ≤21 mm Hg in 92% of those with POAG. The mean IOP in the nonglaucomatous eyes was 14.5±2.5 mm Hg, approximately 2 mm Hg lower than the mean IOP observed in European-derived populations.

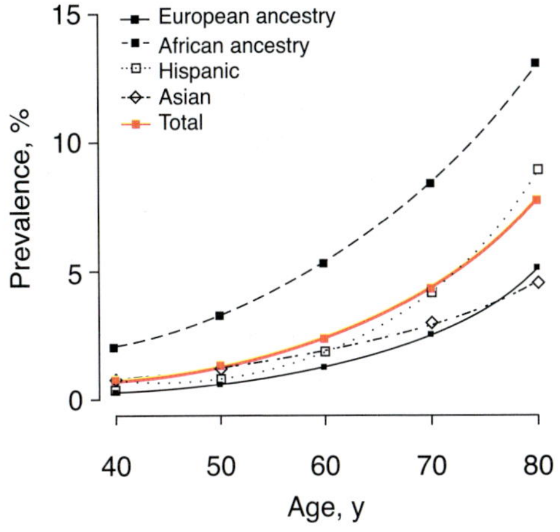

Figure 1-7 The prevalence of primary open-angle glaucoma as a function of age and ethnicity. *(Modified with permission from Elsevier. Courtesy of Tham YC, Li X, Wong TY, Quigley HA, Aung T, Cheng CY. Global prevalence of glaucoma and projections of glaucoma burden through 2040: a systematic review and meta-analysis.* Ophthalmology. *2014;121(11):2081–2090.)*

A meta-analysis estimated the global prevalence of POAG in 2013 to be 3% among persons 40–80 years of age. In this age group, the highest prevalence of POAG, an estimated 4.2%, was found in Africa. The same study estimated the prevalence of POAG in North America to be approximately 3.3%.

Leske MC, Connell AM, Wu SY, et al. Incidence of open-angle glaucoma: the Barbados Eye Studies. The Barbados Eye Studies Group. *Arch Ophthalmol.* 2001;119(1):89–95.

Tielsch JM, Sommer A, Katz J, Royall RM, Quigley HA, Javitt J. Racial variations in the prevalence of primary open-angle glaucoma. The Baltimore Eye Survey. *JAMA.* 1991; 266(3):369–374.

Varma R, Ying-Lai M, Francis BA, et al; Los Angeles Latino Eye Study Group. Prevalence of open-angle glaucoma and ocular hypertension in Latinos: the Los Angeles Latino Eye Study. *Ophthalmology.* 2004;111(8):1439–1448.

Risk factors

Population-based studies and prospective glaucoma clinical trials have identified a number of risk factors that are associated with POAG diagnosis and progression. The most widely accepted risk factors include higher IOP; lower ocular perfusion pressure; older age; lower central corneal thickness (thinner cornea); high myopia; and racial, ethnic, and genetic background. The lifetime risk of glaucoma increases from approximately 3% to 22% with a single affected first-degree relative. Other possible risk factors are discussed in Chapter 7.

Primary Angle-Closure Glaucoma

Prevalence

The prevalence of primary angle-closure glaucoma (PACG) varies among racial and ethnic groups. A meta-analysis estimated the prevalence in Asia to be 1.1% among individuals aged 40–80 years; the prevalence is even higher in East Asia. Among people of European ancestry >40 years, the prevalence is estimated to be between 0.1% and 0.4%. The estimated prevalence in African populations ranges from 0.1% to 0.6%. The highest-known prevalence, estimated to be between 2.5% and 4.8%, is found in Inuit populations >40 years in Alaska and Greenland.

Estimates of the prevalence of PACG vary among different Asian populations. Among participants aged ≥50 years in Guangzhou, China, the prevalence of PACG was 1.5%; and the proportion of these participants with unilateral blindness was 43%, compared with 17% for participants with POAG in the same population-based survey. In the Tajimi Study, the prevalence of PACG was 0.6%.

Risk factors

Age, race, and ethnicity are risk factors for PACG. The prevalence of PACG may vary by sex, with a significantly higher prevalence observed in women in most studies. Hyperopia and a family history of angle closure are also important risk factors. Other risk factors are discussed in Chapter 9.

Cho HK, Kee C. Population-based glaucoma prevalence studies in Asians. *Surv Ophthalmol.* 2014;59(4):434–447.

Gedde SJ, Chen PP, Muir KW; American Academy of Ophthalmology Preferred Practice Pattern Glaucoma Panel. Primary Angle-Closure Disease Preferred Practice Pattern. *Ophthalmology.* 2021;128(1):P30–P70. doi:10.1016/j.ophtha.2020.10.021

Genetics

In general, early-onset forms of glaucoma are rare and can follow patterns of simple mendelian inheritance with pathogenic variants (mutations) that are highly penetrant. Previously, genes with such disease-causing alleles were identified by linkage analysis in large, multigenerational families that showed either autosomal dominant or autosomal recessive patterns of inheritance. Genetic regions associated with glaucoma are named according to the type of glaucoma—*GLC1* for open-angle glaucoma, *GLC2* for angle-closure glaucoma, and *GLC3* for congenital glaucoma—followed by a letter to indicate the sequence of discovery: *GLC1A, GLC1B, GLC1C,* and so on. Table 1-2 lists important mendelian genes associated with glaucoma, for which genetic testing may be of clinical utility.

In contrast, common forms of adult-onset glaucoma such as POAG are rarely associated with these genes. Nonetheless, heritability estimates for POAG vary between 0.3 and 0.8, suggesting a strong genetic component, likely the result of many alleles, each with a small contribution. Current approaches using genome-wide association studies (GWAS) and whole-exome sequencing have successfully identified some of these polygenic disease-causing alleles.

Juvenile Open-Angle Glaucoma

Juvenile open-angle glaucoma (JOAG) is defined by onset before 40 years of age, an open anterior chamber angle, and an absence of secondary features. The myocilin gene (*MYOC,* previously *TIGR,* located within the chromosomal region called *GLC1A*) was the first glaucoma gene discovered. Autosomal dominant pathogenic variants in *MYOC* account for up to 36% of cases of JOAG and 4% of POAG. There is evidence that mutant myocilin

Table 1-2 Clinically Important Glaucoma Loci

Phenotype	Locus	Gene Name (Gene Symbol)	Inheritance Pattern
Juvenile open-angle glaucoma	*GLC1A*	Myocilin *(MYOC);* previously *TIGR*	Autosomal dominant
Normal-tension glaucoma	*GLC1E*	Optineurin *(OPTN)*	Autosomal dominant
	GLC1P	TANK binding kinase 1 *(TBK1)*	Autosomal dominant
Primary congenital glaucoma	*GLC3A*	Cytochrome P450 family 1 subfamily B member 1 *(CYP1B1)*	Autosomal recessive
	GLC3C/ GLC3D	Latent transforming growth factor beta binding protein 2 *(LTBP2)*	Autosomal recessive
	GLC3E	TEK receptor tyrosine kinase (*TEK,* also known as *TIE2*)	Autosomal dominant
		Angiopoietin 1 *(ANGPT1)*	Autosomal dominant
Axenfeld-Rieger syndrome	*IRID1*	Forkhead box C1 *(FOXC1)*	Autosomal dominant
	RIEG1	Paired like homeodomain 2 *(PITX2)*	Autosomal dominant
		C3 and PZP like alpha-2-macroglobulin domain containing 8 *(CPAMD8)*	Autosomal recessive
Aniridia		Paired box 6 *(PAX6)*	Autosomal dominant
Peters anomaly (usually sporadic)		*PITX2*	Autosomal dominant
		FOXC1	Autosomal dominant
		PAX6	Autosomal dominant
		CYP1B1	Autosomal recessive

accumulates in cells rather than being secreted, possibly resulting in endoplasmic reticulum stress and toxicity to the trabecular meshwork.

Familial Normal-Tension Glaucoma

Familial normal-tension glaucoma (NTG) is associated with variants in optineurin *(OPTN)* and copy number variations involving TANK binding kinase 1 *(TBK1).* These genetic abnormalities are associated with early-onset autosomal dominant familial NTG and account for approximately 2%–3% of cases. *OPTN* and *TBK1* encode proteins that interact with each other and are involved in autophagy.

Primary Congenital Glaucoma

Primary congenital glaucoma (PCG) is rare, but it represents the most common form of childhood glaucoma, with an incidence ranging from 1:1250 to 1:10,000 depending on the population studied. Although most cases are sporadic, up to 40% of cases are inherited. Pathogenic variants have been identified in 4 genes. Recessive pathogenic variants in *CYP1B1,* the gene encoding cytochrome P450 1B1, are the most common cause of PCG identified to date. Cytochrome P450 1B1 appears to be required for development and proper function of the trabecular meshwork. Recessive pathogenic variants in *LTBP2* also cause PCG. This gene encodes a protein, latent transforming growth factor beta binding protein 2, that is associated with microfibrils, cell adhesion, and extracellular matrix maintenance. Other ophthalmic diseases associated with *LTBP2* variants include Weill-Marchesani syndrome, microspherophakia, and ectopia lentis. Pathogenic variants in TEK receptor tyrosine kinase (*TEK;* also known as *TIE2*) and angiopoietin 1 *(ANGPT1)* result in maldevelopment of the Schlemm canal in mouse models and are inherited as a dominant trait with variable expressivity in some patients with PCG.

Axenfeld-Rieger Syndrome

Axenfeld-Rieger syndrome is a spectrum of abnormalities of ocular and systemic development, often associated with glaucoma. Linkage analysis has led to the discovery of autosomal dominant pathogenic variants in 2 genes, paired like homeodomain 2 *(PITX2)* and forkhead box C1 *(FOXC1)*. Both genes encode transcription factors that regulate embryonic development.

Aniridia

Aniridia is an autosomal dominant or sporadic ocular developmental disorder characterized by iris hypoplasia and frequently associated with glaucoma. The autosomal dominant form is associated with missense variants in the paired box 6 gene *(PAX6)*, whereas the sporadic form is associated with large deletions or rearrangements involving the same gene, which encodes a transcription factor important for ocular development. Sporadic aniridia due to large deletions of band 11p13, which includes *PAX6*, can be associated with a syndrome comprising *W*ilms tumor, *a*niridia, *g*enitourinary anomalies, and *r*ange of developmental delays (WAGR syndrome). Patients with large deletions of 11p13 involving the adjacent Wilms tumor suppressor gene *(WT1)* are at risk for developing Wilms tumor of the kidney. Therefore, individuals with sporadic aniridia should undergo chromosomal deletion analysis of 11p13 to determine whether screening for Wilms tumor is required.

Genome-Wide Association Studies

Common adult-onset forms of glaucoma are generally associated with complex genetic inheritance patterns. GWAS have been used to identify many genetic loci associated with POAG, PACG, and pseudoexfoliation syndrome. GWAS have also led to the discovery of genetic risk alleles for IOP and certain glaucomatous optic nerve features. In most cases, GWAS alleles appear to increase the risk of glaucoma by affecting IOP. Genes that seem to work at the level of the optic nerve and/or RGC include SIX homeobox 6 *(SIX6)* and CDKN2B antisense RNA 1 *(CDKN2B-AS1)*, which encodes a long noncoding RNA (lncRNA).

Pseudoexfoliation Syndrome

Pseudoexfoliation syndrome is characterized by the presence of an abnormal fibrillar material that can be visualized on various structures in the anterior segment. The fibrillar material may impair aqueous humor outflow and elevate IOP. In one study, disease-associated genetic variants in lysyl oxidase like 1 *(LOXL1)* were present in up to 99% of pseudoexfoliation syndrome cases and 80% of controls. The enzyme lysyl oxidase is involved in elastin metabolism. As elastin is an important component of the lamina cribrosa, an abnormality in elastin function may result in increased susceptibility of the optic nerve to injury. Other factors, including environmental factors such as sun exposure and low ambient temperature, are thought to contribute to the risk of developing pseudoexfoliation syndrome.

Genetic Testing

Genetic counseling and diagnostic testing may be relevant for patients with early-onset glaucoma or ocular developmental abnormalities associated with a high risk of developing glaucoma. Testing for pathogenic variants in the genes listed in Table 1-2 can be useful to determine patterns of inheritance, identify children at risk early in the disease course, estimate risk to future offspring, and establish future gene therapy strategies. In adult-onset POAG, genotyping the various GWAS-identified loci may help predict disease and/or progression, although the clinical utility of this remains unclear.

Khawaja AP, Cooke Bailey JN, Wareham NJ, et al; UK Biobank Eye and Vision Consortium; NEIGHBORHOOD Consortium. Genome-wide analyses identify 68 new loci associated with intraocular pressure and improve risk prediction for primary open-angle glaucoma. *Nat Genet.* 2018;50(6):778–782. doi:10.1038/s41588-018-0126-8

Lewis CJ, Hedberg-Buenz A, DeLuca AP, Stone EM, Alward WLM, Fingert JH. Primary congenital and developmental glaucomas. *Hum Mol Genet.* 2017;26(R1):R28–R36.

Wiggs JL, Pasquale LR. Genetics of glaucoma. *Hum Mol Genet.* 2017;26(R1):R21–R27.

Environmental and Other Factors in Glaucoma

Evidence that environmental factors can play a role in the etiology of glaucoma arises from studies of twins in which the disease was not uniformly manifest in monozygotic twins. These data suggest that while genetic factors contribute to the development of glaucoma, environmental and behavioral factors are also important. Using longitudinal epidemiologic studies (eg, the TwinsUK Registry, the US Department of Veterans Affairs Normative Aging Study, and the Nurses' Health Study), researchers have identified a number of environmental and other factors that may modulate the risk of glaucoma, including sun and low ambient temperature exposure (for pseudoexfoliation syndrome), estrogen exposure, cholesterol levels, statin use, and lead exposure. In addition, components of healthy living, including exercise, consumption of green leafy vegetables, and the avoidance of air pollutants, may be beneficial in reducing the risk of glaucoma. Social and demographic factors influencing glaucoma and other ocular diseases are discussed in BCSC Section 1, *Update on General Medicine.*

Kang JH, Loomis S, Wiggs JL, Stein JD, Pasquale LR. Demographic and geographic features of exfoliation glaucoma in 2 United States–based prospective cohorts. *Ophthalmology.* 2012;119(1):27–35.

Stein JD, Pasquale LR, Talwar N, et al. Geographic and climatic factors associated with exfoliation syndrome. *Arch Ophthalmol.* 2011;129(8):1053–1060.

CHAPTER 2

Intraocular Pressure and Aqueous Humor Dynamics

This chapter includes a related video. Go to aao.org/bcscvideo_section10 or scan the QR code in the text to access this content.

Highlights

- The average rate of aqueous humor production by the ciliary processes is 2–3 µL/min in awake individuals (diurnal) and decreases by approximately 50% during sleep (nocturnal). Aqueous drains through the trabecular meshwork and uveoscleral pathways.
- An understanding of aqueous humor dynamics is essential for the evaluation and management of glaucoma.
- The parameters that contribute to intraocular pressure (IOP) are described by the modified Goldmann equation; they include aqueous humor production rate, uveoscleral outflow rate, outflow facility, and episcleral venous pressure.
- The distribution of IOP in the population is skewed toward higher pressures, but glaucoma can occur at any pressure level.
- Various tonometry methods can be used to estimate IOP, but all currently used methods have sources of error. No device can accurately measure intracameral pressure in all eyes.

Aqueous Humor Production, Composition, and Outflow

Aqueous Humor Production and Composition

Aqueous humor, or *aqueous,* is produced by the ciliary processes (Fig 2-1), enters the posterior chamber, and then flows through the pupil into the anterior chamber (see Chapter 1, Figure 1-6). The average rate of aqueous humor production is 2–3 µL/min in awake individuals (diurnal), decreasing by about 50% during sleep (nocturnal). Because the anterior segment volume is approximately 200–300 µL, the eye's total volume of aqueous humor is turned over about every 100 minutes.

Posterior chamber
BM (ILM)
I
Nonpigmented epithelial cell
Nucleus
M
ZO
GJ
(Apical Surfaces)
D
Pigmented epithelial cell
Nucleus
MG
BM
Ciliary stroma
A
B
C
a
a
b
b
c
e
d
d
c
e
e
c
f
g
f
h
g
h

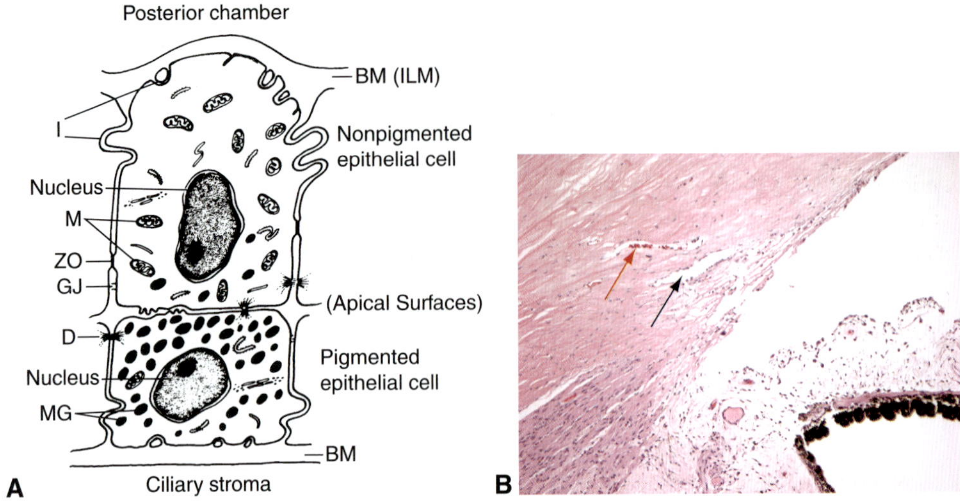

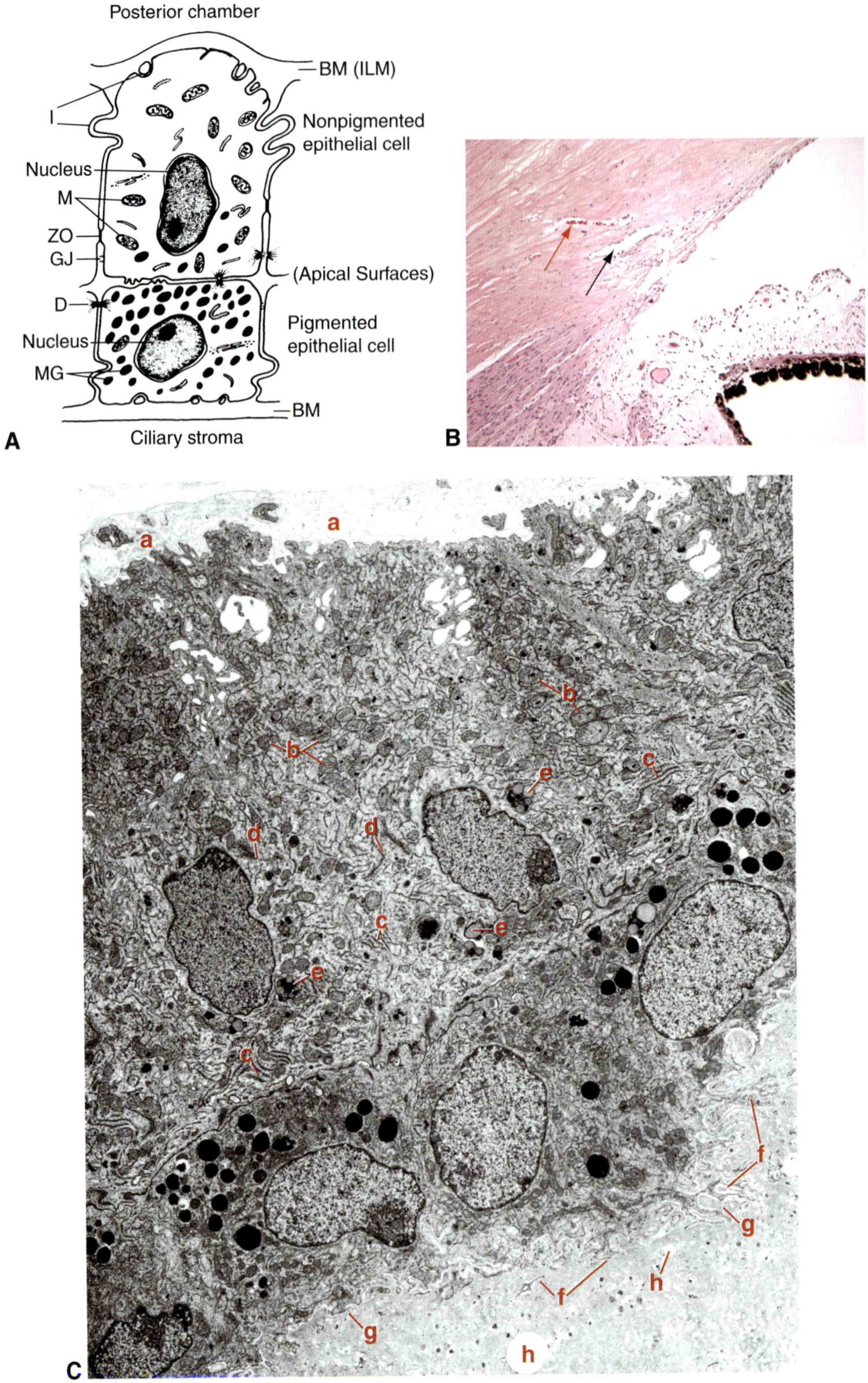

Figure 2-1

The ciliary body contains approximately 80 ciliary processes, each of which is composed of a double layer of epithelium over a core of stroma and a rich supply of fenestrated capillaries (see Fig 2-1). These capillaries are supplied mainly by branches of the major arterial circle of the iris. The apical surfaces of the 2 cell layers—the outer, pigmented epithelium and the inner, nonpigmented epithelium—face each other and are joined by tight junctions, an important component of the blood–aqueous barrier. The nonpigmented epithelial cells, which protrude into the posterior chamber, contain numerous mitochondria, zonula occludens (tight junctions), and microvilli; these cells are thought to be the site of aqueous production. The ciliary processes provide a large surface area for secretion.

Aqueous humor enters the posterior chamber from the ciliary processes by the following physiologic mechanisms:

- active secretion
- ultrafiltration
- simple diffusion

Active secretion refers to transport that requires energy to move sodium, chloride, bicarbonate, and other ions (currently unknown) against an electrochemical gradient. Active secretion is independent of pressure and accounts for the majority of aqueous humor production. This process takes place in the double-layered ciliary epithelium and involves, at least in part, activity of the enzyme carbonic anhydrase II. *Ultrafiltration* refers to a pressure-dependent movement along a pressure gradient. In the ciliary processes, the hydrostatic pressure difference between capillary pressure and intraocular pressure (IOP)

Figure 2-1 *(continued)* Anatomical details of the anterior chamber angle and ciliary body. **A,** The 2 layers of the ciliary epithelium, showing apical surfaces in apposition to each other. Basement membrane (BM) lines the double layer and constitutes the internal limiting membrane (ILM) on the inner surface. The nonpigmented epithelium is characterized by large numbers of mitochondria (M), zonula occludens (ZO), and lateral and surface interdigitations (I). The pigmented epithelium contains numerous melanin granules (MG). Additional intercellular junctions include desmosomes (D) and gap junctions (GJ). **B,** Light micrograph of the anterior chamber angle shows the Schlemm canal *(black arrow),* adjacent to the trabecular meshwork in the sclera. One of the external collector vessels can be seen *(red arrow)* adjacent to the Schlemm canal. **C,** Pars plicata of the ciliary body, showing the 2 epithelial layers in the eye of an older person. The nonpigmented epithelial cells measure approximately 20 μm high by 12 μm wide. The cuboidal pigmented epithelial cells are approximately 10 μm high. The thickened ILM *(a)* is laminated and vesicular; such thickened membranes are characteristic of older eyes. The cytoplasm of the nonpigmented epithelium is characterized by its numerous mitochondria *(b)* and the cisternae of the rough-surfaced endoplasmic reticulum *(c)*. A poorly developed Golgi apparatus *(d)* and several lysosomes and residual bodies *(e)* are shown. Melanin granules in the pigmented epithelium, located mainly in the apical portion, measure approximately 1 μm in diameter. The basal surface is irregular, with many fingerlike processes *(f)*. The basement membrane of the pigmented epithelium *(g)* and a smooth granular material containing vesicles *(h)* and coarse granular particles are seen at the bottom of the figure. The appearance of the basement membrane is typical of older eyes and can be discerned with the light microscope (×5700). *(Part A reproduced with permission from Shields MB.* Textbook of Glaucoma. *3rd ed. Williams & Wilkins; 1992. Part B courtesy of Nasreen A. Syed, MD. Part C modified with permission from Hogan MJ, Alvarado JA, Weddell JE.* Histology of the Human Eye. *Saunders; 1971:283.)*

favors fluid movement into the eye, whereas the oncotic gradient between the two resists fluid movement. The relationship between secretion and ultrafiltration is not known. *Diffusion* involves the passive movement of ions, based on charge and concentration, down the concentration or ionic gradient across a membrane.

In humans and other diurnal animals, the ascorbate concentration is higher in aqueous humor than in plasma. In the healthy eye, the blood–aqueous barrier restricts the passage of plasma proteins into the aqueous. As a result, the aqueous humor is essentially protein-free (1/200–1/500 of the protein found in plasma), allowing optical clarity. Albumin accounts for approximately half of the total protein. The composition of the aqueous humor is altered as it flows from the posterior chamber, through the pupil, and into the anterior chamber. This alteration occurs across the hyaloid face of the vitreous, the surface of the lens, the blood vessels of the iris, and the corneal endothelium; and it is secondary to other dilutional exchanges and active processes. See Chapter 9 in BCSC Section 2, *Fundamentals and Principles of Ophthalmology,* for in-depth discussion of aqueous humor composition and production.

Suppression of Aqueous Humor Formation

Various classes of drugs can suppress formation of aqueous humor. The mechanisms of action of these drugs are discussed in Chapter 12.

Inhibition of the enzyme carbonic anhydrase II suppresses aqueous humor formation. However, the precise role of carbonic anhydrase has been vigorously debated. Its function may be to provide the bicarbonate ion, which, evidence suggests, is actively secreted in human eyes. Carbonic anhydrase may also provide bicarbonate or hydrogen ions for an intracellular buffering system.

Blockade of β_2-receptors, the most prevalent adrenergic receptors in the ciliary epithelium, may reduce aqueous humor formation and affect active secretion by causing a decrease either in the efficiency of Na^+,K^+-ATPase (also called the *sodium-potassium pump*) or in the number of pump sites. For additional discussion of Na^+,K^+-ATPase and the "pump-leak" hypothesis, see BCSC Section 2, *Fundamentals and Principles of Ophthalmology.* Stimulation of α_2-receptors also reduces aqueous humor formation, possibly by means of a decrease in ciliary body blood flow, mediated through inhibition of cyclic adenosine monophosphate (cAMP); the exact mechanism is unclear.

Aqueous Humor Outflow

Aqueous humor outflow occurs by 2 major mechanisms: the pressure-sensitive *trabecular meshwork* pathway and the pressure-insensitive *uveoscleral* pathway.

Trabecular meshwork outflow

Aqueous humor exiting the eye through the trabecular meshwork, or *conventional,* pathway first crosses the trabecular meshwork, enters the Schlemm canal, and passes through collector channels in the outer wall of the canal, which drain either directly into aqueous veins or into the vessels of the intrascleral plexus, which then drain into aqueous veins.

From there, aqueous humor returns to the systemic circulation via the episcleral venous system and the superior ophthalmic veins, ultimately draining into the cavernous sinus.

The *trabecular meshwork* is classically divided into 3 layers: uveal, corneoscleral, and juxtacanalicular (Fig 2-2). The *uveal trabecular meshwork* is adjacent to the anterior chamber and is arranged in bands that extend from the iris root and the ciliary body to the peripheral cornea. The *corneoscleral meshwork* consists of perforated sheets that extend from the scleral spur to the lateral wall of the scleral sulcus. The *juxtacanalicular meshwork,* thought to be the major site of outflow resistance, is adjacent to and forms the inner wall of the Schlemm canal. Aqueous humor moves both across and between the endothelial cells lining the inner wall of the Schlemm canal.

The trabecular meshwork is composed of multiple layers, each of which consists of a collagenous connective tissue core covered by a continuous endothelial layer. The trabecular meshwork is the site of pressure-sensitive aqueous humor outflow and functions as a one-way valve, permitting aqueous humor to leave the eye by bulk flow but limiting flow in the other direction, independent of energy. The cells of the trabecular meshwork are phagocytic, and in the presence of inflammation and after laser trabeculoplasty, phagocytosis may increase.

In most older adults, the trabecular meshwork cells contain a large number of pigment granules in their cytoplasm, giving the entire meshwork a pigmented appearance, the degree of which can vary with location in the meshwork and among individuals. There are approximately 200,000–300,000 trabecular meshwork cells per eye. With age, the number of trabecular meshwork cells decreases, and the basement membrane beneath them thickens, potentially increasing outflow resistance. An interesting effect of all types of laser trabeculoplasty is that it induces division of trabecular cells and causes a change in the production of cytokines and other structurally important elements of the extracellular matrix.

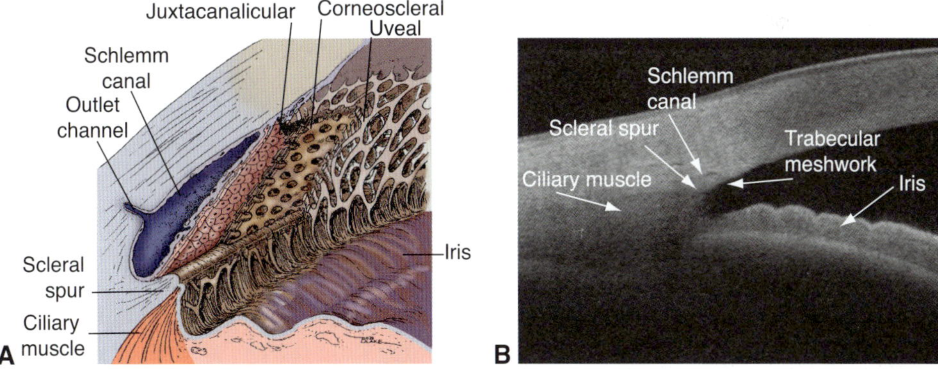

Figure 2-2 Trabecular meshwork and Schlemm canal. **A,** Three layers of the trabecular meshwork (shown in cutaway views): uveal, corneoscleral, and juxtacanalicular. **B,** Anterior segment optical coherence tomography image of the trabecular meshwork and Schlemm canal. *(Part A modified with permission from Shields MB.* Textbook of Glaucoma. *3rd ed. Williams & Wilkins; 1992. Part B courtesy of Syril K. Dorairaj, MD.)*

The *Schlemm canal,* similar to lymphatic channels, is completely lined with an endothelial layer that rests on a discontinuous basement membrane. The canal is a single channel, typically with a diameter of approximately 200–300 μm, although this can vary considerably, with narrowings that can obstruct flow. The exact path of aqueous flow across the inner wall of the Schlemm canal is uncertain. Intracellular and intercellular pores suggest bulk flow, while so-called giant vacuoles that have direct communication with the intertrabecular spaces suggest active transport. However, these vacuoles may be artifacts of tissue preparation and microscopy. The outer wall of the Schlemm canal is formed by a single layer of endothelial cells that do not contain pores. See Chapter 2 in BCSC Section 2, *Fundamentals and Principles of Ophthalmology,* for additional discussion and illustrations of the trabecular meshwork and Schlemm canal.

A complex system of *collector channels* connects the Schlemm canal to the aqueous veins, which drain into the episcleral veins, forming the distal portion of the trabecular meshwork outflow system *(distal outflow system)* (Video 2-1). As previously mentioned, the episcleral veins subsequently drain into the superior ophthalmic veins. These, in turn, ultimately drain into the cavernous sinus.

VIDEO 2-1 Aqueous humor flow through the distal outflow system as seen using indocyanine green aqueous angiography.
Courtesy of Alex Huang, MD, PhD.
Available at: aao.org/bcscvideo_section10

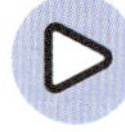

The trabecular meshwork pathway is dynamic. With increasing IOP, the cross-sectional area of the Schlemm canal decreases, while the trabecular meshwork expands. Similarly, in the distal outflow system, the amount of aqueous humor flow through individual vessels appears to vary dynamically, a concept referred to as *segmental outflow,* which may have implications for the success of trabecular bypass procedures. However, no compelling evidence thus far supports the performance of location-dependent procedures.

Andrew NH, Akkach S, Casson RJ. A review of aqueous outflow resistance and its relevance to microinvasive glaucoma surgery. *Surv Ophthalmol.* 2020;65(1):18–31.

Uveoscleral outflow

In the healthy eye, any outflow not passing through the trabecular meshwork is termed *uveoscleral* (also called *unconventional* or *pressure-insensitive*) *outflow.* Although it is pressure insensitive, uveoscleral outflow is the bulk flow that depends on a pressure gradient that remains relatively constant with changes in IOP. Various mechanisms are probably involved in uveoscleral outflow. Aqueous humor leaving the eye via the uveoscleral pathway passes from the anterior chamber into the interstitial spaces between the ciliary muscle bundles and then into the supraciliary and suprachoroidal spaces. From there, the exact path of the aqueous humor exiting the eye is unclear. It may include passage through the intact sclera or along the nerves and vessels that penetrate it, or it may involve absorption into the vortex veins. Lymphatic vessels have also been identified in the ciliary body, and aqueous humor drainage through a uveolymphatic pathway has also been proposed.

Johnson M, McLaren JW, Overby DR. Unconventional aqueous humor outflow: a review. *Exp Eye Res.* 2017;158:94–111.

Aqueous Humor Dynamics

An understanding of aqueous humor dynamics is essential for the evaluation and management of glaucoma. Aqueous humor dynamics involves the measurement of parameters that affect IOP. The modified *Goldmann equation* is a mathematical model of the relationship between IOP and the parameters that contribute to its level in the eye at steady state:

$$P_0 = (F - U)/C + P_v$$

where P_0 is the IOP in millimeters of mercury (mm Hg), F is the rate of aqueous humor production in microliters per minute (µL/min), U is the rate of aqueous humor drainage through the pressure-insensitive uveoscleral pathway in microliters per minute (µL/min), C is the facility of outflow through the pressure-sensitive trabecular meshwork pathway in microliters per minute per millimeter of mercury (µL/min/mm Hg), and P_v is the episcleral venous pressure in millimeters of mercury. Although there are 5 parameters in the equation, only 4 need to be measured—the fifth parameter can then be calculated. Resistance to outflow *(R)* is the inverse of facility *(C)*. Figure 2-3 illustrates the effect of outflow facility *(C)* on IOP. Because aqueous production is usually normal in patients with glaucoma, outflow must also be unaffected. However, *resistance* to outflow is often increased, leading to the increase in eye pressure necessary to maintain that outflow. For typical eye pressures encountered by clinicians, outflow facility is probably between 0.2 and 0.3 µL/min/mm Hg—the flat part of the curve shown in Figure 2-3, where large changes in outflow facility lead to small changes in IOP.

Measurement of Aqueous Humor Production

The rate of aqueous humor production by the ciliary processes cannot be measured noninvasively, but it is assumed to be equal to the aqueous humor outflow rate in an eye

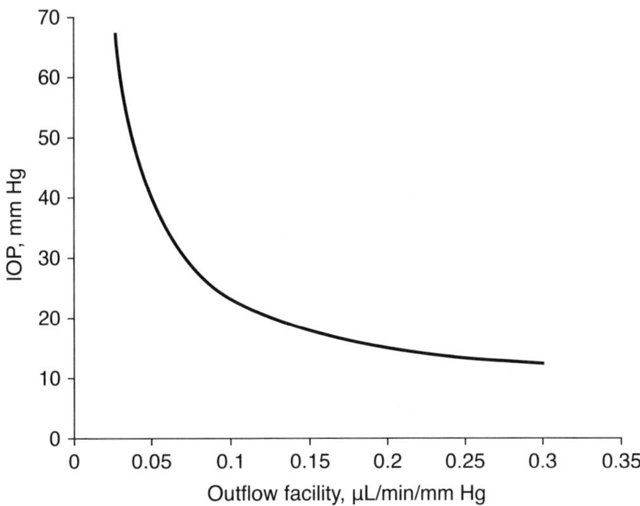

Figure 2-3 The effect of outflow facility on intraocular pressure (IOP), based on the modified Goldmann equation (assuming a constant aqueous humor production rate of 2.5 µL/min, uveoscleral outflow rate of 35%, and episcleral venous pressure of 7 mm Hg). *(Courtesy of Arthur J. Sit, MD.)*

at steady state. The most common method used to measure the rate of aqueous humor outflow is *fluorophotometry.* For this test, fluorescein is administered topically, its gradual dilution in the anterior chamber is measured optically, and the change in fluorescein concentration over time is then used to calculate aqueous flow. As previously noted, the normal flow rate is approximately 2–3 µL/min in awake individuals, and the aqueous volume is turned over at a rate of approximately 1% per minute.

The rate of aqueous humor production varies according to our circadian rhythm and is reduced by approximately half during sleep, as previously mentioned. It also decreases with age. The rate is affected by a variety of factors, including the following:

- integrity of the blood–aqueous barrier
- blood flow to the ciliary body
- neurohumoral regulation of vascular tissue and the ciliary epithelium

Aqueous humor production may decrease after trauma or intraocular inflammation and after the administration of certain systemic drugs (eg, general anesthetics and some systemic hypotensive agents), as well as aqueous humor suppressants used for treatment of glaucoma. Carotid occlusive disease may also decrease aqueous humor production.

Brubaker RF. Flow of aqueous humor in humans [The Friedenwald Lecture]. *Invest Ophthalmol Vis Sci.* 1991;32(13):3145–3166.

Measurement of Outflow Facility

The facility of outflow (*C* in the Goldmann equation) is the mathematical inverse of outflow resistance and varies widely in healthy eyes, with a mean ranging from 0.22 to 0.30 µL/min/mm Hg. Outflow facility decreases with age and is affected by ocular surgery, trauma, certain medications, and endocrine factors. Patients with glaucoma and elevated IOP typically have decreased outflow facility. In healthy eyes, approximately 50% of conventional outflow resistance is in the trabecular meshwork; the remainder is in the distal outflow system. However, in primary open-angle glaucoma with elevated IOP or in ocular hypertension, most of the pathologic change occurs in the juxtacanalicular tissue of the trabecular meshwork and the inner wall of the Schlemm canal.

Tonography is a method used to measure the facility of aqueous humor outflow. In this technique, a weighted Schiøtz tonometer or the probe tip of a pneumotonometer is placed on the cornea, acutely elevating the IOP. Outflow facility (in µL/min/mm Hg) can be computed from the rate at which the pressure declines with time, reflecting the ease with which aqueous humor leaves the eye to reestablish a steady state.

However, tonography depends on a number of assumptions (eg, ocular rigidity, stability of aqueous humor formation, and constancy of ocular blood volume) and is subject to many sources of error, such as poor patient fixation and eyelid squeezing. These problems reduce the accuracy and reproducibility of tonography for an individual patient. In general, tonography is best employed as a research tool and is rarely used clinically.

Kazemi A, McLaren JW, Lin SC, et al. Comparison of aqueous outflow facility measurement by pneumatonography and digital Schiøtz tonography. *Invest Ophthalmol Vis Sci.* 2017; 58(1):204–210.

Vahabikashi A, Gelman A, Dong B, et al. Increased stiffness and flow resistance of the inner wall of Schlemm canal in glaucomatous human eyes. *Proc Natl Acad Sci USA.* 2019;116(52):26555–26563.

Measurement of Episcleral Venous Pressure

The episcleral veins are the ultimate destination for aqueous humor draining through the trabecular meshwork pathway. Thus, the pressure in these veins, the *episcleral venous pressure (EVP),* represents the lowest-possible IOP in an intact eye with normal aqueous humor production. EVP is a dynamic parameter, varying with alterations in body position and systemic blood pressure. It is often increased in syndromes with facial hemangiomas (eg, Sturge-Weber [encephalofacial angiomatosis]), carotid-cavernous sinus fistulas, and cavernous sinus thrombosis. Also, it may be affected by some medications, including topical Rho kinase inhibitors. EVP may be partially responsible for the elevated IOP seen in thyroid eye disease.

EVP can be measured noninvasively by *venomanometry,* in which a transparent flexible membrane is placed against the sclera and the pressure is slowly increased. The pressure that begins to collapse an episcleral vein corresponds to EVP; however, visualizing this endpoint can be difficult. The use of automated pressure measurements, video recording of the vein collapse, and image analysis software can help to precisely identify the endpoint and associated EVP. The usual range of values is 6–9 mm Hg, but higher values have been reported when different endpoints and measurement techniques are used. According to the Goldmann equation, IOP acutely rises approximately 1 mm Hg for every 1-mm-Hg increase in EVP. However, elevation of EVP can cause reflux of blood into the Schlemm canal, altering the normal outflow of aqueous humor. As a result, the change in IOP may be greater or less than that predicted by the Goldmann equation.

Sit AJ, McLaren JW. Measurement of episcleral venous pressure. *Exp Eye Res.* 2011;93(3): 291–298.

Measurement of Uveoscleral Outflow Rate

Uveoscleral outflow rate cannot be measured noninvasively and, therefore, is usually calculated from the Goldmann equation after determination of the other parameters. There is evidence that outflow via the uveoscleral pathway is substantial in human eyes, accounting for roughly 50% of total aqueous outflow, although invasive studies using tracers tend to report lower values. Some studies indicate that uveoscleral outflow decreases with age and is reduced in patients with glaucoma. It is increased by cycloplegia, adrenergic agents, and prostaglandin $F_{2\alpha}$ analogues but decreased by miotics. It is also increased by suprachoroidal stents and by cyclodialysis clefts.

Bill A, Phillips CI. Uveoscleral drainage of aqueous humour in human eyes. *Exp Eye Res.* 1971;12(3):275–281.

Brubaker RF. Measurement of uveoscleral outflow in humans. *J Glaucoma.* 2001;10(5 Suppl 1): S45–S48.

Intraocular Pressure

IOP Distribution and Relation to Glaucoma

Pooled data from large epidemiologic studies indicate that the mean IOP in the general population of European ancestry is approximately 15.5 mm Hg, with a standard deviation (SD) of 2.6 mm Hg. Studies also show a nonnormal (non-Gaussian) distribution of IOP in the population, with a skew toward higher pressures, especially in individuals older than 40 years (Fig 2-4). In addition, IOP has been found to be genetically influenced.

The value 21 mm Hg (2 SDs above the mean) was traditionally used both to separate normal from abnormal pressures and to define which patients required ocular hypotensive therapy. However, it is now understood that glaucoma is a multifactorial disease process for which IOP is an important risk factor. Many patients with glaucoma consistently have IOPs ≤21 mm Hg, and most individuals with IOP >21 mm Hg do not develop glaucoma. Consequently, screening for glaucoma based solely on the criterion of IOP >21 mm Hg misses up to half of the people with glaucoma and optic nerve damage in the screened population.

General agreement has been reached that, for the population as a whole, there is no clear level below which IOP can be considered "normal" or safe and above which IOP can be considered "elevated" or unsafe. IOP is a continuous risk factor across its entire range: the higher the IOP, the greater the risk for glaucoma. Although other risk factors affect an individual's susceptibility to glaucoma, all current treatments are designed to reduce IOP.

Sommer A, Tielsch JM, Katz J, et al. Relationship between intraocular pressure and primary open-angle glaucoma among white and black Americans. The Baltimore Eye Survey. *Arch Ophthalmol.* 1991;109(8):1090–1095.

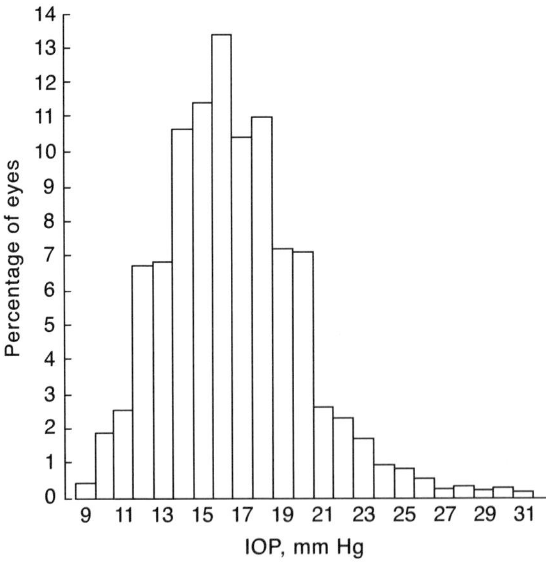

Figure 2-4 Frequency distribution of IOP: 5220 eyes in the Framingham Eye Study. *(Modified from Colton T, Ederer F. The distribution of intraocular pressures in the general population.* Surv Ophthalmol. *1980;25(3):123–129. With permission from Elsevier.)*

Variations in IOP

Intraocular pressure is affected by a variety of factors, including the time of day (see the section "Circadian variation"), body position, respiration, exercise, systemic medications, and topical medications (Table 2-1).

Body position significantly affects IOP, and the lowest IOP measurements are obtained when a person is seated with the neck in a vertical, neutral position. IOP is higher when an individual is recumbent rather than upright, predominantly because of an increase in EVP. Some people have an exaggerated rise in IOP when recumbent; this tendency may be important in the pathogenesis of certain forms of glaucoma. Alcohol consumption causes a transient decrease in IOP. Cannabis also decreases IOP but has not proved clinically useful as a hypotensive agent because of its short duration of action and its side effects; moreover, the reduction in systemic blood pressure that it causes may negate any protective effect of IOP lowering in terms of optic nerve perfusion. In most studies, caffeine has

Table 2-1 Factors That Affect Intraocular Pressure

Factors that may increase intraocular pressure

- Elevated episcleral venous pressure
  - Bending over or being in a supine position
  - Breath holding
  - Elevated central venous pressure
  - Intubation
  - Orbital venous outflow obstruction
  - Playing a wind instrument
  - Valsalva maneuver
  - Wearing a tight collar or tight necktie
- Pressure on the eye
  - Blepharospasm
  - Eye rubbing
  - Eyelid squeezing and crying, especially in young children
- Elevated body temperature (associated with increased aqueous humor production)
- Hormonal influences
  - Hypothyroidism
  - Thyroid eye disease
- Drugs unrelated to glaucoma therapy
  - Anticholinergics, topiramate: may precipitate angle closure
  - Corticosteroids
  - Ketamine (evidence for slight increase or no change)
  - Lysergic acid diethylamide (LSD)

Factors that may decrease intraocular pressure

- Aerobic exercise
- Anesthetic drugs
  - Depolarizing muscle relaxants such as succinylcholine
  - Inhalational anesthetics
- Metabolic or respiratory acidosis (decreases aqueous humor production)
- Hormonal influences
  - Pregnancy
- Drugs unrelated to glaucoma therapy
  - Alcohol
  - Heroin
  - Marijuana (cannabis)

not been shown to have an appreciable effect on IOP. There is little variation in IOP with age in healthy individuals.

Pujari R, Jampel H. Treating glaucoma with medical marijuana: peering through the smoke. *Ophthalmol Glaucoma.* 2019;2(4):201–203.

Circadian variation

In individuals without glaucoma, IOP varies by 2–6 mm Hg over a 24-hour period, as aqueous humor production, outflow facility, and uveoscleral outflow change. Higher mean IOP is associated with wider fluctuation in pressure. The time at which peak IOP occurs varies among individuals. However, 24-hour IOP measurement performed with individuals in their habitual body positions (standing or sitting during the daytime and supine at night) indicates that most people (with or without glaucoma) have peak pressures during sleep, in the early-morning hours (despite the reduction in aqueous humor production that occurs during sleep). This peak corresponds with a decrease in outflow facility and uveoscleral outflow. During waking hours, peak pressure often occurs soon after awakening. While eye drops can have variable effects on circadian variation, it is thought that glaucoma surgery often results in decreased variation.

Clinical Pearl In selected patients, measurement of IOP outside office hours may be useful in determining why optic nerve damage continues to occur despite apparently adequately controlled pressure.

Liu JH, Zhang X, Kripke DF, Weinreb RN. Twenty-four-hour intraocular pressure pattern associated with early glaucomatous changes. *Invest Ophthalmol Vis Sci.* 2003;44(4): 1586–1590.

Nau CB, Malihi M, McLaren JW, Hodge DO, Sit AJ. Circadian variation of aqueous humor dynamics in older healthy adults. *Invest Ophthalmol Vis Sci.* 2013;54(12):7623–7629.

IOP fluctuation and glaucoma

A considerable body of literature demonstrates an association between IOP fluctuation and the risk of glaucoma progression. However, the data are largely retrospective, based on post hoc analyses of IOP variations between visits in large clinical trials. IOP fluctuation is also closely correlated with the level of mean IOP and appears to be a more important risk factor in certain groups of patients, including those with low IOP. Glaucoma surgery results in less IOP fluctuation than does medical therapy, but the clinical significance of this finding has not been demonstrated. Moreover, the specific measures of variability that may best predict glaucoma progression are unknown, and the technology to effectively measure IOP fluctuation in a short time frame remains limited.

Caprioli J, Coleman AL. Intraocular pressure fluctuation a risk factor for visual field progression at low intraocular pressures in the Advanced Glaucoma Intervention Study. *Ophthalmology.* 2008;115(7):1123–1129.

Musch DC, Gillespie BW, Niziol LM, Lichter PR, Varma R; CIGTS Study Group. Intraocular pressure control and long-term visual field loss in the Collaborative Initial Glaucoma Treatment Study. *Ophthalmology.* 2011;118(9):1766–1773.

Clinical Measurement of IOP

Tonometry is the noninvasive measurement of IOP. Many different methods of tonometry have been developed, and each has advantages and disadvantages. All currently used methods have sources of error, and no device can accurately measure intracameral pressure in all eyes.

Tonometry

Applanation tonometry

Applanation tonometry, the most widely used method, is based on the Imbert-Fick principle, which states that the pressure inside an ideal dry, infinitely thin-walled sphere equals the force necessary to flatten its surface divided by the area of the flattening:

$$P = F/A$$

where P = pressure, F = force, and A = area. In applanation tonometry, the cornea is flattened, and IOP is determined by measuring the applanating force and the area flattened.

The *Goldmann applanation tonometer,* the most widely used tonometer in clinical practice and research, measures the force necessary to flatten an area of the cornea 3.06 mm in diameter (Fig 2-5). At this diameter, the material resistance of the cornea to flattening is counterbalanced by the capillary attraction of the tear film meniscus to the tonometer head. Furthermore, the IOP (in mm Hg) equals the flattening force (in gram-force) multiplied by 10. A split-image prism allows the examiner to accurately determine the flattened area. Topical anesthetic is administered, and fluorescein dye is instilled in the tear film to outline the area of flattening. Fluorescein semicircles, or *mires,* visible through the split-image prism move with the ocular pulse, and the endpoint is reached when the inner edges of the semicircles touch each other at the midpoint of their excursion (Fig 2-6). By properly aligning the mires, the examiner can ensure the appropriate area of corneal applanation to obtain the most accurate IOP reading.

The *Perkins tonometer* is a counterbalanced applanation tonometer that, like the Goldmann tonometer, uses a split-image prism and requires instillation of fluorescein dye in the tear film. It is portable and can be used with the patient either upright or supine.

Applanation tonometry is safe, and the measurements obtained are relatively accurate in most clinical situations. Because applanation does not displace much fluid (approximately 0.5 µL) or substantially increase the pressure in the eye, IOP measurement by this method is relatively unaffected by ocular rigidity, compared with indentation (Shiøtz) tonometry.

The accuracy of applanation tonometry can be reduced in certain situations (Table 2-2). An inadequate amount of fluorescein in the tear film can lead to poor visualization of the mires and the measurement endpoint, resulting in inaccurate readings. Tear film thickness can also affect accuracy. A common misconception is that an excessively thick tear film leads to erroneous readings because extremely thick mires require greater force to reach the measurement endpoint. However, this is incorrect, as the inner edges of the mires will touch when an area 3.06 mm in diameter is applanated, regardless of

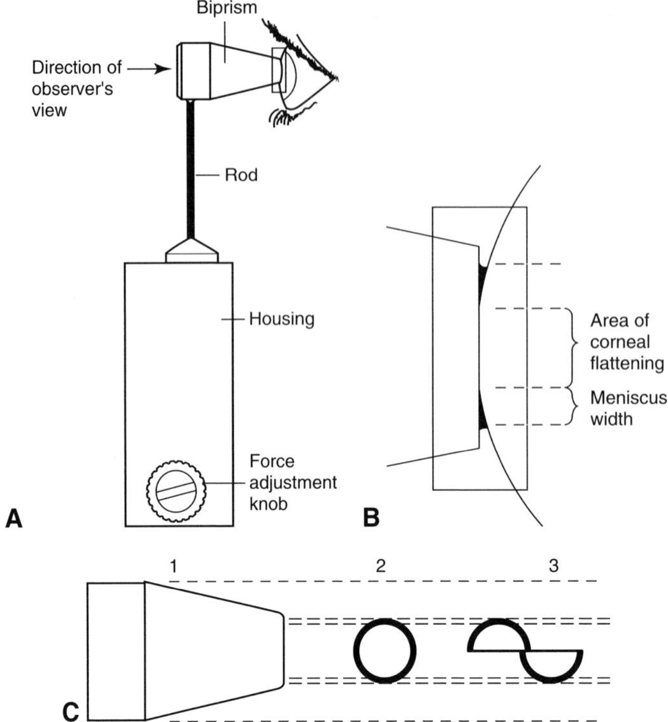

Figure 2-5 Goldmann-type applanation tonometry. **A,** Basic features of the tonometer, shown in contact with the patient's cornea. **B,** The enlargement shows the tear film meniscus created by contact of the split-image prism ("biprism" above) and cornea. **C,** The view through the split-image prism *(1)* reveals a circular meniscus *(2)*, which is converted into 2 semicircles *(3)* by the prisms. *(Redrawn with permission from Shields MB.* Textbook of Glaucoma. *3rd ed. Williams & Wilkins; 1992.)*

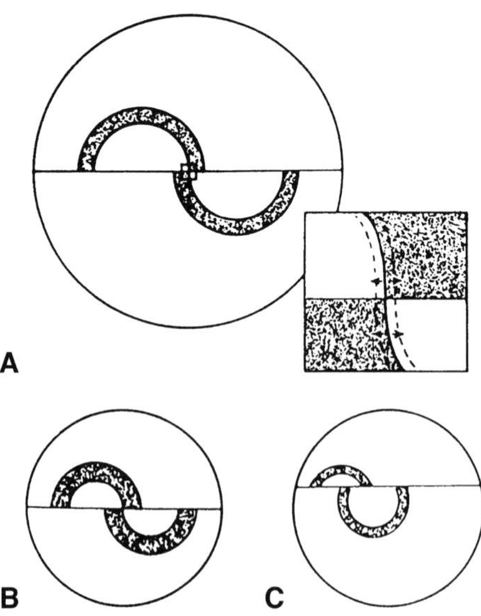

Figure 2-6 Mires viewed through the split-image prism of the Goldmann-type applanation tonometer. **A,** Proper width and position of the mires. The enlargement depicts excursions of the mires, which are caused by ocular pulsations. **B,** The mires are too wide. **C,** Improper vertical and horizontal alignment. *(Reproduced with permission from Shields MB.* Textbook of Glaucoma. *3rd ed. Williams & Wilkins; 1992.)*

Table 2-2 Possible Sources of Nonrepresentative IOP in Tonometry[a]

Factors That May Cause Artifactually Low IOP	Factors That May Cause Artifactually High IOP	Factors That May Increase IOP During Measurement
Corneal biomechanical properties (eg, rigidity)	Corneal biomechanical properties (eg, rigidity)	Breath holding or Valsalva maneuver
Corneal irregularity (eg, ectasia)	Corneal irregularity (eg, ectasia)	Extraocular muscle force applied to a restricted globe[a]
Inaccurately calibrated tonometer	Inaccurately calibrated tonometer	Straining to reach the slit lamp
High corneal astigmatism	High corneal astigmatism	Pressure on the globe
Inadequate amount of fluorescein in tear film	Excessive amount of fluorescein in tear film or extremely thick tear film	Squeezing of the eyelids
Technician errors	Technician errors	Tight collar or tight necktie (may be a meaningful increase in IOP if worn frequently)
Thin central cornea	Thick central cornea	
Measurement done over a soft contact lens	Corneal scarring or band keratopathy	
Corneal edema		

IOP = intraocular pressure.
[a] May depend on the method used to measure IOP.

the mire thickness. Rather, accuracy is reduced because the surface tension changes with alterations in tear film thickness. Because the cornea is curved, an increasing tear film thickness will form a meniscus with a larger curvature radius, with a lower surface tension. The low surface tension inadequately counterbalances the corneal resistance, resulting in an artificially high IOP reading. Conversely, a very thin tear film has a small radius of curvature with a high surface tension that exceeds the corneal resistance, yielding a falsely low IOP reading.

In eyes with marked corneal astigmatism, the fluorescein pattern seen by the clinician through the split-image prism appears elliptical, and the IOP may be artificially high or low. To obtain an accurate reading in an astigmatic eye, the clinician should rotate the prism so that the red mark on the prism holder is set at the least-curved meridian of the cornea (along the negative axis). Alternatively, 2 pressure readings taken 90° apart can be averaged.

Corneal edema predisposes to inaccurately low readings, whereas pressure measurements taken over a corneal scar will be falsely high. Tonometry performed over a soft contact lens gives artificially low values.

Whitacre MM, Stein R. Sources of error with use of Goldmann-type tonometers. *Surv Ophthalmol.* 1993;38(1):1–30.

Tonometry and central corneal thickness Measurements obtained with the most common types of tonometers are affected by central corneal thickness (CCT). Goldmann tonometer readings are most accurate when the CCT is 520 μm. Thicker corneas resist the deformation inherent in most methods of tonometry, resulting in an overestimation of IOP, whereas thinner corneas may give an artificially low reading. IOP may also be underestimated after laser or other types of keratorefractive surgery if these procedures resulted in a CCT significantly less than that assumed for Goldmann tonometry.

The relationship between measured IOP and CCT is not linear, so correction factors are only estimates at best. In addition, the biomechanical properties of individual corneas may vary, and the stiffness or elasticity of the cornea may affect IOP measurement. Currently, there is no validated correction factor for the effect of CCT on applanation tonometers; therefore, the correction methods proposed in the literature are not applicable to clinical use. A thin central cornea is a known risk factor for progression from ocular hypertension to glaucoma. However, it has not been determined whether this increased risk of glaucoma is attributable only to underestimation of IOP or whether a thin central cornea is a biomarker for another risk factor independent of IOP measurement.

Brandt JD, Beiser JA, Kass MA, Gordon MO; Ocular Hypertension Treatment Study Group. Central corneal thickness in the Ocular Hypertension Treatment Study (OHTS). *Ophthalmology.* 2001;108(10):1779–1788.

Gordon MO, Beiser JA, Brandt JA, et al. The Ocular Hypertension Treatment Study: baseline factors that predict the onset of primary open-angle glaucoma. *Arch Ophthalmol.* 2002;120(6):714–720.

Mackay-Marg–type tonometry

Mackay-Marg–type tonometers use an annular ring to gently flatten a small area of the cornea. As the area of flattening increases, the pressure in the center of the ring increases as well and is measured with a transducer. The IOP is equivalent to the pressure when the center of the ring is just covered by the flattened cornea.

Portable electronic devices of the Mackay-Marg type (eg, Tono-Pen, Reichert Technologies; Fig 2-7A) contain a strain gauge to measure the pressure at the center of an annular ring placed on the cornea. The instrument tip is tapped against the surface of the cornea, obtaining several measurements that are then used by the device to provide an IOP measurement along with the coefficient of variation. These devices are particularly useful in patients with corneal scars or edema, as the measurement tip is small enough to be applied only on areas of normal cornea. It also can be used to obtain measurements regardless of the patient's body position. However, some studies suggest that the Tono-Pen tends to overestimate low IOPs and underestimate high IOPs.

Eisenberg DL, Sherman BG, McKeown CA, Schuman JS. Tonometry in adults and children. A manometric evaluation of pneumatonometry, applanation, and TonoPen in vitro and in vivo. *Ophthalmology.* 1998;105(7):1173–1181.

Pneumotonometry

The *pneumatic tonometer,* or *pneumotonometer,* has characteristics of both an applanation tonometer and Mackay-Marg–type devices (Fig 2-7B). It has a cylindrical air-filled chamber and a probe tip covered with a flexible, inert silicone elastomer (Silastic membrane) diaphragm. Because of the constant flow of air through the chamber, there is a small gap between the diaphragm and the probe edge. As the probe tip touches and applanates the cornea, the air pressure increases until this gap is completely closed, at which point the IOP is equivalent to the air pressure.

Similar to the Tono-Pen, the pneumotonometer makes contact with only a small area of the cornea and therefore is especially useful in eyes with corneal scars or localized

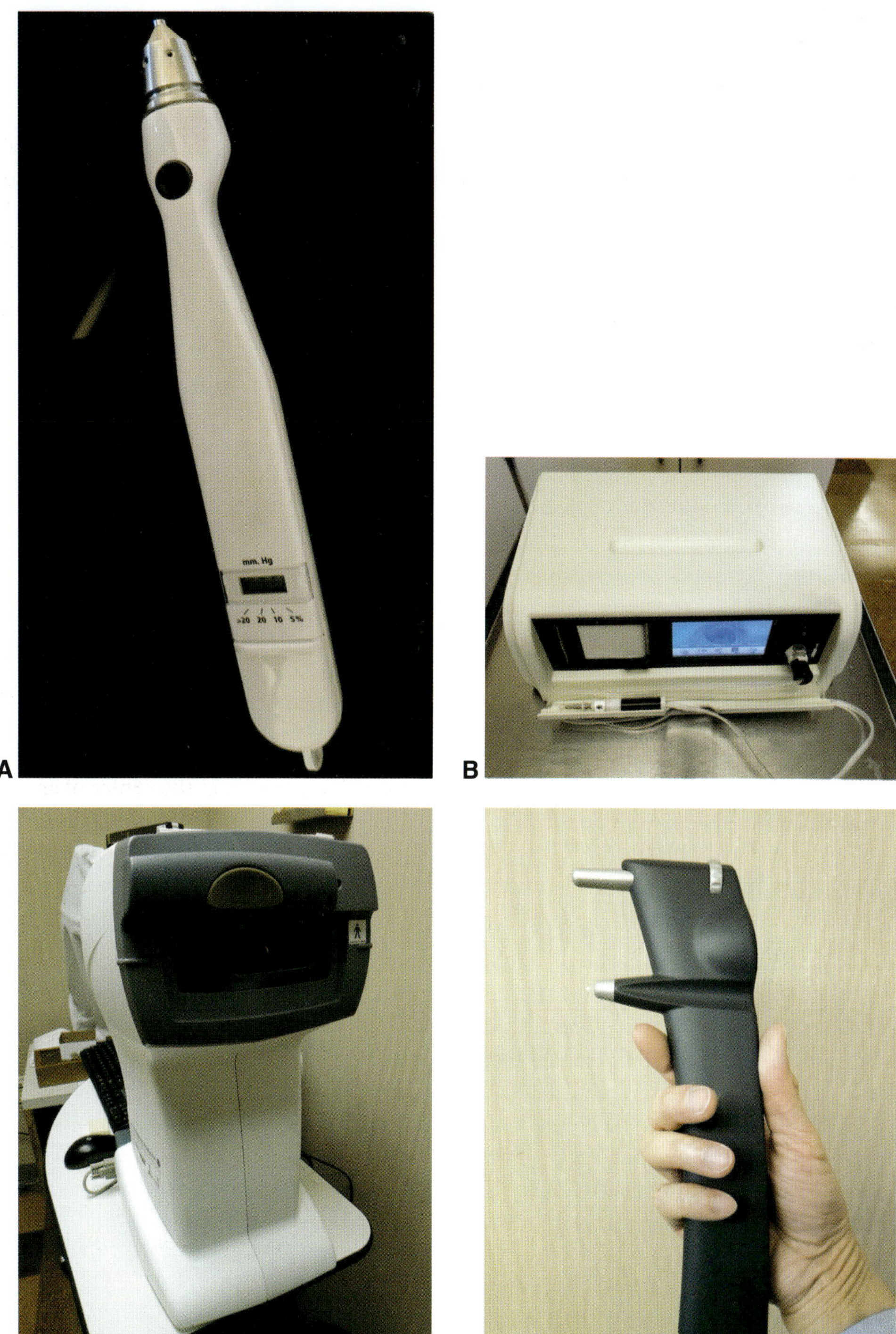

Figure 2-7 Nonapplanation tonometers in common use have advantages and disadvantages compared with Goldmann applanation tonometers. **A,** Tono-Pen (Reichert Technologies). **B,** Pneumatonometer (Reichert Technologies). **C,** Ocular Response Analyzer (Reichert Technologies). **D,** Rebound tonometer (iCare; iCare Finland OY). *(Courtesy of Arthur J. Sit, MD.)*

edema. It can be used with the patient in an upright, lateral decubitus, or supine position. Measurements obtained by placing the probe on the sclera appear to correlate well with those obtained with the probe placed on the cornea. While scleral placement could be useful for patients with severe corneal disease (eg, those with keratoprostheses), there are insufficient data to validate this application of the device. The pneumotonometer can also record IOP continuously while the probe is on the eye and can be used for tonography.

Kapamajian MA, de la Cruz J, Hallak JA, Vajaranant TS. Correlation between corneal and scleral pneumatonometry: an alternative method for intraocular pressure measurement. *Am J Ophthalmol.* 2013;156(5):902–906.e1.

Dynamic contour tonometry

The *dynamic contour tonometer,* a type of nonapplanation contact tonometer, is based on the principle that when the surface of the cornea is aligned with the surface of the instrument tip, the pressure in the tear film between these surfaces is equal to the IOP and can be measured by a pressure transducer. The tip is similar in shape and size to an applanation tonometer tip except that it has a rounded concave surface and a pressure transducer embedded in the center. This allows the device to measure ocular pulse amplitude (the difference between diastolic and systolic IOP) in addition to IOP. Evidence suggests that IOP measurements obtained with dynamic contour tonometry may be more independent of corneal biomechanical properties and thickness than those obtained with applanation tonometry.

Schneider E, Grehn F. Intraocular pressure measurement-comparison of dynamic contour tonometry and Goldmann applanation tonometry. *J Glaucoma.* 2006;15(1):2–6.

Noncontact tonometry

Noncontact (air-puff) tonometers determine IOP by measuring the force of air required to indent and flatten the cornea, thereby avoiding contact with the eye. IOP is measured when the amount of corneal indentation corresponds with the maximum amount of light reflection from the cornea. Readings obtained with these instruments vary widely, and IOP is often overestimated. Noncontact tonometers are often used in large-scale public health programs or by nonmedical health care providers.

The *Ocular Response Analyzer* (ORA, Reichert Technologies; Fig 2-7C) is a type of noncontact tonometer that uses correction algorithms so that its IOP readings more closely match those obtained with applanation techniques, and the effect of corneal biomechanical properties on pressure measurement is reduced. Studies have found that the corneal compensated IOP (IOPcc) has a stronger correlation with glaucoma progression than does IOP measured with Goldmann or rebound tonometry. In addition to measuring IOPcc, the ORA calculates indicators of ocular biomechanical properties, including corneal hysteresis. During the measurement process, the cornea is indented beyond the IOP measurement point. *Corneal hysteresis* is the difference between the IOP measured during the initial corneal indentation and the IOP measured during corneal rebound. Reduced corneal hysteresis has been associated with an increased risk of developing visual field defects in glaucoma suspects and with disease progression in patients with confirmed glaucoma.

Medeiros FA, Meira-Freitas D, Lisboa R, Kuang TM, Zangwill LM, Weinreb RN. Corneal hysteresis as a risk factor for glaucoma progression: a prospective longitudinal study. *Ophthalmology.* 2013;120(8):1533–1540.

Susanna BN, Ogata NG, Daga FB, Susanna CN, Diniz-Filho A, Medeiros FA. Association between rates of visual field progression and intraocular pressure measurements obtained by different tonometers. *Ophthalmology.* 2019;126(1):49–54.

Susanna CN, Diniz-Filho A, Daga FB, et al. A prospective longitudinal study to investigate corneal hysteresis as a risk factor for predicting development of glaucoma. *Am J Ophthalmol.* 2018;187:148–152.

Rebound tonometry

Rebound tonometry determines IOP by measuring the speed at which a small probe propelled against the cornea decelerates and rebounds after impact (Fig 2-7D). Rebound tonometers are portable, and topical anesthesia is not required; these characteristics make them particularly suitable for use in pediatric populations and for home tonometry in some patients. However, rebound tonometry is strongly influenced by CCT, even when compared with applanation tonometry. Thus, care must be taken in the interpretation of IOP measurements in eyes with thick or thin corneas. This method of tonometry has allowed development of a home tonometer (iCare HOME, iCare Finland OY), which can play a role in evaluating eye pressure outside office hours.

Kontiola AI. A new induction-based impact method for measuring intraocular pressure. *Acta Ophthalmol Scand.* 2000;78(2):142–145.

Rao A, Kumar M, Prakash B, Varshney G. Relationship of central corneal thickness and intraocular pressure by iCare rebound tonometer. *J Glaucoma.* 2014;23(6):380–384.

Infection control in clinical tonometry

Infectious agents—including HIV, hepatitis C virus, and adenovirus—can be recovered from tears. To prevent the transfer of such pathogens, tonometers must be cleaned after each use. The tonometer tips (prisms) should be cleaned immediately after the use of Goldmann and Perkins tonometers. The ideal method for disinfection is controversial. Sodium hypochlorite (dilute bleach) offers effective disinfection against adenovirus and herpes simplex virus, the viruses commonly associated with nosocomial outbreaks in eye care. In contrast, alcohol wipes or soaks do not appear to be effective at eradicating all infectious virions. The efficacy of other disinfection protocols has not been adequately evaluated. The prism head should be rinsed with water and dried before reuse to prevent damage to the corneal epithelium. Single-use disposable applanation tonometer tips may be a useful alternative to cleaning. For cleaning other tonometers, refer to the manufacturer's recommendations.

Junk AK, Chen PP, Lin SC, et al. Disinfection of tonometers: a report by the American Academy of Ophthalmology. *Ophthalmology.* 2017;124(12):1867–1875.

Tactile Tension

It is possible to estimate IOP by applying *digital pressure* on the globe, referred to as *tactile tension.* This test may be useful in uncooperative patients. However, the results may be inaccurate even when the test is performed by very experienced clinicians. In general, tactile tensions are useful only for detecting large differences in IOP between a patient's 2 eyes.

CHAPTER 3

Clinical Evaluation: History

This chapter includes a case study. Go to aao.org/bcsccasestudy_section10 or scan the QR code in the text to access this content.

Highlights

- Management of glaucoma is based on accurate categorization of the disease, assessment of disease severity, and likelihood of progression.
- Clinical evaluation of a patient with glaucoma or suspected glaucoma begins with a thorough ocular and medical history and a review of available records.
- Factors known to increase the risk of glaucoma include older age, African or Asian descent or Hispanic ethnicity, and family history of glaucoma.
- The patient's ocular and systemic medical history and medication use are important considerations in diagnosing and managing glaucoma.
- Patients who report a decrease in quality of life due to glaucoma may benefit from evaluation by a low vision specialist or surgical management.

Importance of the Patient History

Appropriate management of glaucoma starts with diagnosing the specific form of the disease in each patient, determining the severity of the optic nerve damage, and predicting the likelihood of progression. Clinical evaluation of the glaucoma patient or suspect begins with a thorough history, including symptoms, onset, duration, and severity (Case Study 3-1). Also important are the past ocular history and a general medical history, including the patient's medications and allergies.

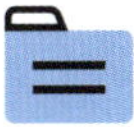

CASE STUDY 3-1 Primary open-angle glaucoma.
Courtesy of Kelly Walton Muir, MD, MHSc and Alice Choi, MD.
Available at: aao.org/bcsccasestudy_section10

Relevant Factors

The points discussed in the following sections are relevant in assessing all patients with glaucoma or suspected glaucoma.

Demographics and family history

- *Age.* Although glaucoma can occur in any age group, the prevalence of most of the common types is increased in older individuals, and the incidence increases with age.
- *Race and ethnicity.* Individuals of African descent or Hispanic ethnicity are at increased risk for primary open-angle glaucoma (POAG), whereas persons of Asian descent are at increased risk for angle-closure glaucoma. Among individuals in Scandinavian countries, pseudoexfoliation syndrome accounts for over 50% of OAG cases.
- *Family history of glaucoma.* A family history of glaucoma increases the risk of this disease. For patients with a positive family history, the disease severity and outcomes experienced by other affected family members, including vision loss and blindness, should be considered, as earlier or more aggressive treatment may be needed.

Symptoms

The most common forms of glaucoma are usually asymptomatic until relatively late stages. However, some types of glaucoma, such as acute angle closure, are generally accompanied by relatively sudden pain, redness, and decreased vision. Patients with anatomically narrow angles and intermittent angle closure may report a history of occasional headaches and halos around lights. Patients with pigment dispersion syndrome may report blurred vision, pain, or halos around lights after exercise; these symptoms may be related to active pigment dispersion and acute intraocular pressure (IOP) elevation.

Ocular history

Certain aspects of the patient's ocular history may be pertinent to glaucoma, including the following:

- *Refractive error.* High myopia is a risk factor for POAG, while hyperopia is a risk factor for angle closure.
- *Ocular trauma.* Ocular trauma can be associated with angle recession and traumatic glaucoma. Of note, patients with traumatic glaucoma may report a history of ocular trauma that occurred decades before the development of IOP elevation.
- *Ocular surgery.* A history of complicated cataract surgery, corneal transplant, or vitrectomy may be associated with an increased risk of glaucoma. For example, full-thickness penetrating keratoplasty is often linked with the development of angle-closure glaucoma. Although refractive surgery is generally not associated with an increased risk of glaucoma, keratorefractive procedures such as laser in situ keratomileusis (LASIK) and photorefractive keratotomy may result in thin corneas, which can lead to artifactually low IOP measurements.

Systemic diseases

The patient's systemic medical history sometimes plays a role in diagnosing and managing glaucoma. Systemic diseases that may be relevant to glaucoma include migraine, vasospasm, sleep apnea, diabetes, cardiovascular disease, thyroid disease, asthma, and chronic obstructive pulmonary disease (COPD). For example, a history of migraine or vasospasm (eg, Raynaud disease) may be more prevalent in patients who have glaucoma and relatively low IOP. Sleep apnea has also been described as a risk factor for glaucoma. Patients with autoimmune thyroid disorders and thyroid eye disease may have elevated episcleral venous pressure. In addition, a history of systemic arterial hypertension and hypotensive therapy is pertinent because treatment-related systemic hypotension may increase the risk of glaucoma progression.

A patient's systemic conditions can affect the choice of medical treatment. For instance, in patients with asthma or COPD, β-blockers may be contraindicated; therefore, a history of these conditions should be actively sought in all patients with glaucoma or suspected glaucoma for whom treatment with topical β-blockers is being considered.

Medication use and allergies

The patient's past or present medication use and their allergies or reactions to particular drugs are also essential to consider in diagnosing or treating glaucoma. Extended use of topical, inhaled, or systemic corticosteroids is a risk factor for increased IOP. Also, certain systemic medications, such as topiramate, may be associated with an increased risk of angle-closure glaucoma (see Chapter 10). In addition, the systemic use of drugs with anticholinergic activity may increase the risk of angle-closure disease in persons with anatomically narrow anterior chamber angles.

It is important to inquire about ocular hypotensive medications that the patient previously used (if any) and reactions or allergies to them. The patient's medication history may influence treatment selection. Patients with a known allergy to a sulfonamide antibiotic may have an increased risk of a subsequent reaction to multiple classes of medications, including carbonic anhydrase inhibitors (CAIs), which may be used to treat glaucoma. Cross-reactivity between sulfonamide antibiotics and sulfonamide nonantibiotics such as CAIs may be as low as 10% because they are different medication classes. Finally, use of certain medications can affect glaucoma treatment. For instance, if a patient is already taking systemic β-blockers for conditions other than glaucoma, the effectiveness of topical β-blockers in lowering IOP will be diminished.

Review of records

A review of records, particularly those documenting past IOP levels, status of the optic nerve, and visual fields, is useful in guiding current glaucoma management. Information on maximum-recorded IOP levels is important in setting an individualized target pressure. Records of optic nerve status and visual fields can be crucial in establishing whether change has occurred over time and if so, how rapid that change has been. In cases of suspected glaucoma, documentation of optic nerve head or retinal nerve fiber layer change over time may establish the diagnosis even in the absence of visual field loss. In patients with previously diagnosed disease, records showing progressive optic nerve damage or visual field loss are indicative of inadequately treated disease. If the glaucoma is not adequately controlled while the patient is on topical ocular hypotensive therapy, the clinician should actively seek to obtain a history of adherence to treatment.

Quality of Life

It is important to ask patients with glaucoma about any effects of the disease (and of glaucoma medications) on their quality of life and activities of daily living, such as driving, walking, reading, and interacting socially. Possible ocular adverse effects of glaucoma medications include dry eyes, blurred vision, redness, and irritation. All of these may affect patient adherence to topical glaucoma medication regimens. Patients who report a progressive decline in quality of life due to glaucoma may require more aggressive interventions to control the disease and may benefit from evaluation by a low vision specialist or surgical management. In patients with severe glaucoma and advanced visual field loss, subjective changes in vision quality may be the only indicator that the disease is not adequately controlled.

Social Determinants of Health

Similar to the way that the history of the present illness, ocular and medical history, and other types of patient information are obtained, ophthalmologists and their health care teams can assess the role of social determinants of health (SDOH) in their patients' lives. For discussion of SDOH and implicit bias, see Chapter 1 in BCSC Section 1, *Update on General Medicine.*

CHAPTER 4

Clinical Evaluation and Imaging of the Anterior Segment

This chapter includes related videos. Go to aao.org/bcscvideo_section10 or scan the QR codes in the text to access this content.

Highlights

- Systematic examination of the anterior segment, including gonioscopy, is necessary to establish an accurate diagnosis for patients with glaucoma or ocular hypertension.
- Detection of angle closure and important secondary causes of ocular hypertension or glaucoma requires careful and complete assessment of anterior segment structures.
- Various anterior segment imaging modalities can add important information to aid in the diagnosis of disease processes associated with glaucoma.

Refractive Error

Determining the refractive status of the eye is important in the evaluation of glaucoma for 2 main reasons. First, correction of significant refractive error is necessary for accurate perimetry. Second, refractive error (both myopia and hyperopia) is associated with glaucoma. For example, *myopia,* especially high myopia, is a risk factor for primary open-angle glaucoma. Also, pigment dispersion syndrome is often associated with moderate myopia. Optic nerve head (also called *optic disc*) and peripapillary anomalies associated with myopia can confound the evaluation of the optic nerve head and retinal nerve fiber layer, both with biomicroscopy and with computerized imaging (see Chapter 5). *Hyperopia* is associated with an increased risk of primary angle closure, and the hyperopic eye generally has a smaller optic nerve head.

Ocular Adnexa

Examination of the ocular adnexa is necessary to identify conditions associated with secondary glaucomas and possible external effects of glaucoma therapy. The entities described in this section are discussed in greater depth and illustrated elsewhere in the BCSC series, particularly Sections 6, 7, and 8.

Examples of diseases associated with glaucoma that can also involve the ocular adnexa include tuberous sclerosis complex (Bourneville disease), juvenile xanthogranuloma, and oculodermal melanocytosis (nevus of Ota). In *tuberous sclerosis,* glaucoma may occur secondary to vitreous hemorrhage, anterior segment neovascularization, or retinal detachment. A typical external sign of tuberous sclerosis is pink to red-brown angiofibromas (see BCSC Section 6, *Pediatric Ophthalmology and Strabismus*), which are often found on the face, including the eyelids and chin. In *juvenile xanthogranuloma,* yellow or orange papules or nodules may be present on the eyelids or face. In *oculodermal melanocytosis,* blue to brown discoloration or darkening occurs on the periocular skin (see Section 7, *Oculofacial Plastic and Orbital Surgery).* It can be unilateral or bilateral and may be subtle, particularly in persons of African, Asian, or Hispanic ancestry.

The presence of subcutaneous eyelid plexiform neurofibromas is a hallmark of the type 1 variant of *neurofibromatosis* (*NF1;* see Section 7, *Oculofacial Plastic and Orbital Surgery*). Although generally uncommon in patients with NF1, glaucoma occurs in 25%–50% of those with an eyelid plexiform neurofibroma and is usually ipsilateral to the eyelid neurofibroma.

Several disease processes with ocular adnexal abnormalities are associated with elevated episcleral venous pressure (EVP) (see Chapter 8). The presence of a facial cutaneous angioma (*nevus flammeus,* or *port-wine birthmark*) (see Section 6, *Pediatric Ophthalmology and Strabismus*) can indicate *encephalotrigeminal angiomatosis (Sturge-Weber syndrome).* The cutaneous hemangiomas of a closely related condition, *Klippel-Trénaunay-Weber syndrome,* extend over an affected limb and may also involve the face, including the eyelids.

Orbital varices (distensible venous malformations of the orbit), arteriovenous fistulas, and superior vena cava syndrome may also be associated with elevated EVP and secondary glaucoma (see Section 7, *Oculofacial Plastic and Orbital Surgery,* for further discussion of many of these conditions). Intermittent unilateral proptosis and dilated eyelid veins are key external signs of *orbital varices. Carotid-cavernous, dural-cavernous,* and other *arteriovenous fistulas* can result in orbital bruits, restricted ocular motility, proptosis, and pulsating exophthalmos. *Superior vena cava syndrome* can cause proptosis, facial and eyelid edema, and conjunctival chemosis.

Thyroid eye disease may also be associated with glaucoma by causing elevated EVP. Ocular adnexal features of this disease include exophthalmos, eyelid retraction, and motility disorders (see Section 7, *Oculofacial Plastic and Orbital Surgery*).

Long-term use of ocular hypotensive prostaglandin analogues may result in ocular adnexal abnormalities, including increased pigmentation of the periocular skin and growth of the eyelashes. Other reported external abnormalities are caused by periorbital fat atrophy and include enophthalmos, deepening of the upper eyelid sulcus, and upper eyelid ptosis. Ocular hypotensive prostaglandin analogues may also cause inferior scleral show and tightening of the eyelids (see Chapter 12).

Pupillary Function

Testing of pupillary function in patients with glaucoma can be helpful in assessing severity of the disease and the effects of glaucoma surgery or medications. Pupil diameter can be affected by parasympathomimetic agents and adrenergic agonists (see Chapter 12).

A diminished pupillary reaction to light due to slowed conduction in the optic nerve fibers *(relative afferent pupillary defect; RAPD)* is often noted in eyes with asymmetric glaucoma damage; however, if an RAPD cannot be reconciled with the overall clinical picture of glaucoma, the presence of a nonglaucomatous optic neuropathy must be ruled out. In some clinical situations, assessing the pupils for the presence of an RAPD is impossible, and a subjective comparison between the eyes of the perceived brightness of a test light may be helpful. See BCSC Section 5, *Neuro-Ophthalmology,* for further discussion of RAPDs.

Slit-Lamp Biomicroscopy

The slit lamp allows visualization of cross sections of ocular structures such as the conjunctiva, cornea, and anterior chamber. Biomicroscopy of the anterior segment is performed

- to detect signs of underlying ocular conditions that may be associated with glaucoma or ocular hypertension
- to evaluate the eye in preparation for glaucoma surgery
- to monitor the results of a previously performed glaucoma surgery

BCSC Section 8, *External Disease and Cornea,* discusses slit-lamp technique and the examination of the external eye in greater depth.

Conjunctiva

Acute intraocular pressure (IOP) elevation and long-term use of many ocular hypotensive medications may cause conjunctival hyperemia. Allergic or hypersensitivity reactions to medications (especially α_2-adrenergic agonists) or their preservatives can result in a follicular conjunctivitis. Potential adverse effects of topical hypotensive drugs include decreased tear production, foreshortening of the conjunctival fornices and, in severe cases, pseudopemphigoid with conjunctival scarring. An assessment for subconjunctival scarring or other conjunctival abnormalities should be done before filtering surgery is performed. The presence or absence of any filtering bleb should be noted. If a bleb is present, it is characterized as either focal or diffuse, and its size, position, and degree of elevation are noted, along with the amount of vascularization and the thickness of the overlying conjunctiva. If a leak is suspected, a Seidel test is performed (Fig 4-1; see also Chapter 13, Video 13-6). The presence of "sweating" (minimal diffuse leakage through a thin conjunctiva seen with observation over a few seconds) may be considered acceptable.

Clinical Pearl The Seidel test is used to detect an aqueous humor leak. A sterile topical anesthetic solution is instilled to prevent a blinking response. Concentrated sodium fluorescein is applied to the area where the leak is suspected. A moistened fluorescein strip or 2% sodium fluorescein solution is used.

Immediately after application of fluorescein, the examiner looks for fluorescence using a slit-lamp biomicroscope with a cobalt blue filter:

- When a high concentration of fluorescein is present, fluorescence is not seen because of quenching.
- When the fluorescein is diluted by leakage of aqueous, fluorescence is detected (see Fig 4-1).

Episclera and Sclera

Dilation of the episcleral vessels may indicate elevated EVP, which can be idiopathic or can occur in the secondary glaucomas associated with non-ocular disease processes (see the section Ocular Adnexa in this chapter and Chapter 8). Sentinel vessels may be found in eyes harboring an intraocular tumor, which can cause unilateral glaucoma. The clinician should note any thinning or staphylomatous areas. Patchy slate-gray pigmentation of the sclera is present in oculodermal melanocytosis, and affected patients are at increased risk for developing glaucoma and ocular melanoma. Also, scleritis may be associated with elevated IOP.

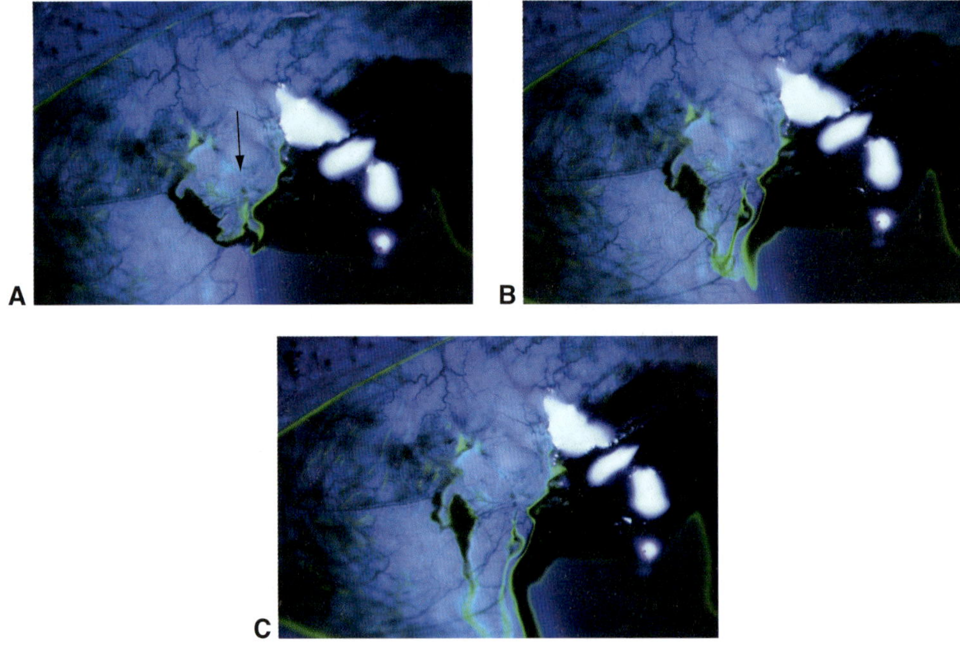

Figure 4-1 Seidel test. After application of a concentrated fluorescein solution, quenching blocks fluorescence unless there is an aqueous humor leak that dilutes the fluorescein. The dark area on the right of these images represents an area of highly concentrated fluorescein. As aqueous humor leaks (*arrow,* part **A**), the fluorescein is diluted, and an enlarging rivulet of fluorescence is detected **(A–C).** *(Courtesy of Angelo P. Tanna, MD.)*

Cornea

Corneal enlargement associated with breaks in Descemet membrane *(Haab striae)* is commonly found in pediatric glaucoma patients who had onset of IOP elevation before 4 years of age. Glaucomas associated with other corneal abnormalities are described in Chapters 10 and 11. *Punctate epithelial erosions,* especially in the inferonasal interpalpebral region, are often indicative of a toxic reaction to medication. *Microcystic epithelial edema* is commonly associated with severely elevated IOP, particularly when the IOP increase is acute.

The following corneal endothelial abnormalities can provide important clues to underlying conditions in secondary IOP elevation or glaucoma:

- Krukenberg spindle (vertically oriented pigment deposition on the corneal endothelium): in pigment dispersion syndrome
- deposition of pseudoexfoliative material: in pseudoexfoliation syndrome
- keratic precipitates (KPs), especially stellate KPs associated with herpesvirus infections: in uveitis
- irregular and vesicular lesions: in posterior polymorphous corneal dystrophy
- fine, repeated irregularities of the corneal endothelium ("hammered silver" appearance): in iridocorneal endothelial syndrome (ICE)

In addition to the above abnormalities, the clinician should note the presence of traumatic or surgical corneal scars, as glaucoma may be associated with corneal trauma or surgery. For all patients suspected of having glaucoma, the central corneal thickness should be measured, as a thin central cornea is a risk factor for glaucoma and results in underestimation of IOP by most tonometers (see Chapters 2 and 7).

Anterior Chamber

When evaluating the anterior chamber, the examiner should note the uniformity of depth of the chamber. In the Van Herick method of estimating angle width, the examiner projects a narrow slit beam onto the cornea at approximately a 60° angle, just anterior to the limbus (Video 4-1). However, the results can be misleading: this method is not sensitive enough to detect angle closure and is not a substitute for gonioscopy (see Gonioscopy section).

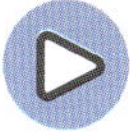

VIDEO 4-1 Gonioscopy: Van Herick technique.
Courtesy of Wallace L. M. Alward, MD, and Reid A. Longmuir, MD.
Available at: aao.org/bcscvideo_section10

Primary angle closure, iris bombé, and *plateau iris syndrome/configuration* can result in an anterior chamber that is shallow or flat peripherally. In contrast, in *malignant glaucoma* and other forms of non–pupillary block angle closure with a posterior "pushing" mechanism, both the central and peripheral anterior chamber are shallow or flat. In many circumstances, especially in the assessment of acute unilateral IOP elevation (when the cornea is often edematous, limiting the view of the anterior chamber and angle), examination of the fellow eye can provide useful information.

In *pigment dispersion syndrome,* the anterior chamber is often deep, and the iris configuration is often concave. In this condition, friction between the posteriorly bowed iris and the lens zonular fibers causes pigment granules to be liberated from the iris epithelium, and these granules then obstruct the trabecular meshwork.

The presence of white or red blood cells, circulating pigment, or inflammatory debris (such as fibrin) should be noted. The degree of inflammation (flare and cells) and presence of pigment should be determined before the instillation of topical medications.

Iris

The iris should be examined before pupillary dilation. The clinician should note the following (including examples of causes):

- heterochromia: in Fuchs uveitis syndrome or iris melanoma
- iris atrophy: after surgery or trauma; in ICE syndrome
- ectropion uveae (the presence of pigmented iris epithelial cells on the anterior iris surface): in ICE syndrome, neovascular glaucoma, congenital ectropion uveae
- corectopia (displacement of the pupil): in ectopia lentis et pupillae, ICE syndrome; following trauma or surgery
- nevi or nodules: in iris nevus syndrome, neurofibromatosis type 1, uveitis
- pseudoexfoliative material: in pseudoexfoliation syndrome
- transillumination defects: in pigment dispersion syndrome
- presence and patency of an iridotomy or iridectomy
- any surgically induced iris abnormalities

Iris color should also be noted, especially in patients being considered for treatment with a prostaglandin analogue (see Chapter 12).

Early stages of neovascularization of the anterior segment may appear as either fine tufts at the pupillary margin or a fine network of vessels on the surface of the iris adjacent to the iris root. Early rubeosis may not be visible if the IOP is elevated. The clinician should also examine the iris for evidence of ocular trauma, such as iris sphincter tears, iridodialysis (tear in the iris root), or iridodonesis (abnormal iris motion caused by poor or absent lens zonular support).

The contour of the iris can provide clues about the underlying mechanism of angle closure and the presence of pigment dispersion syndrome. Irregularities in the iris contour may suggest choroidal effusion or hemorrhage. Other conditions that can cause contour irregularities include an iris or ciliary body cyst and, in rare cases, uveal melanoma; ultrasonography is required to characterize such lesions, and either type can lead to IOP elevation.

Lens

Findings from the lens examination may help the clinician determine the etiology of a lens-related glaucoma and may guide management. The clinician should examine the lens both before and after pupillary dilation, evaluating its size, shape, clarity, stability, and anterior capsule. Assessment before dilation provides useful information about the effect of lens opacity, posterior capsule opacification, or lens subluxation on visual function. A posterior subcapsular cataract may be indicative of prior long-term corticosteroid use. After mydriasis, it is important to observe for signs of exfoliative or pseudoexfoliative material on the anterior lens capsule. A yellow-brown or rust-colored discoloration of the lens epithelium in an eye with siderosis and glaucoma may indicate the presence of an intraocular foreign body.

Gonioscopy

Proper management of glaucoma requires the clinician to determine whether the angle is open or closed, as well as whether other pathologic findings, such as angle recession or peripheral anterior synechiae (PAS), are present. Gonioscopy is an essential diagnostic technique for evaluating the anterior chamber angle and its structures (Table 4-1). However, this method has been underused in clinical practice, and opportunities to provide more accurate diagnoses and appropriate management may be missed as a consequence.

Gonioscopy is necessary to visualize angle structures. Because light reflected from angle structures undergoes total internal reflection at the air–tear film interface, visualizing these structures without the aid of an optical device is not possible. At that interface, the critical angle (approximately 48°) is reached, and light is totally reflected back into the corneal stroma, preventing direct visualization. During gonioscopy, the examiner prevents total internal reflection by placing a plastic or glass prism against the cornea. The small space between the prism and cornea is filled by the patient's tears, saline solution, or a clear viscous substance. Figures 4-2 and 4-3 show schematic and clinical views of the angle as seen with gonioscopy.

Direct and Indirect Gonioscopy

Gonioscopy techniques fall into 2 broad categories, direct and indirect (Fig 4-4). *Direct gonioscopy* is performed with a binocular microscope, fiber-optic illuminator, or slit-pen light together with a direct goniolens, such as the Koeppe, Swan-Jacob, Barkan, Wurst, or Richardson type. The goniolens is placed on the eye; and saline solution, methylcellulose, or an ophthalmic viscoelastic is used to fill the space between the cornea and the

Table 4-1 Gonioscopic Examination

Tissue	Features and Pathologic Findings
Posterior cornea	Pigmentation, keratic precipitates
Schwalbe line	Thickening, anterior displacement
Trabecular meshwork	Pigmentation, peripheral anterior synechiae, inflammatory or neovascular membranes
Scleral spur	Iris processes
Ciliary body band	Angle recession, cyclodialysis cleft
Iris	Contour, rubeosis, atrophy, cysts, tumors, iridodonesis, iridodialysis
Zonular fibers	Pigmentation, rupture (may be visible after dilation)

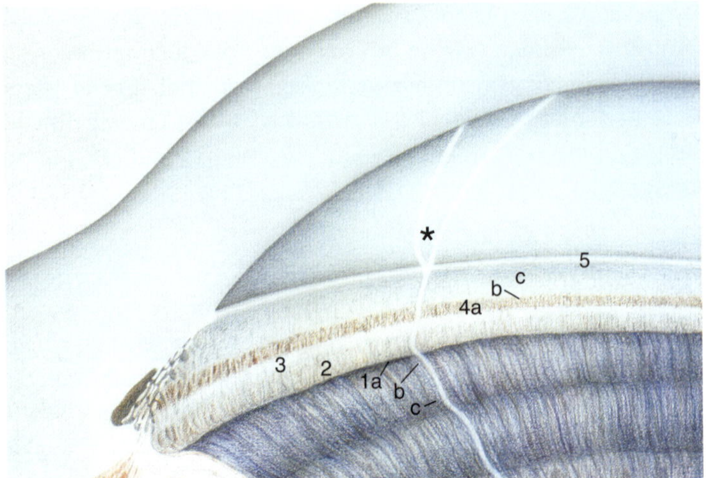

Figure 4-2 Gonioscopic appearance of a normal anterior chamber angle. *1,* Peripheral iris: *a,* insertion; *b,* curvature; *c,* angular approach. *2,* Ciliary body band. *3,* Scleral spur. *4,* Trabecular meshwork: *a,* posterior; *b,* mid; *c,* anterior. *5,* Schwalbe line. *Asterisk,* Corneal wedge (parallelepiped corneal wedge).

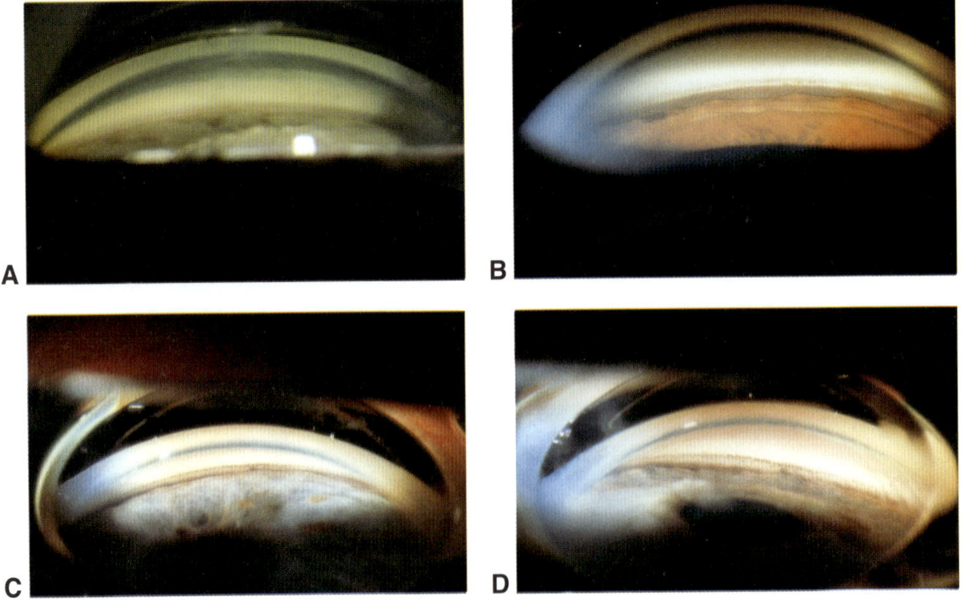

Figure 4-3 Normal and narrow angles. **A,** Normal open angle. Gonioscopic photograph shows trace pigmentation of the posterior trabecular meshwork and normal insertion of the iris into a narrow ciliary body band. The Goldmann lens was used. **B,** Normal open angle. This gonioscopic view using the Goldmann lens shows mild pigmentation of the posterior trabecular meshwork. A wide ciliary body band with posterior insertion of the iris can also be seen. **C,** Narrow angle. This gonioscopic view using the Zeiss lens without indentation shows pigment in the inferior angle; visualization of angle structures is poor. **D,** Narrow angle. Gonioscopy with a Zeiss lens with indentation shows peripheral anterior synechiae in the posterior trabecular meshwork. Pigment deposits on the Schwalbe line can also be seen. This is the same angle as shown in part C. *(Part A courtesy of Angelo P. Tanna, MD; parts B–D courtesy of Elizabeth A. Hodapp, MD.)*

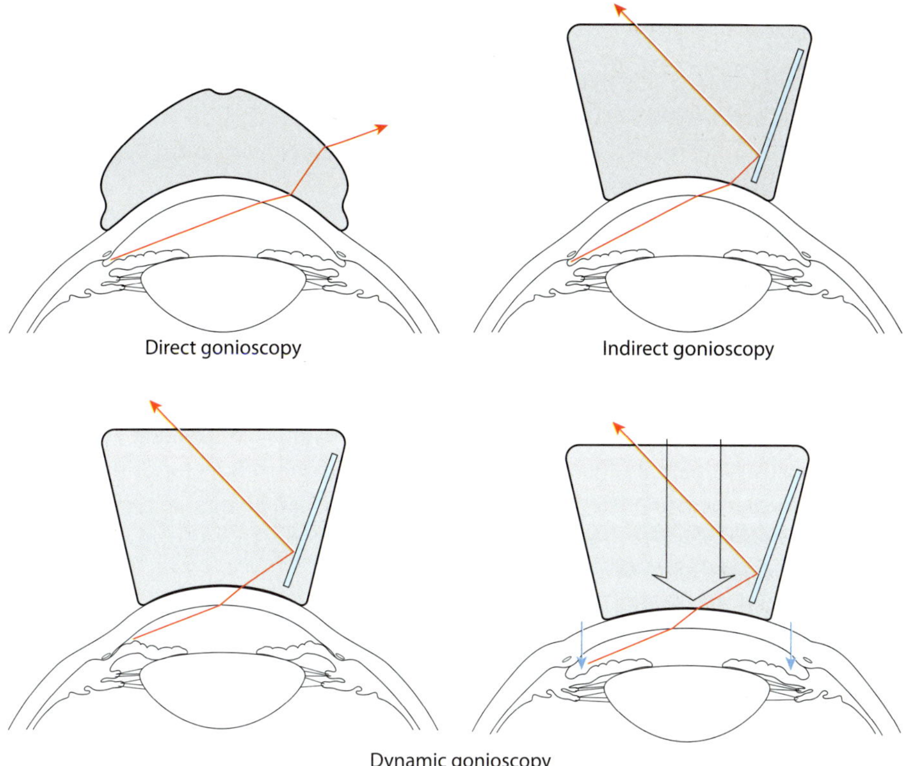

Figure 4-4 Direct and indirect gonioscopy. Gonioscopic lenses eliminate the air–tear film interface and total internal reflection. With a direct lens, the light reflected from the anterior chamber angle is observed directly, whereas with an indirect lens, the light is reflected by a mirror within the lens. Posterior pressure on the cornea with an indirect lens forces open an appositionally closed or narrow anterior chamber angle (dynamic gonioscopy). *(Illustration by Mark Miller.)*

goniolens, acting as an optical coupler between the 2 surfaces. The goniolens provides direct visualization of the anterior chamber angle (ie, light reflected from the angle is visualized directly). With direct gonioscopy, the clinician has a direct (not reflected) view of the angle structures, which is essential when angle surgery (eg, goniotomy or placement of a stent in the Schlemm canal) is performed. Direct gonioscopy is most easily accomplished with the patient in a supine position, and it is commonly used in the operating room for examining the eyes of infants under anesthesia.

In *indirect gonioscopy,* light reflected from the angle passes into the gonioscopy lens and is reflected by 1 or more mirrors within the lens. This method, which is employed more frequently in the clinic than in the operating room, may be used with the patient upright, with illumination and magnification provided by a slit-lamp biomicroscope (Video 4-2). The indirect goniolens yields an inverted and slightly foreshortened image of the angle opposite the mirror. Although the image is inverted, the right–left orientation of a horizontal mirror and the up–down orientation of a vertical mirror remain unchanged. The foreshortening, combined with the upright position of the patient, makes the angle appear somewhat shallower than it does on direct gonioscopy. The Goldmann

1- or 3-mirror gonioscopy lens requires a viscous fluid such as methylcellulose for optical coupling with the cornea. Of note, posterior pressure on the goniolens, especially if it is tilted, indents the sclera and may falsely narrow the angle. Among indirect gonioscopy lenses, the Goldmann-type 1- and 3-mirror lenses provide the clearest visualization of the anterior chamber angle structures, and they may be modified with antireflective coatings for use during laser procedures.

VIDEO 4-2 Gonioscopy: general techniques.
Courtesy of Wallace L. M. Alward, MD, and Reid A. Longmuir, MD.
Available at: aao.org/bcscvideo_section10

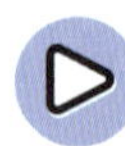

The Posner, Sussman, and Zeiss 4-mirror gonioscopy lenses allow all 4 quadrants of the anterior chamber angle to be visualized without rotating the goniolens during examination. Because these lenses have approximately the same radius of curvature as the cornea, they are optically coupled by the patient's tears. The posterior diameter of these lenses is smaller than the corneal diameter; thus, posterior pressure can be used to force open a narrow angle by means of a technique called *dynamic gonioscopy* (also known as *compression* or *indentation gonioscopy*). With dynamic gonioscopy, the clinician puts gentle pressure on the cornea with the goniolens, which forces aqueous humor into the angle, causing it to open to a greater degree than its native state in the absence of PAS (see Fig 4-4). With indirect gonioscopy, the examiner can optimize the view of the anterior chamber angle by repositioning the patient's eye (having the patient look toward the mirror being viewed by the examiner) or by slightly tilting the goniolens. However, pressure on the cornea will artificially open a truly narrow or closed angle. The examiner can detect this pressure by noting the induced Descemet membrane folds.

When an area of the angle is closed, one cannot initially differentiate between appositional angle closure and angle closure due to PAS. Dynamic gonioscopy is essential for distinguishing iridocorneal apposition from synechial closure. Many clinicians prefer the Posner, Sussman, and Zeiss 4-mirror lenses because of their ease of use and the ability to perform dynamic gonioscopy.

Gonioscopic Assessment and Documentation

In performing both direct and indirect gonioscopy, the clinician must recognize the landmarks of the anterior chamber angle. It is important to perform gonioscopy with dim room lighting and a thin, short light beam in order to minimize the amount of light entering the pupil. An excessive amount of light can cause increased pupillary constriction that could falsely open the angle, changing the peripheral angle appearance and potentially preventing the identification of a narrow or occluded angle. The scleral spur and the Schwalbe line, 2 important angle landmarks, are most consistently identified. A convenient gonioscopic technique to determine the exact position of the Schwalbe line is the *parallelepiped,* or *corneal wedge, technique* (Video 4-3; see also Fig 4-2). This technique allows the examiner to determine the exact junction of the cornea and the trabecular meshwork. Using a narrow slit beam and sharp focus, the examiner sees 2 curvilinear reflections, 1 from the external surface of the cornea and its junction with the sclera and the other from the internal surface of the cornea. The 2 reflections meet at the Schwalbe line (see Fig 4-2). The scleral spur appears as a thin, pale stripe between the ciliary body face and the pigmented zone of the trabecular meshwork. The inferior portion of the angle is generally wider and is the easiest place in which to locate the landmarks. After verifying the landmarks, the clinician should examine the entire angle in an orderly manner (see Table 4-1).

VIDEO 4-3 Gonioscopy: an introduction to the corneal wedge.
Courtesy of Wallace L. M. Alward, MD, and Reid A. Longmuir, MD.
Available at: aao.org/bcscvideo_section10

As previously mentioned, proper management of glaucoma requires the clinician to determine not only whether the angle is open or closed but also whether other pathologic findings, such as angle recession or PAS, are present. In angle closure, the peripheral iris obstructs the trabecular meshwork—that is, the meshwork is not visible on gonioscopy. The width of the angle is determined by the site of the iris insertion on the ciliary face, the convexity of the iris, and the prominence of the peripheral iris roll. In many cases, the angle appears to be open but very narrow. It is often difficult to distinguish a narrow but open angle from an angle with partial closure; dynamic gonioscopy is useful in this situation (Video 4-4; see also Figs 4-3, 4-4).

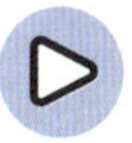

VIDEO 4-4 Gonioscopy: indentation technique.
Courtesy of Wallace L. M. Alward, MD, and Reid A. Longmuir, MD.
Available at: aao.org/bcscvideo_section10

Although gonioscopy is considered the reference standard method for angle assessment, it should be noted that this method is subjective and has limited reproducibility.

Grading

The best method for describing the angle is to use a standardized grading system. A number of gonioscopic grading systems have been developed, all of which facilitate a standardized description of the degree to which the angle is open or closed. However, certain details about the angle will be lost with some grading systems. The most commonly used gonioscopic grading systems are the Shaffer and Spaeth systems. A quadrant-by-quadrant narrative description of the angle noting localized findings such as neovascular tufts, angle recession, or PAS may also be used to document serial gonioscopic findings.

The *Shaffer system* describes the angle between the trabecular meshwork and the iris in degrees. Angles are graded on a scale of 0 to 4, with grade 1 (10°) or lower denoting angles at high risk for angle closure.

The *Spaeth gonioscopic grading system* expands on this schema to also include a description of the peripheral iris contour and the apparent insertion of the iris root, forming the 3 main factors assessed in this system (Fig 4-5). In addition, the clinician can comment on the degree of pigmentation and the effects of dynamic gonioscopy on the angle configuration, including the possible presence of PAS.

Blood and vessels

Ordinarily, the Schlemm canal cannot be seen on gonioscopy; however, it can easily be visualized if blood enters the canal. This can occur when EVP exceeds IOP, most commonly because of compression of the episcleral veins by the lip of the goniolens (Fig 4-6).

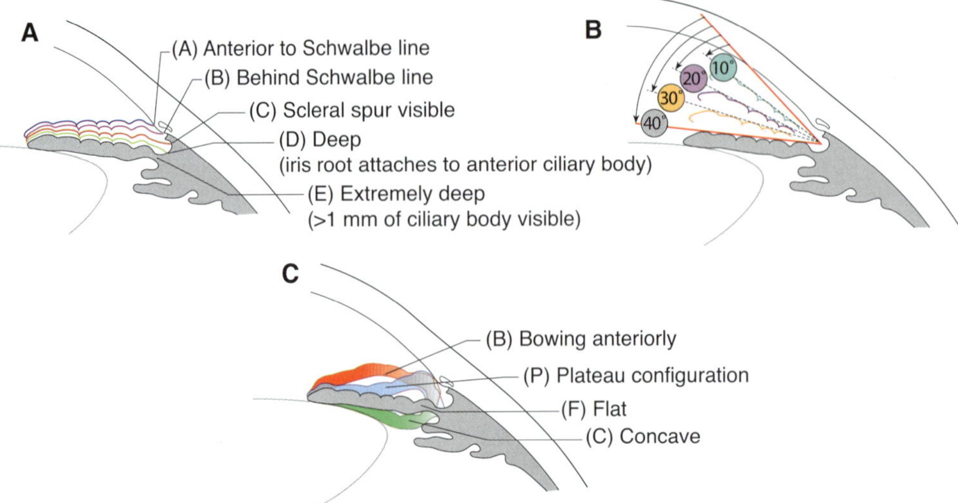

Figure 4-5 The Spaeth gonioscopic grading system for the anterior chamber angle, based on 3 variables: the apparent (not actual) site of iris attachment to the inner surface of the cornea, sclera, or ciliary body **(A);** the angular width of the angle recess **(B);** and the configuration of the peripheral iris **(C).** The system also accommodates the degree of angle pigmentation, grading it on a scale of 0 (no pigment) to 4+ (intense pigment). *(Illustration by Mark Miller.)*

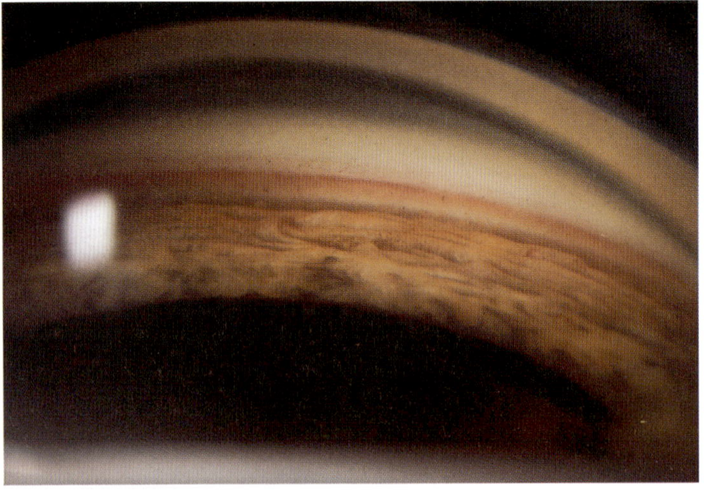

Figure 4-6 Goniophotograph showing blood in the Schlemm canal, visible through the semi-opaque trabecular meshwork. Elevated episcleral venous pressure resulted in blood reflux into the canal. *(Courtesy of G. A. Cioffi, MD.)*

Pathologic causes of blood in the canal include hypotony and elevated EVP, as in carotid-cavernous fistula or encephalotrigeminal angiomatosis (Sturge-Weber syndrome).

Normal blood vessels in the angle include radial iris vessels, portions of the arterial circle of the ciliary body, and vertical branches of the anterior ciliary arteries. Normal vessels are oriented either radially along the iris or circumferentially (in a serpentine manner) in the ciliary body face. Vessels that cross the scleral spur to reach the trabecular meshwork are usually abnormal (Fig 4-7). The vessels seen in Fuchs uveitis syndrome are fine, branching, unsheathed, and meandering. In neovascular glaucoma, the vessels cross the ciliary body and scleral spur and arborize over the trabecular meshwork. Contraction of the myofibroblasts accompanying these vessels leads to formation of PAS.

Iris processes and peripheral anterior synechiae

It is important to distinguish PAS from iris processes, which are often found in an otherwise normal anterior chamber angle. Iris processes are open and lacy and follow the normal curve of the angle. Angle structures are visible in the open spaces between the iris processes. Synechiae are more solid or sheetlike (Fig 4-8). They are composed of iris stroma and obliterate the angle recess.

Pigmentation

Pigmentation of the trabecular meshwork increases with age and tends to be more marked in individuals with darkly pigmented irides. Pigmentation can be segmental and is usually most marked in the inferior angle. The pigmentation pattern of an individual angle changes over time, especially in conditions such as pigment dispersion syndrome. Heavy pigmentation of the trabecular meshwork suggests pigment dispersion or pseudoexfoliation syndrome. In *pigment dispersion syndrome,* over time, active release of pigment may cease, and the trabecular meshwork pigmentation dissipates. This occurs most rapidly in the inferior angle, resulting in relatively heavier pigmentation of the superior angle—sometimes the only remaining sign of previous pigment dispersion syndrome.

Pseudoexfoliation syndrome may be associated with deposition of pigment granules on the anterior iris surface and increased pigmentation in the anterior chamber angle, as iridolenticular friction causes pigment release from the iris epithelium, leading to peripupillary transillumination defects. In addition, anterior to the Schwalbe line, a line of pigment deposition, known as the *Sampaolesi line,* is often present in pseudoexfoliation syndrome (see Chapter 8, Fig 8-3). Other conditions that can cause increased angle pigmentation include uveal melanoma, trauma, surgery, inflammation, angle closure, and hyphema.

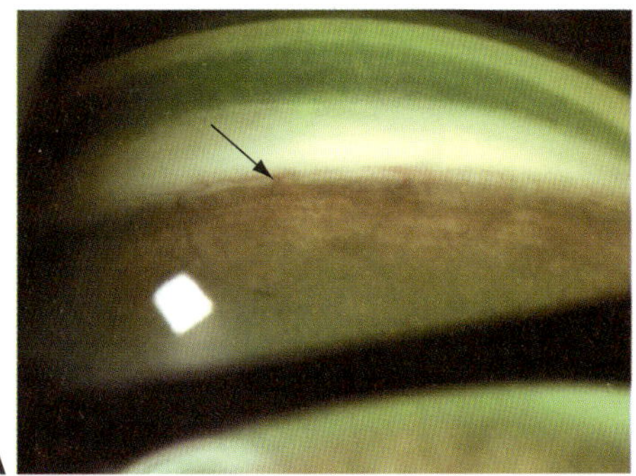

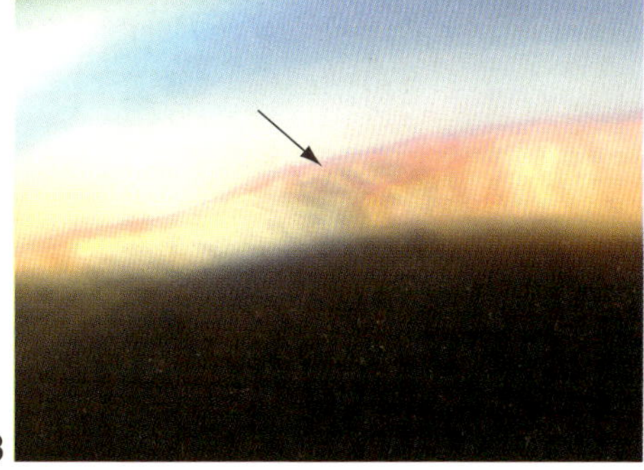

Figure 4-7 Goniophotographs showing neovascularization of the angle *(arrows).* **A,** Anatomically open angle. **B,** Closed angle. *(Part A courtesy of Keith Barton, MD; part B courtesy of Ronald L. Gross, MD.)*

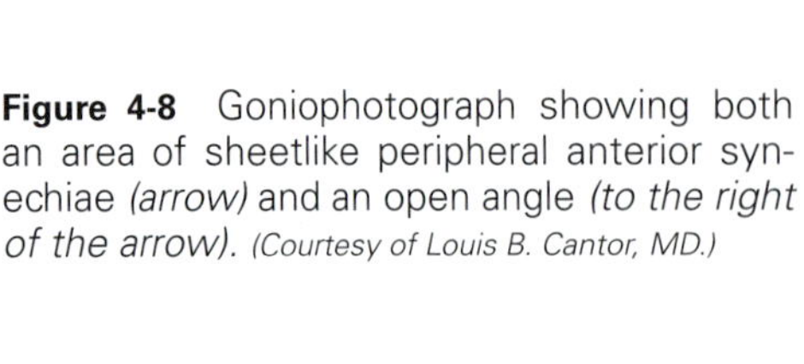

Figure 4-8 Goniophotograph showing both an area of sheetlike peripheral anterior synechiae *(arrow)* and an open angle *(to the right of the arrow)*. (Courtesy of Louis B. Cantor, MD.)

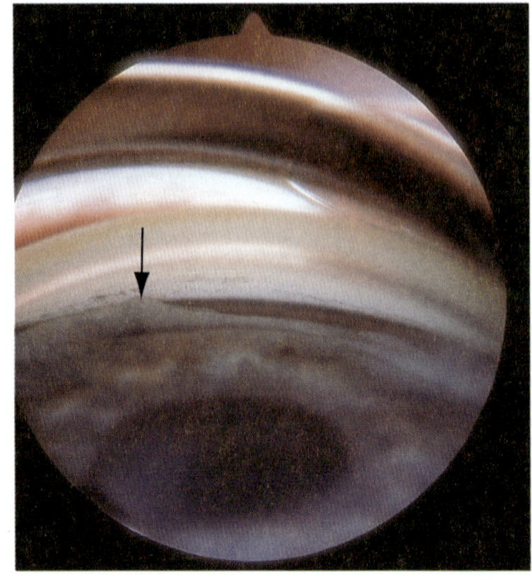

Effects of trauma

Posttraumatic angle recession may be associated with monocular open-angle glaucoma. The gonioscopic criteria for diagnosing angle recession include the following:

- an abnormally wide ciliary body band (Fig 4-9)
- increased prominence of the scleral spur
- torn iris processes
- marked variation of ciliary face width and angle depth in different quadrants of the same eye

In evaluating for angle recession, the clinician may find it helpful to compare one part of the angle to other areas of the angle in the same eye or to the same part of the angle in the fellow eye. Figure 4-10 illustrates a variety of gonioscopic findings caused by blunt trauma. If the ciliary body separates from the scleral spur *(cyclodialysis cleft)*, it will appear gonioscopically as a deep angle recess with a gap between the scleral spur and the ciliary body. Detection of a very small cleft may require ultrasound biomicroscopy.

Other findings

Various other findings may be visible by gonioscopy, including the following:

- angle recession
- anteriorly rotated ciliary processes (sometimes visible after dilation)
- goniotomy or trabeculotomy cleft
- inflammatory angle precipitates (analogous to KPs)
- intraocular lens haptics
- iridodialysis
- iris or ciliary body tumors or cysts
- hyphema or hypopyon
- surgical devices such as aqueous drainage tubes and stents
- peripheral lens abnormalities such as severe zonular dehiscence (sometimes visible after dilation)

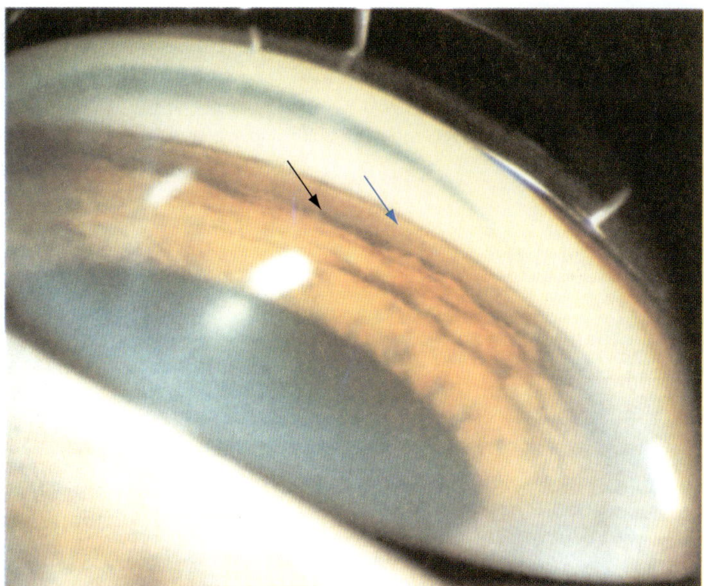

Figure 4-9 Goniophotograph showing angle recession. Note the widening of the ciliary body band *(black arrow). Blue arrow* points to the scleral spur for reference. *(Modified from Wright KW, ed.* Textbook of Ophthalmology; *1997.)*

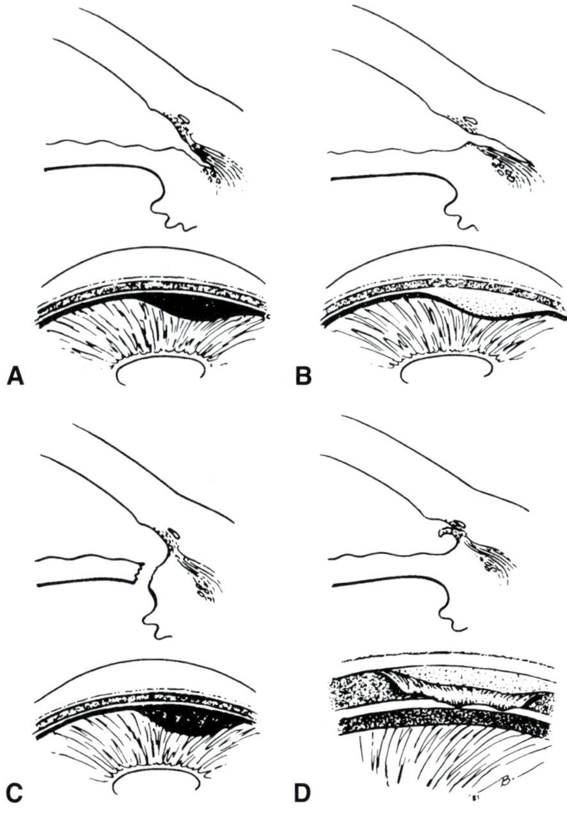

Figure 4-10 Forms of anterior chamber angle injury associated with blunt trauma, showing cross-sectional and corresponding gonioscopic appearance. **A,** Angle recession (tear between longitudinal and circular muscles of the ciliary body). **B,** Cyclodialysis cleft (separation of the ciliary body from the scleral spur) with widening of the suprachoroidal space. **C,** Iridodialysis (tear in the iris root). **D,** Trabecular damage (tear in the anterior portion of the meshwork, creating a flap that is hinged at the scleral spur). *(Reproduced with permission from Shields MB.* Textbook of Glaucoma. *3rd ed. Williams & Wilkins; 1992.)*

- retained anterior chamber foreign body or crystalline lens material
- sclerostomy site for trabeculectomy

Alward WLM, Longmuir RA. *Color Atlas of Gonioscopy.* 2nd ed. American Academy of Ophthalmology; 2008. Accessed December 19, 2023. aao.org/education/disease-review/color-atlas-of-gonioscopy

Anterior Segment Imaging

Ultrasound Biomicroscopy

Ultrasound biomicroscopy (UBM) is used to evaluate the angle, other anterior segment structures, and implanted devices that cannot be directly visualized or fully assessed with slit-lamp biomicroscopy (see Chapter 9, Video 9-1). Similarly, UBM can be useful in evaluating the angle of eyes with corneal opacities that prevent gonioscopic examination. UBM has also been used to assess the iris contour in pigment dispersion syndrome, helping to clarify the underlying mechanism of this condition (see Chapter 8).

Structures, conditions, and implanted devices that can be evaluated by UBM include:

- iris and ciliary body
  - plateau iris (Fig 4-11A)
  - choroidal effusion
  - tumors, cysts (Fig 4-11B)
- implanted devices, specifically, their position
  - glaucoma drainage devices and stents
  - intraocular lens (haptics)
- foreign bodies or retained lens material

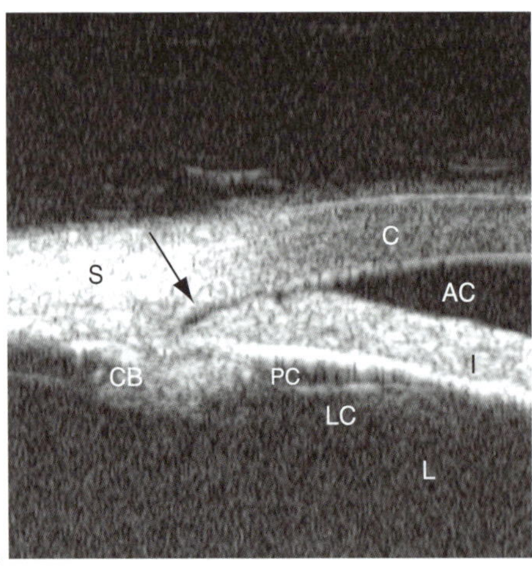

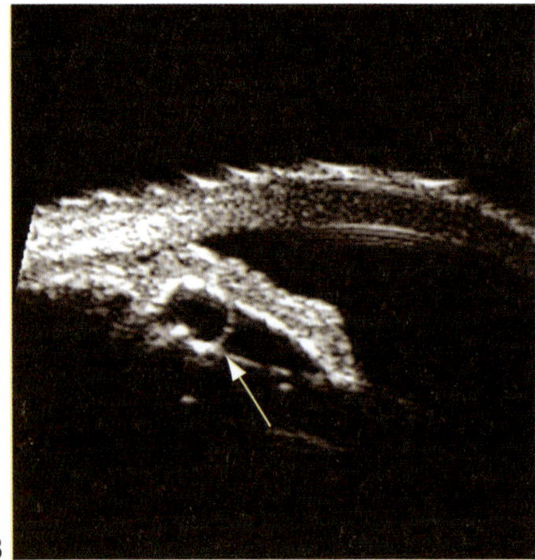

Figure 4-11 Ultrasound biomicroscopy imaging. **A,** Narrow angle due to plateau iris, with anatomical structures labeled, including the scleral spur *(arrow).* **B,** An area of angle closure as a result of a peripheral iris pigment epithelial cyst *(arrow).* AC = anterior chamber; C = cornea; CB = ciliary body; I = iris; L = lens; LC = lens capsule; PC = posterior chamber; S = sclera. *(Part A courtesy of Shan C. Lin, MD; part B courtesy of Angelo P. Tanna, MD.)*

Table 4-2 Comparison of Anterior Segment Imaging Modalities

Modality	Technology	Resolution, µm	Penetrates Pigmented Tissue?	Requires Coupling Medium?	Requires Highly-Trained Technician?	Testing Speed
Ultrasound biomicroscopy	Sound reflection	25–50	Yes	Yes	Yes	Slow
Anterior segment optical coherence tomography	Optical reflection	5–30	No	No	No	Rapid

Conventional ocular ultrasonography is typically performed using a transducer that operates at 10–20 MHz. While they do not penetrate as deeply through tissue, higher frequencies provide better resolution for meaningful anterior segment evaluation. Thus, anterior segment UBM is performed using 35–60 MHz (or an even higher frequency for imaging the Schlemm canal) linear probes. These probes must be positioned very close to the eye with a fluid interface (often contained within a disposable probe cover) for acoustic coupling (Table 4-2). The high ultrasound frequency sound waves penetrate less deeply—approximately 5 mm for a probe operating at 50 MHz.

The information provided by UBM is complementary to that obtained by gonioscopy and can help elucidate the underlying mechanism in some cases of angle closure (see Chapters 9 and 10). Assessment of UBM images for angle closure begins with identifying the scleral spur and determining the degree of angle crowding (see Fig 4-11). The mechanism(s) of angle closure can be inferred based on a qualitative assessment of the iris contour, peripheral iris thickness, ciliary body anatomy (size, position, and degree of rotation), anterior chamber depth, lens thickness, and lens vault (Fig 4-12; see also Chapter 9). Various quantitative parameters that characterize some of these anatomical features on UBM are under investigation with optical coherence tomography (OCT; see the following section). The most important ones are illustrated in Figure 4-12. Automated quantitative analysis is available on some commercially available UBM platforms; however, the operator usually must identify the scleral spur in order for the software program to provide metrics related to angle openness: iris thickness, lens vault, and others.

Anterior Segment Optical Coherence Tomography

Anterior segment OCT (AS-OCT) allows high-resolution imaging of the anterior segment, including the anterior chamber angle (Fig 4-13). It is a noncontact modality that can be performed relatively rapidly. A major limitation of this modality is that, in contrast with UBM, AS-OCT does not allow visualization of the ciliary sulcus and ciliary body (see Table 4-2). Also, as with UBM, AS-OCT does not always yield images that allow reliable identification of angle landmarks, particularly the scleral spur, which is critical for most of the calculated anterior segment measurements. Moreover, neither modality can differentiate between appositional and synechial angle closure; this differentiation is possible only with dynamic gonioscopy.

Gonioscopy remains the reference standard method for evaluating the anterior chamber angle, but it has limitations. A skilled examiner and patient cooperation are required,

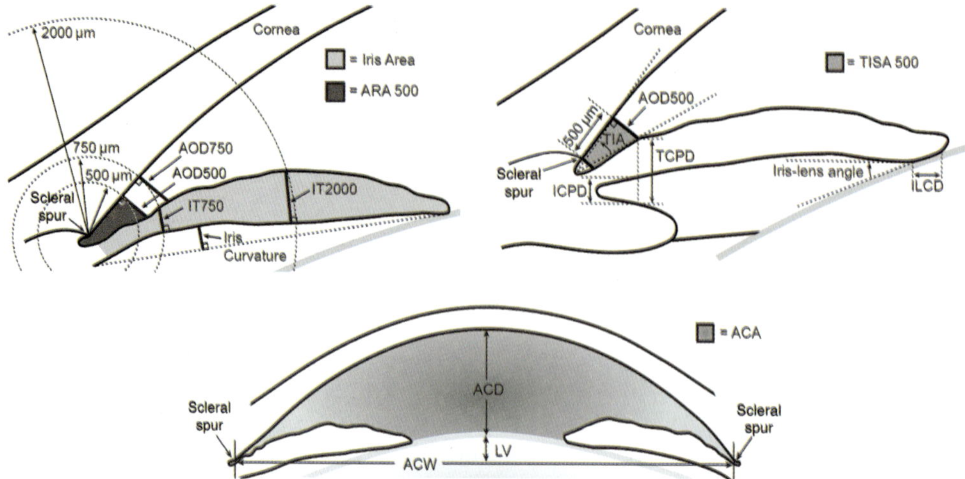

Figure 4-12 Schematic diagrams depicting anterior segment parameters captured by ultrasound biomicroscopy and anterior segment optical coherence tomography (OCT). ACA = anterior chamber area; ACD = anterior chamber depth; ACW = anterior chamber width; AOD = angle opening distance; ARA = angle recess area; ICPD = iris–ciliary process distance; ILCD = iris–lens contact distance; IT = iris thickness; LV = lens vault; TCPD = trabecular–ciliary process distance; TIA = trabecular iris angle; TISA = trabecular–iris space area. *(Reproduced from Chansangpetch S, Rojanapongpun P, Lin SC. Anterior segment imaging for angle closure.* Am J Ophthalmol. *2018;188:xvi–xxix. Copyright 2018, with permission from Elsevier.)*

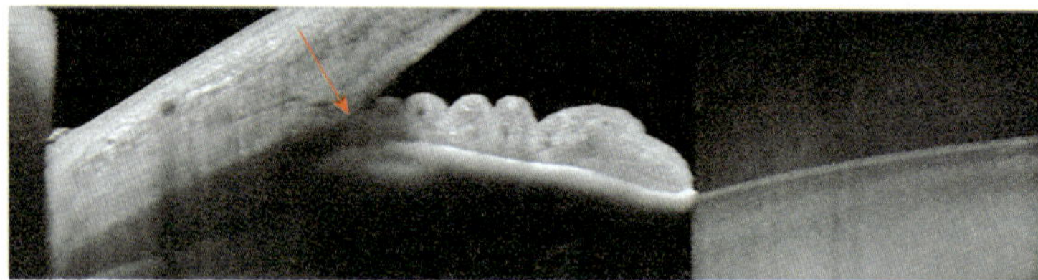

Figure 4-13 Anterior segment OCT scan demonstrating iridotrabecular contact *(arrow)*. *(Courtesy of Angelo P. Tanna, MD.)*

and the results can be subjective. The illumination required to obtain an adequate view of angle structures can cause miosis, resulting in the relative opening of the angle compared with its status at lower levels of ambient light. These limitations are at least partially overcome with AS-OCT; however, correct identification of the scleral spur is not always possible, complicating interpretation of angle configuration.

AS-OCT has the potential to add meaningful information that can aid clinicians in detecting angle-closure disease. The principles for evaluation of the angle are similar to those previously described for UBM, as are many of the quantitative parameters (see Fig 4-12). As with UBM, automated quantitative analysis is available on some platforms. With the new generation of 3-dimensional AS-OCT devices, this modality has the ability to detect and quantify areas of iridotrabecular contact. Videos 4-5 and 4-6 show an eye with an occludable angle before and after cataract surgery.

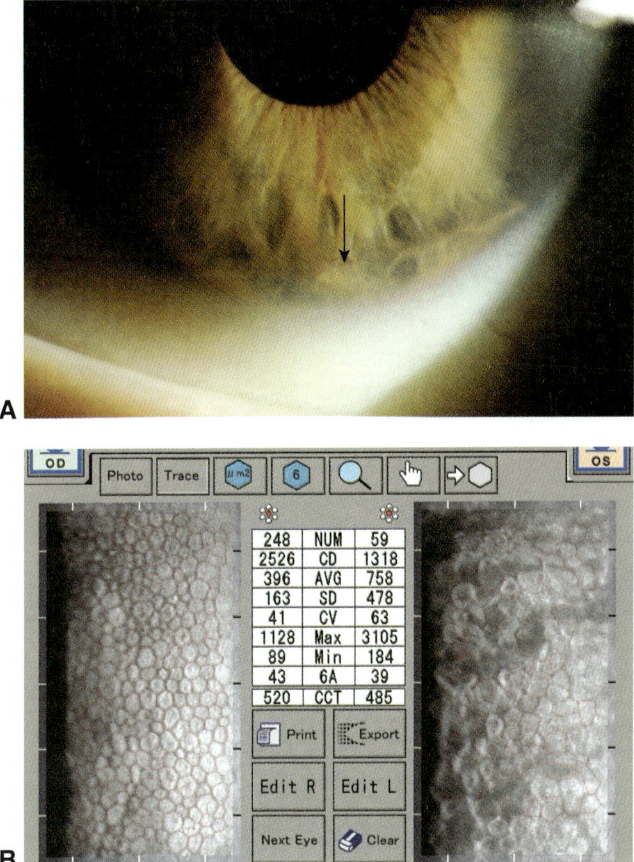

Figure 4-14 Iridocorneal endothelial syndrome. **A,** Slit-lamp view, with mild distortion of the inferior iris and peripheral anterior synechiae *(arrow)*. **B,** Specular microscopy images from the same patient. The right-eye image shows tightly packed endothelial cells with a normal hexagonal shape, while the left-eye image shows endothelial cells that are reduced in number and pleomorphic. Many cells exhibit a dark specular reflex. *(Courtesy of Angelo P. Tanna, MD.)*

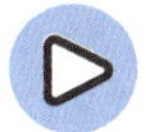

VIDEO 4-5 High-resolution anterior segment OCT: 3D imaging of an occludable angle before cataract surgery.
Courtesy of Shan C. Lin, MD.
Available at: aao.org/bcscvideo_section10

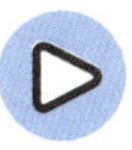

VIDEO 4-6 High-resolution anterior segment OCT: 3D imaging of an occludable angle after cataract surgery.
Courtesy of Shan C. Lin, MD.
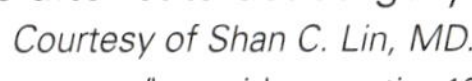
Available at: aao.org/bcscvideo_section10

Chansangpetch S, Rojanapongpun P, Lin SC. Anterior segment imaging for angle closure. *Am J Ophthalmol.* 2018;188:xvi–xxix.

Specular Microscopy

Specular microscopy allows noncontact, noninvasive imaging of the corneal endothelial cell layer (Fig 4-14). Most commercially available devices automatically identify the endothelial cells and analyze the images to provide the user with quantitative assessments of endothelial cell density (ECD) and morphology. ECD is often monitored in the context of clinical trials of surgically implanted devices such as aqueous drainage devices and stents. Any glaucoma device surgically implanted in the anterior chamber can lead to progressive reduction in ECD through direct mechanical effects or alteration of aqueous flow near the endothelium.

Specular microscopy is useful for the diagnosis and monitoring of various disorders of the posterior cornea, such as posterior polymorphous corneal dystrophy and ICE syndrome. In these diseases, the endothelial cell count is reduced, and the cells lose their normal hexagonal shape (see Fig 4-14). See BCSC Section 8, *External Disease and Cornea,* for further discussion of specular microscopy.

CHAPTER 5

Clinical Evaluation and Imaging of the Posterior Segment: Optic Nerve Head, Retinal Nerve Fiber Layer, and Macula

Highlights

- Glaucomatous damage tends to affect the inferior and superior poles of the optic nerve head, especially in the early stages of disease.
- Clinical determination of the cup–disc ratio is an imprecise method for documenting the extent of optic nerve damage in patients with glaucoma.
- Optical coherence tomography (OCT) provides quantitative measurements of peripapillary retinal nerve fiber layer thickness, optic nerve head topography, and macular layer thicknesses.
- Glaucomatous damage can affect the macular region, leading to central and paracentral visual field loss that may not be detected by conventional perimetry but can be identified in OCT scans of the macula.

Clinical Examination of the Optic Nerve Head and Retinal Nerve Fiber Layer

See Chapter 1 for detailed descriptions of optic nerve anatomy and glaucoma pathophysiology.

Optic Nerve Head

Clinical examination of the optic nerve head (ONH; also known as *optic disc*—the terms are used interchangeably in the literature) is typically performed using a *slit-lamp biomicroscope* combined with a handheld lens (60, 78, or 90 diopters). A slit beam, rather than diffuse illumination, is useful for identifying subtle changes in ONH contour. This optical system provides high magnification, illumination, and a stereoscopic view. In addition, the height of the slit beam can be adjusted to enable quantitative measurement of ONH diameter. The ONH is viewed, and the height of the slit beam is adjusted so that it is the same as the vertical diameter of the ONH. The ONH diameter can then be calculated with adjustment for the magnification of the lens used for measurement. A healthy ONH ranges from approximately 1.5 to 1.7 mm in diameter. Note that the patient's refractive error will affect this measurement, leading to underestimation in patients with myopia and overestimation in patients with hyperopia.

The *direct ophthalmoscope* can also be used for clinical examination of the ONH. However, this instrument may not provide sufficient stereoscopic detail for detection of subtle changes in ONH topography. The head-mounted *indirect ophthalmoscope* can be used to examine the ONH in young children and in patients who cannot cooperate during slit-lamp biomicroscopy. In addition, lower-power lenses are helpful when slit-lamp biomicroscopy is not possible and a more detailed view of the optic nerve is needed. Although the optic nerve can be evaluated using an indirect ophthalmoscope, optic nerve cupping (or excavation) and pallor appear less pronounced with this method than with slit-lamp methods, and the magnification offered by an indirect ophthalmoscope is often insufficient to detect subtle or localized details that are important in glaucoma evaluation. Thus, indirect ophthalmoscopy is not recommended for routine use in assessing the ONH.

The ONH is usually round or slightly oval in shape and contains a central cup *(optic cup)*. The tissue between the cup and the ONH margin is known as the *neural rim* or *neuroretinal rim*. The size of the physiologic cup is developmentally determined and is related to the size of the ONH. A larger disc area leads to a larger cup size for a given number of ganglion cell axons. For example, a cup–disc ratio of 0.7 in a large ONH may be normal, whereas a cup–disc ratio of 0.3 in a very small ONH may be pathologic. Thus, assessment of ONH size is important; in healthy individuals, a small ONH (vertical disc diameter <1.5 mm) has a small cup, whereas a large ONH (vertical disc diameter >2.2 mm) has a large cup. Black individuals, on average, have larger disc areas and larger cup–disc ratios than White individuals, although substantial overlap exists. For these reasons, the cup–disc ratio alone is insufficient to assess the ONH for glaucomatous damage.

It can be difficult to differentiate a large physiologic or normal cup from acquired *glaucomatous cupping* of the ONH. For example, early cupping changes in glaucomatous optic neuropathy are subtle (Table 5-1).

Diffuse neuroretinal rim thinning associated with generalized enlargement of the cup may be an early sign of glaucomatous damage. However, diffuse loss can be difficult to

Table 5-1 Ophthalmoscopic Signs of Glaucoma

Generalized	Focal	Less Specific
Large optic cup Asymmetry of the optic cup between the eyes Progressive enlargement of the optic cup	Focal loss or notching of the neuroretinal rim Vertical elongation of the optic cup Retinal nerve fiber layer hemorrhage Segmental nerve fiber layer loss	Exposure of the lamina cribrosa Nasal displacement of vessels Baring of circumlinear vessels Beta (β) zone peripapillary atrophy

identify without prior images of the ONH. Comparison with the fellow eye may be helpful because cup–disc ratio asymmetry >0.2 between the 2 eyes is unusual in healthy eyes without ONH size asymmetry (Fig 5-1). The vertical cup–disc ratio typically ranges from 0.1 to 0.4, although up to 5% of individuals without glaucoma have cup–disc ratios >0.6 (ie, physiologic cupping). Cup–disc ratio asymmetry values >0.2, which occur in fewer than 1% of individuals without glaucoma, may be related to ONH size asymmetry. Increased physiologic cup size may be a familial trait; it is also present in individuals with high myopia. In these individuals, oblique optic nerve insertion into the globe causes the ONH to appear tilted. Examinations of other family members may clarify whether a large cup is inherited or acquired.

Focal loss of the neuroretinal rim often initially occurs at the inferior and superior poles of the optic nerve in patients with early glaucomatous optic neuropathy (Fig 5-2).

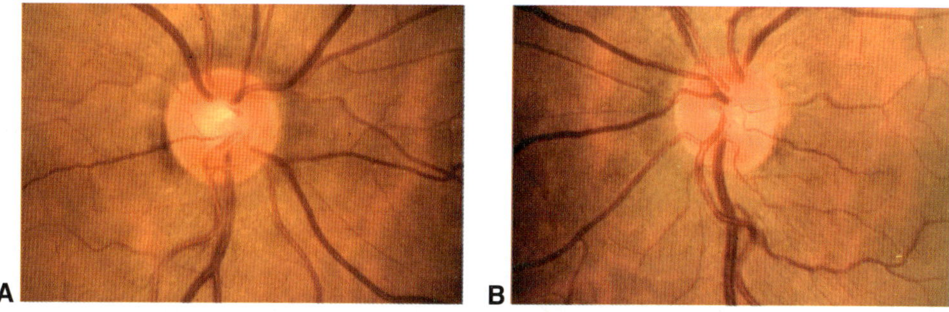

Figure 5-1 Asymmetry of optic nerve cupping. Note the generalized enlargement of the optic cup in the right eye **(A)** compared with the healthy left eye **(B).** *(Courtesy of G. A. Cioffi, MD.)*

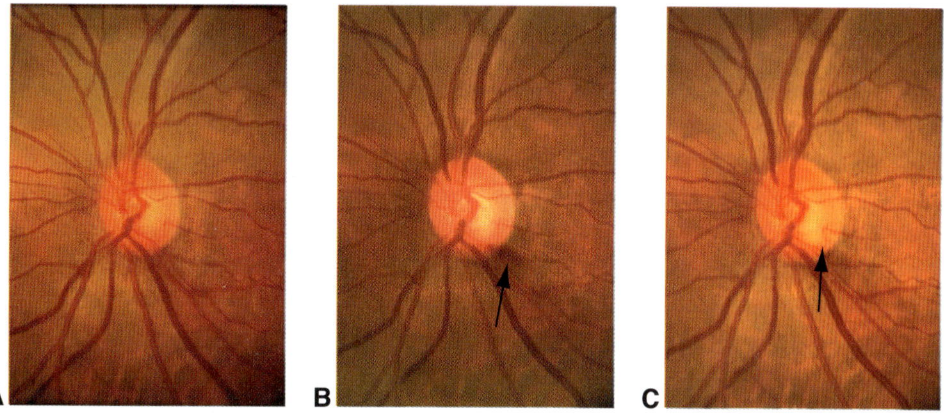

Figure 5-2 Progressive optic nerve head (ONH) excavation in a patient with uncontrolled open-angle glaucoma over a 3-year period. The overall size of the ONH is small. **A,** The overall cup size is larger than expected for a small ONH, and the inferior neuroretinal rim is thinner than the superior rim, suggesting early glaucomatous optic neuropathy. **B,** Progressive thinning of the inferior neuroretinal rim is apparent at the 5 o'clock position, and optic disc hemorrhage is present in the same location *(arrow).* **C,** Further inferior neuroretinal rim loss is evident at the 5 o'clock position, where a notch is present *(arrow).* *(Courtesy of Angelo P. Tanna, MD.)*

This preferential loss of rim tissue leads to a vertically elongated cup in glaucomatous nerves (Fig 5-3). To help identify subtle neuroretinal rim thinning, a convention known as the *ISNT rule* may be useful. In healthy eyes, the Inferior neuroretinal rim is generally the thickest, followed by the Superior, Nasal, and Temporal rims. The absence of this pattern may indicate focal loss of rim tissue. However, violations of the ISNT rule are not highly specific; they may also be observed in healthy eyes.

Deep localized notching, in which the lamina cribrosa is visible at the ONH margin, is sometimes called an *acquired optic disc pit* (Fig 5-4). Patients with acquired optic disc pits have a particularly high risk of disease progression. Even in healthy eyes, laminar pores may be visible as grayish dots at the base of the physiologic cup. In glaucomatous optic neuropathy, ONH excavation is characterized by extensive exposure (within the optic nerve cup) of the underlying lamina cribrosa and its pores or striations (Fig 5-5). Backward bowing, strain, and compression of the lamina cribrosa cause damage to the laminar pores and beams. Glaucomatous damage to the lamina may also cause tearing of connective tissue bundles between pores, leading to the coalescence of small pores and formation of larger pores. During cup enlargement, nasal migration of the central retinal artery and central retinal vein is often apparent.

Retinal nerve fiber layer (RNFL) hemorrhages, which can be a sign of glaucoma, usually appear as linear red streaks on or near the ONH surface (Fig 5-6). However, their

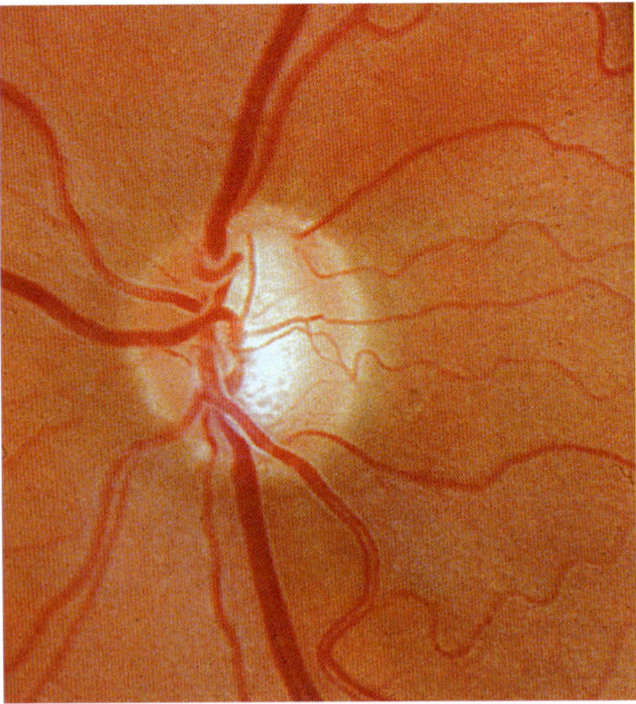

Figure 5-3 Vertical elongation of the optic cup in the left eye of a patient with moderately advanced glaucoma. Localized thinning of the inferior and superior neuroretinal rim with exposure of the inferior lamina cribrosa is also shown. *(Courtesy of Felipe A. Medeiros, MD, PhD.)*

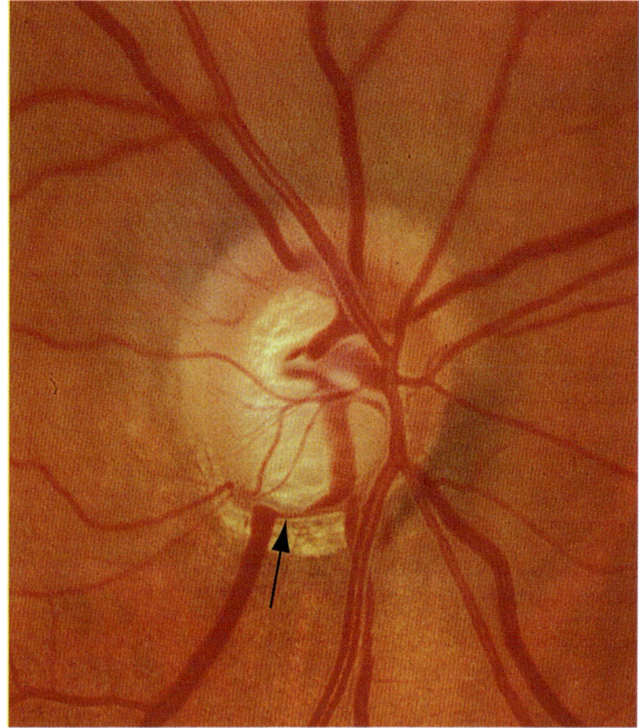

Figure 5-4 Acquired optic disc pit in the inferior temporal region *(arrow)*. Note the absence of rim tissue. *(Courtesy of Felipe A. Medeiros, MD, PhD.)*

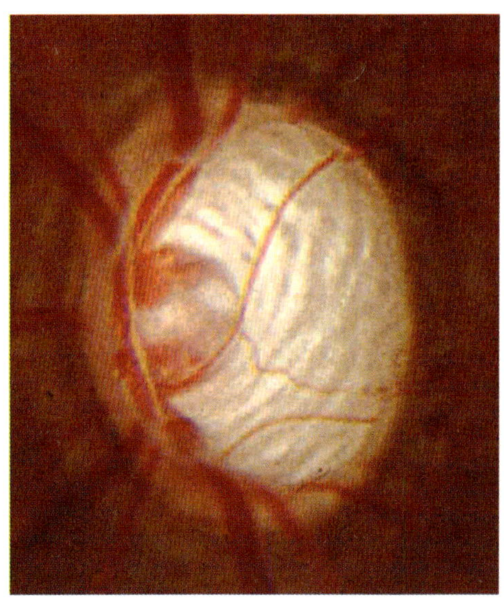

Figure 5-5 Striations of the lamina cribrosa in an optic nerve with severe glaucomatous damage. *(Courtesy of Felipe A. Medeiros, MD, PhD.)*

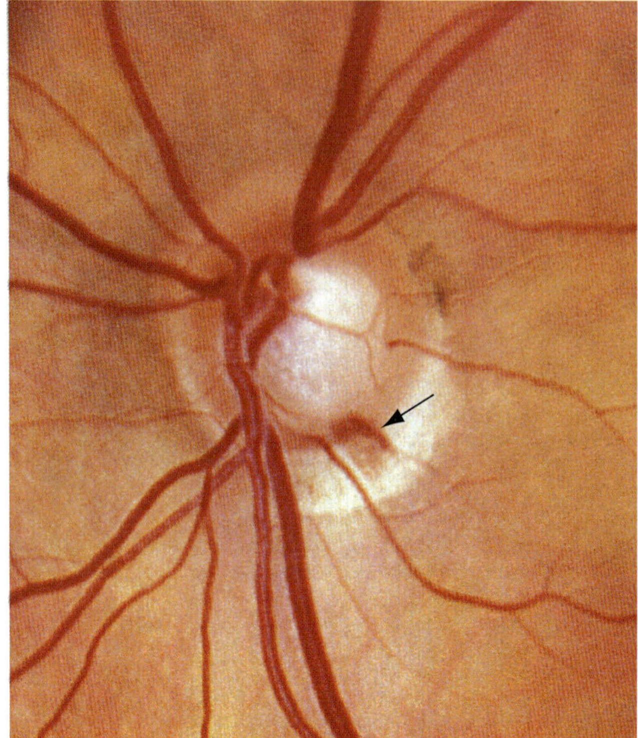

Figure 5-6 Flame-shaped optic disc hemorrhage *(arrow)* in a patient with open-angle glaucoma. *(Courtesy of Angelo P. Tanna, MD.)*

appearance can be highly variable; hemorrhages may be difficult to detect unless the clinician specifically searches for them. During the course of disease, one-third of patients with glaucoma may develop optic disc hemorrhages, which typically resolve over several weeks to a few months. Some patients with glaucoma have repeated episodes of optic disc hemorrhage, whereas others have none. Optic disc hemorrhages constitute an important prognostic sign for the development or progression of visual field loss; their presence in any patient warrants follow-up. Optic disc hemorrhages are often followed by localized notching of the neuroretinal rim and visual field loss. The hemorrhages may also be caused by posterior vitreous detachment, diabetes, retinal vein occlusion, and anticoagulation therapy.

Retinal Nerve Fiber Layer

In healthy eyes, optimal direct visualization of the RNFL is achieved using red-free (green) illumination. Nerve fibers extend from the peripheral retina to converge at the ONH; these fibers appear as fine striations created by the bundles of axons. In healthy eyes, RNFL brightness and striations are most visible superiorly and inferiorly. In eyes with progressive glaucomatous optic neuropathy, the RNFL thins and becomes less visible. The loss may be diffuse (generalized) or focal (Fig 5-7). Diffuse loss is characterized

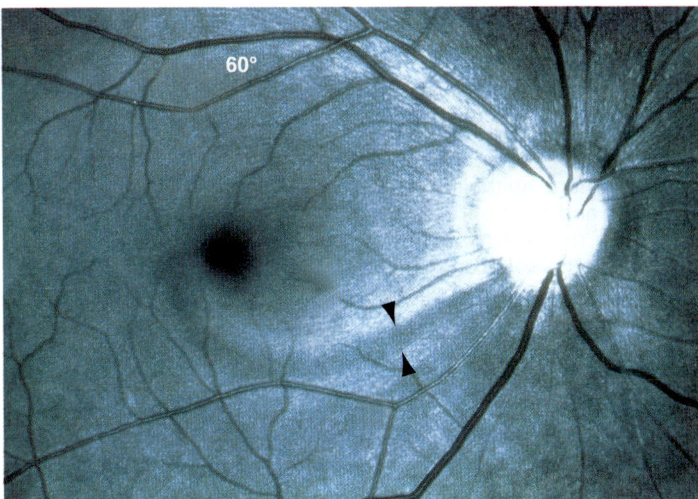

Figure 5-7 Photograph of the nerve fiber layer showing a nerve fiber bundle defect *(arrowheads)*. *(Courtesy of Felipe A. Medeiros, MD, PhD.)*

by a general decrease in RNFL brightness, along with a reduction of the usual difference between the superior and inferior poles relative to the temporal and nasal regions. In contrast, focal RNFL loss is characterized by wedge-shaped dark areas that extend from the ONH in an arcuate pattern. In glaucoma, diffuse nerve fiber loss is more common than focal loss (ie, nerve fiber bundle defects); however, diffuse loss is more difficult to observe.

The RNFL can be clearly visualized in high-contrast black-and-white photographs; good-quality photographs can allow experienced clinicians to recognize even early disease. However, such photographs are difficult to obtain and have been largely abandoned in clinical practice because modern imaging methods enable quantification of RNFL thickness. Slit-lamp techniques and direct ophthalmoscopy can be used to observe the RNFL. Optimal ONH evaluation can be achieved by clinical examination using a red-free filter and a wide slit beam at the slit lamp, in combination with quantitative nerve fiber layer imaging.

Atypical Optic Nerves

Peripapillary atrophy can be classified into 2 general types: alpha (α) zone and beta (β) zone. Alpha zone peripapillary atrophy is present in most nonglaucomatous eyes, as well as eyes with glaucoma. It is characterized by a region of irregular hypopigmentation and hyperpigmentation of the retinal pigment epithelium (RPE). With respect to glaucoma, beta zone peripapillary atrophy is a less specific sign of the disease but is particularly important. This type of peripapillary atrophy results from atrophy of the RPE and choriocapillaris, leading to increased visibility of the large choroidal vessels and sclera (Fig 5-8). Beta zone peripapillary atrophy is more common and extensive in eyes with glaucoma than in healthy eyes. The area of atrophy is spatially correlated with the area of neuroretinal rim loss; atrophy is greatest in the corresponding area where the neuroretinal rim is

Assessment of Image and Segmentation Quality

Similar to applications of other imaging methods, it is important to assess the quality of OCT scans before evaluating the structures involved. The first step of this assessment consists of noting quality measurements provided by the machine. Because these measures vary across device manufacturers, the user needs to understand how each manufacturer defines "good," "borderline," and "poor" scan quality. Scans with poor quality should be evaluated with caution.

The second step of quality assessment consists of evaluating the automated segmentation of retinal layers and ONH structures. Similar to the previously mentioned variability in quality measurements, each vendor has a unique approach to the segmentation of anatomical structures; thus, the success of a particular algorithm is device specific. In general, it is important to confirm that the layers and structures relevant to glaucoma have been correctly segmented. Images or regions of images for which the segmentation algorithm failed should be excluded from consideration.

OCT device–related sources of error can influence measurements and provide false findings of glaucoma detection or progression. For example, low signal strength related to cataract progression, posterior capsule opacification, high myopia, corneal opacity, poor tear film, and other factors that affect signal strength may provide an artifactually low nerve fiber layer measurement suggesting that glaucoma is present or progressing. Segmentation defects due to the effects of blinking, effects of patient movement, and other image capture artifacts can all produce low nerve fiber layer measurements and false detection of glaucoma.

Evaluation of the Retinal Nerve Fiber Layer

Retinal nerve fiber layer thickness measurements are typically acquired in the peripapillary area at a fixed radius around the ONH. Most commercially available OCT devices acquire RNFL thickness measurements in a 3.45-mm-diameter circle around the ONH. This approach helps to avoid variability and artifacts caused by ONH size, myopia, and peripapillary atrophy when measures are made closer to the ONH.

Although considerable interindividual variability exists, RNFL thickness measurements are generally lower in glaucomatous eyes than in healthy eyes. Measurement parameters presented in OCT reports include the global average peripapillary RNFL thickness (ie, the average of all thickness measurements in the peripapillary circle) and the average RNFL thicknesses in quadrants (superior, inferior, temporal, nasal) or clock-hour sectors. Figure 5-9 shows an example of OCT-based RNFL analysis in a patient with glaucomatous RNFL loss in the right eye and normal RNFL thickness in the left eye. The sensitivity and specificity of glaucomatous damage detection vary according to the parameter evaluated and the characteristics of the study population. In general, the parameters with the best diagnostic accuracy are the global average peripapillary RNFL thickness and the average peripapillary RNFL thicknesses in the inferior and superior quadrants, which correspond to the superior and inferior areas of the optic nerve most commonly affected in glaucoma.

Although sectoral RNFL parameters may increase the likelihood of detecting localized RNFL damage in glaucoma, these parameters may exhibit greater fluctuation because

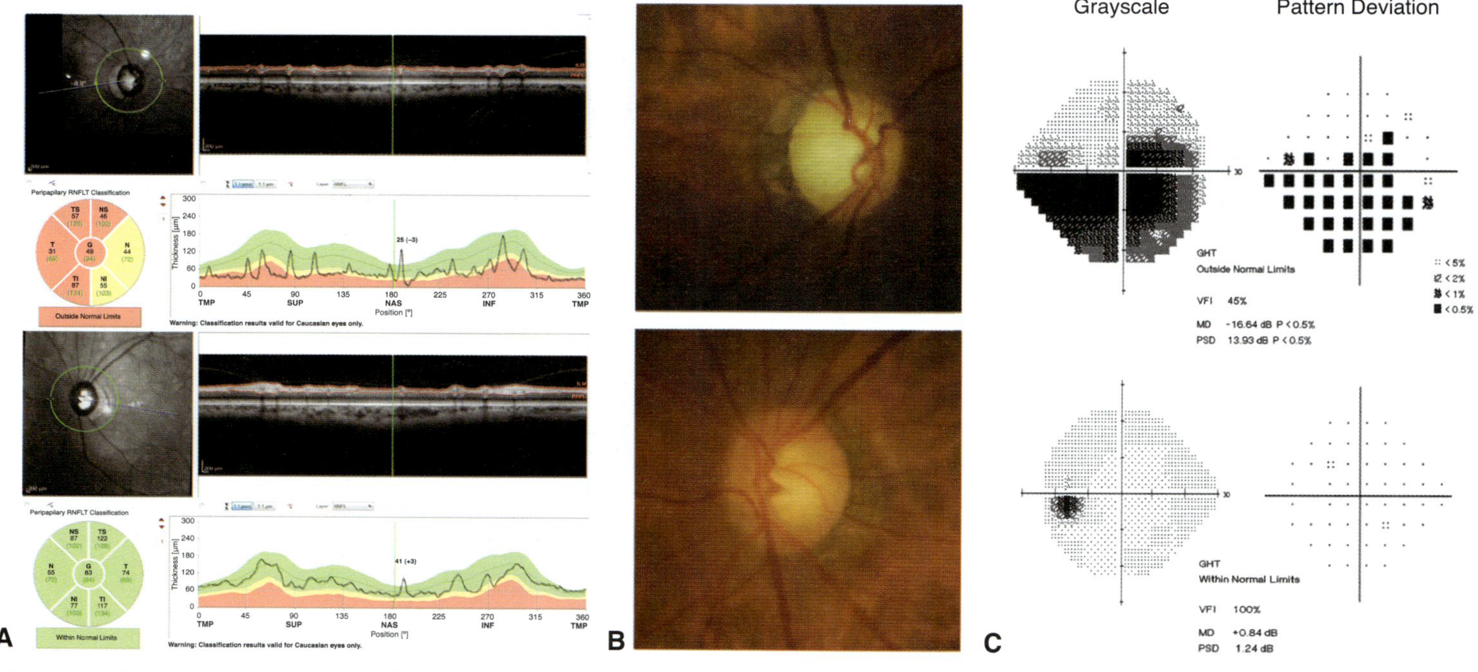

Figure 5-9 Example of retinal nerve fiber layer (RNFL) analysis with optical coherence tomography (OCT). *Top,* The right eye displays diffuse RNFL thinning **(A),** consistent with the neuroretinal rim thinning and enlarged cup visible in photographs of the ONH **(B)** and with the visual field loss that is evident on standard automated perimetry **(C).** *Bottom,* The left eye displays normal RNFL thickness on OCT **(A),** normal ONH morphology **(B),** and normal visual field **(C).** *(Courtesy of Felipe A. Medeiros, MD, PhD.)*

they consist of measurements averaged over relatively small areas. In contrast, the global average RNFL thickness has generally been shown to be the most reproducible parameter; its reproducibility enhances the ability to detect progression over time. However, this reproducibility may be offset by less robust discovery of localized RNFL defects, which are averaged out in the calculation. Importantly, most OCT devices can acquire and construct a 3-dimensional map of peripapillary RNFL thickness; such maps may facilitate the identification of localized arcuate RNFL defects that may be missed with global summary parameters.

Evaluation of the Optic Nerve Head

Optical coherence tomography devices can also provide topographic measurements of the ONH, including measurements of the ONH area, neuroretinal rim area, and cup–disc ratio. These parameters and the methods for calculating them differ across platforms. The improved resolution of OCT and the sophistication of segmentation algorithms for anatomical structures have resulted in the clinically useful delineation of ONH structures.

Modern OCT devices generally define the ONH border as the site of Bruch membrane termination. The circle defining this landmark around the ONH is the *Bruch membrane opening (BMO).* The border of the optic cup is then defined as the ring of points along the anterior border of the nerve fiber layer closest to and inside the BMO; this border is known as the *minimum rim width (MRW).* When these 2 borders are identified by OCT device algorithms, the region of the ONH between the BMO and MRW is defined as the neuroretinal rim thickness. This measure is more anatomically appropriate for assessment of glaucoma, compared with the ONH border determined via biomicroscopy (ie, typically the scleral opening). The BMO-MRW may be more sensitive than other rim-based parameters in terms of glaucoma diagnosis. Figure 5-10 shows an example of an OCT report with calculations of BMO-MRW measurements.

Evaluation of the Macular Ganglion Cell Layer

There is increasing interest in evaluating the macular region to identify glaucomatous damage. Because much of the total macular thickness consists of RNFL and ganglion cell bodies, this region is particularly attractive for assessment of structural glaucomatous damage. The macular retinal ganglion cell layer contains >50% of all ganglion cells in the retina. The results of relatively recent investigations have also suggested that, contrary to previous belief, glaucomatous damage frequently affects the macular region during an early stage of disease, leading to central and para-central visual field loss that cannot be detected by conventional perimetry. OCT enables quantitative assessment of either the entire macular thickness or the thickness of specific layers that may be important in glaucoma.

The retinal layers used in measurements of macular thickness for glaucoma evaluation vary among OCT platforms. Commonly used parameters include the thickness of the ganglion cell layer combined with the inner plexiform layer, as well as the *ganglion cell complex,* which is composed of the RNFL, the ganglion cell layer, and the inner plexiform layer. In eyes with myopic ONHs or large areas of peripapillary atrophy, which can

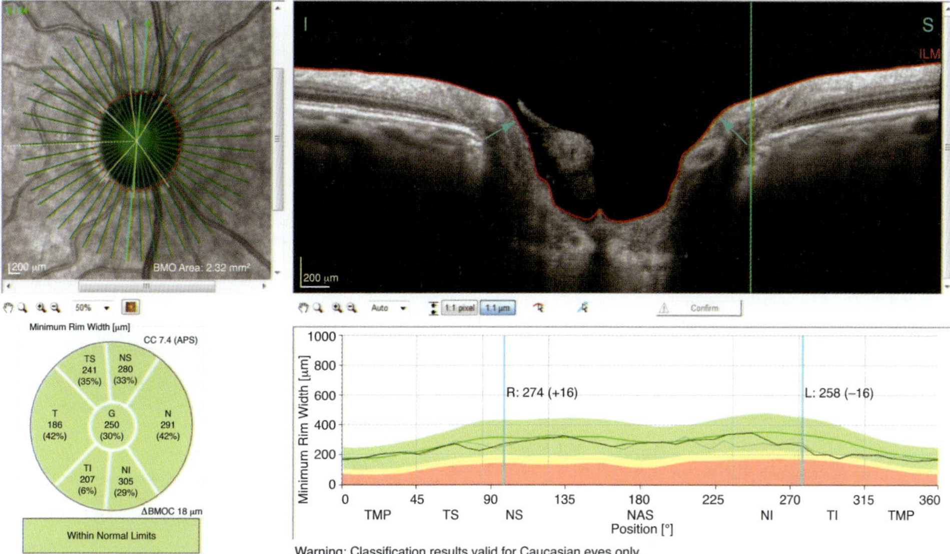

Figure 5-10 OCT scans showing the results of Bruch membrane opening–minimum rim width (BMO-MRW) segmentation. The OCT scan on the right shows how the BMO-MRW boundary is determined. The boundary corresponds to the minimum distance extending from the border of the Bruch membrane to the internal limiting membrane *(arrows).* Global and sectoral ONH, cup, and rim measurements are then calculated and compared with a normative database. *(Courtesy of Felipe A. Medeiros, MD, PhD.)*

produce artifacts on peripapillary RNFL images, macular imaging may help to diagnose and monitor glaucomatous damage. Figure 5-11 shows an example of macular damage detected in a glaucomatous eye with OCT, along with corresponding RNFL scans and ONH photographs.

Detection of Glaucoma

The results of studies comparing the diagnostic abilities of various RNFL, ONH, and macular parameters have been inconsistent, possibly because of differences in the criteria used to select patients with glaucoma and control participants, as well as differences in the characteristics of the included populations. All diagnostic accuracy studies require the use of reference criteria when affected patients (ie, cases) and control participants are being selected. In most studies, the reference criteria for glaucoma cases are glaucomatous visual field loss with "compatible" optic nerve damage. If the reference criteria include clinician assessment of the ONH, there is a greater likelihood that patients with obvious ONH abnormalities (eg, in the rim or cup), rather than patients with RNFL abnormalities, will be included as glaucoma cases in the study. Reference criteria for control participants frequently require a "normal" ONH, which is equivalent to a clinically normal neuroretinal rim and cup. These selection criteria can bias studies toward favoring accurate topographic ONH parameters. Furthermore, potential control participants with anomalous

OD
OS
OD - OS Asymmetry
OS - OD Asymmetry
Retina thickness [µm]
Retina thickness difference [µm]
Hemisphere asymmetry
Average thickness [µm]
S - I
I - S
Superior (S)
305
Total 296
Inferior (I)
288
Superior (S)
317
Total 298
Inferior (I)
280
A
IR 30° ART [HR]
Asymmetry
OD - OS
Circle diameter: 3.5 mm
BMO Area: 1.58 mm²
BMO Area: 1.41 mm²
S
−28
N
0
T
13
I
−5
NS
−16
TS
−38
N
−4
G
−5
T
13
NI
−20
TI
11
OCT ART (98) Q: 24 [HS]
OCT ART (85) Q: 22 [HS]
200 µm
Within normal limits (>5%)
Borderline (<5%)
Outside normal limits (<1%)
RNFL thickness (3.5 mm) [µm]
TMP TS NS NAS NI TI TMP
Position [°]
S 78
T 62
N 79
I 66
CC 7.7 (APS)
TS 66 <1%
NS 92 (26%)
T 62 (28%)
N 78 (51%)
TI 39 <1%
NI 93 (33%)
Segmentation unconfirmed
Classification OD
Outside normal limits
S 106
N 79
T 49
I 71
NS 108 (55%)
TS 103 (22%)
N 82 (65%)
T 49 (3%)
NI 113 (69%)
TI 28 <1%
Classification OS
Outside normal limits
B

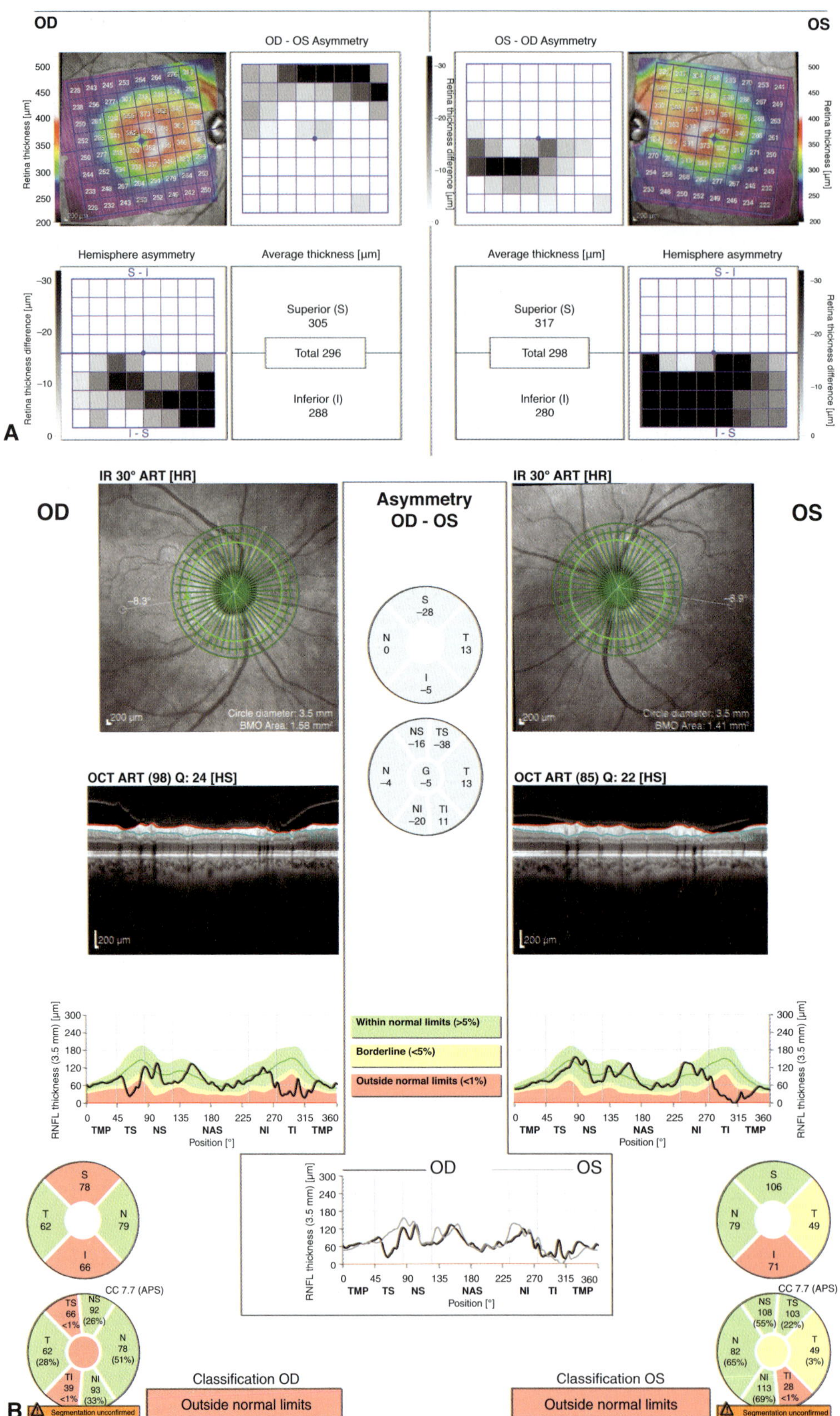

Figure 5-11

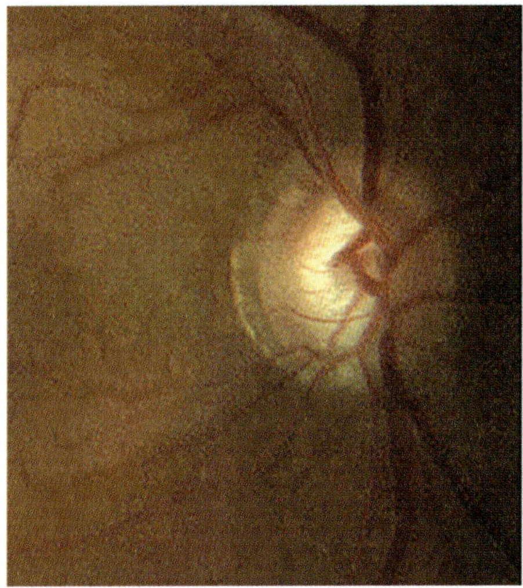

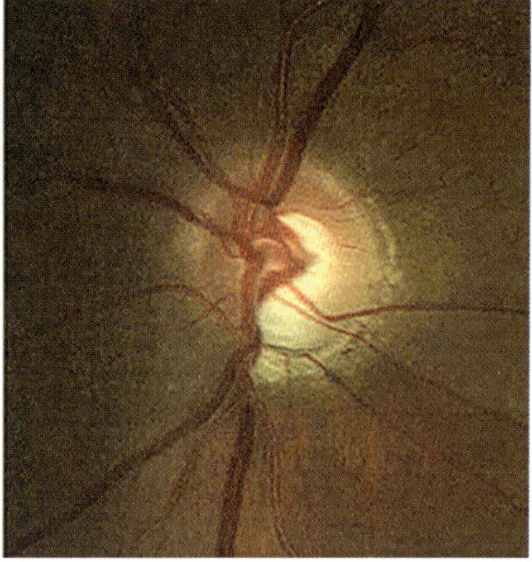

Figure 5-11 *(continued)* Macular thickness maps from a patient with glaucoma. **A,** Hemisphere asymmetry plots show differences in thickness between corresponding superior and inferior regions in each eye; oculus dexter (OD)–oculus sinister (OS)/OS-OD asymmetry plots show differences between the right and left eyes. Note that the right eye displays thinning in the inferior arcuate region, which is most visible in the hemisphere asymmetry graph. The OD-OS asymmetry plot for the right eye shows a superior arcuate defect. The OS-OD asymmetry plot for the left eye reveals an extensive inferior arcuate defect involving the paracentral region. **B,** Peripapillary RNFL scans of the same eyes. The right eye exhibits localized losses in both the superior and inferior temporal regions, which correspond to the damage visible in the macular scan. The left eye exhibits damage that is limited to the inferior temporal region, consistent with the macular scan. **C,** ONH photographs showing rim thinning in the superior and inferior temporal regions of the right eye. The left eye demonstrates notching and complete loss of the rim in the inferior temporal location, but the superior rim appears to be well preserved. *(Courtesy of Felipe A. Medeiros, MD, PhD.)*

ONH characteristics, such as nonglaucomatous tilted discs, are often excluded from such studies and from normative databases.

Although imaging technologies generally facilitate glaucoma detection, their diagnostic performance decreases for detecting early disease, compared with moderate or advanced disease. Most studies evaluating the diagnostic accuracy of OCT devices have evaluated the ability to differentiate between healthy eyes and eyes with well-defined glaucomatous visual field defects, rather than eyes with early disease.

Some studies have prospectively investigated the ability of OCT to identify glaucoma in individuals with suspected disease (according to conventional examination) at the time of enrollment. In 1 study, OCT-based assessment of the RNFL detected abnormalities in one-third of participants up to 5 years before the first appearance of a visual field defect on standard automated perimetry. Importantly, other studies have shown that RNFL thickness measurements are predictive of future visual field loss in glaucoma suspects. Figure 5-12 shows an eye in which OCT measurements of RNFL thickness were abnormal before the development of visual field defects.

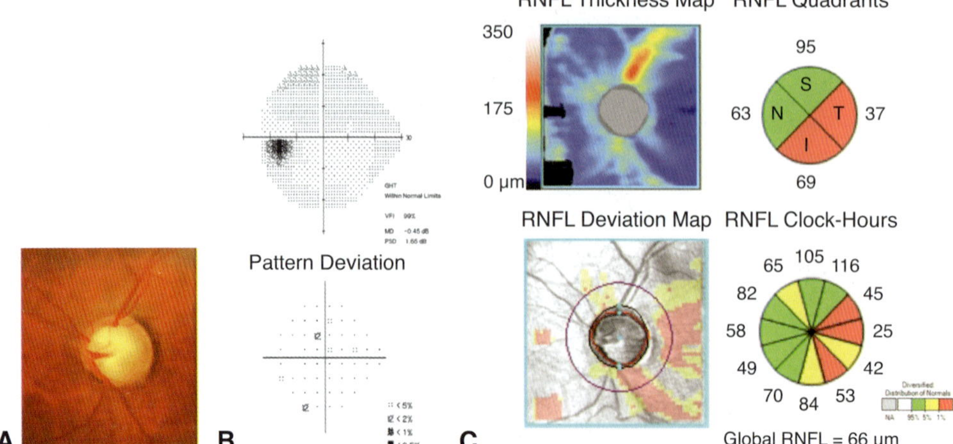

Figure 5-12 Structural damage may precede a detectable visual field defect. **A,** Photograph of the ONH shows marked neuroretinal rim thinning and an enlarged cup. **B,** Standard automated perimetry shows that the visual field remains within normal limits. **C,** RNFL analysis with OCT shows loss of the RNFL, which is worse in the inferior and temporal regions. *(Courtesy of Felipe A. Medeiros, MD, PhD.)*

Bussel II, Wollstein G, Schuman JS. OCT for glaucoma diagnosis, screening and detection of glaucoma progression. *Br J Ophthalmol.* 2014;98(Suppl 2):ii15–ii19.

Lisboa R, Leite MT, Zangwill LM, Tafreshi A, Weinreb RN, Medeiros FA. Diagnosing preperimetric glaucoma with spectral domain optical coherence tomography. *Ophthalmology.* 2012;119(11):2261–2269.

Detection of Glaucoma Progression

Imaging is important in the longitudinal monitoring of structural damage. Several studies have shown that imaging parameters such as measurements of RNFL, neural rim, and macular thicknesses can detect progressive glaucomatous damage. These parameters can also facilitate quantitative assessment of glaucoma progression, which is essential for establishing appropriate treatment. Although many patients with glaucoma will show some evidence of progression if observed long enough, the rate of deterioration can substantially vary: whereas most patients display relatively slow progression, others have aggressive disease with rapid deterioration that eventually causes impairment. The use of imaging may assist in the detection of patients with rapid progression that requires more aggressive intervention.

Several studies have used OCT to evaluate the clinical value of using RNFL, ONH, and macular measurements to assess glaucoma progression. Although glaucomatous changes reflect the loss of retinal ganglion cells, the temporal relationship among changes in the ONH, RNFL, and macula remains poorly understood. Overall, RNFL, ONH, and macular parameters show faster rates of loss in glaucomatous eyes compared with the typical age-related changes observed in control eyes; however, considerable variability exists with reported rates of change. Figure 5-13 shows progressive RNFL loss in the inferotemporal region.

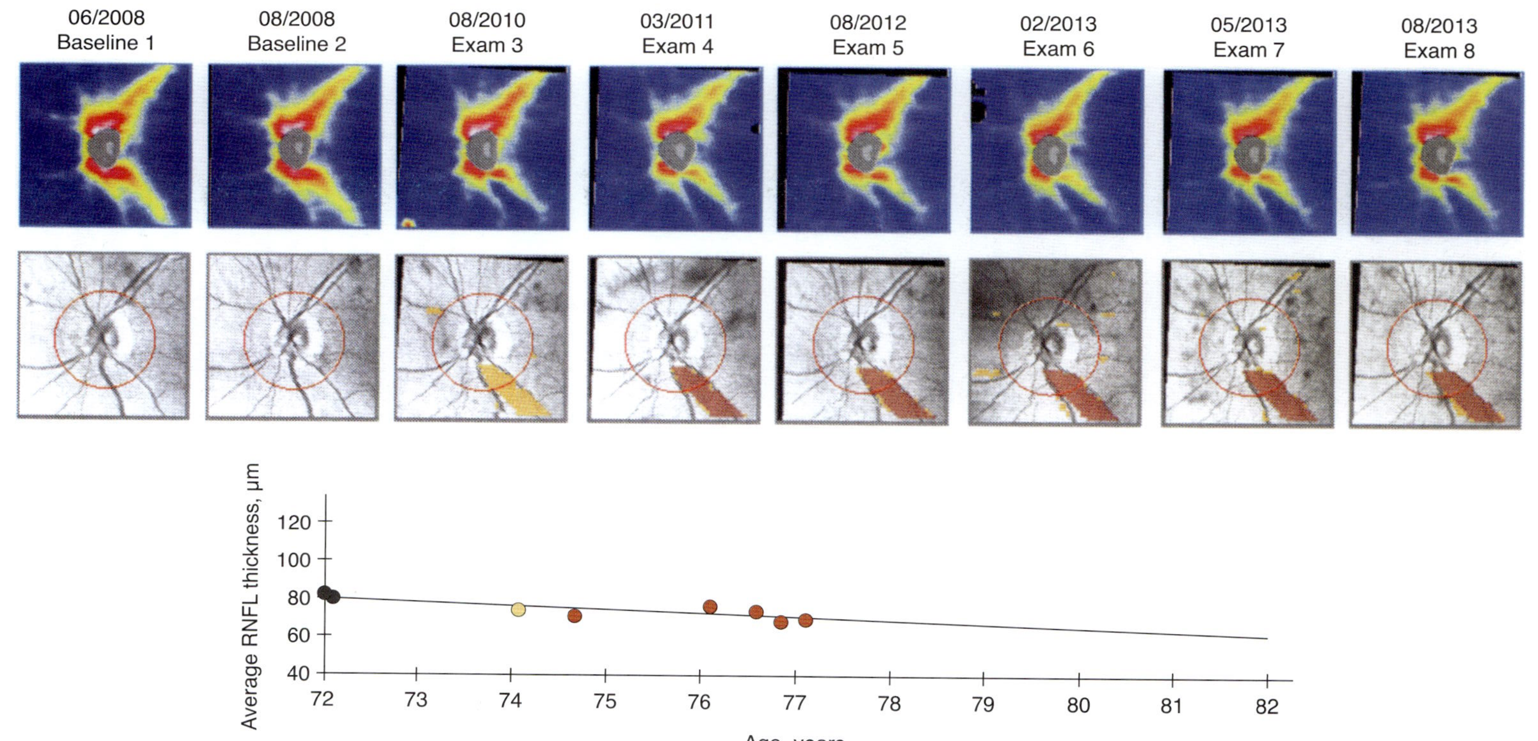

Figure 5-13 OCT images showing progressive RNFL loss in the inferotemporal region. The plot at the bottom of the figure shows the rate of change in average peripapillary RNFL thickness. *(Courtesy of Felipe A. Medeiros, MD, PhD.)*

Detection of disease progression fundamentally depends on the ability to distinguish among true change (ie, disease-induced change), inherent test–retest variability, and changes attributable to normal aging. Several studies have shown that RNFL, ONH, and macular thickness measurements obtained by OCT have excellent short-term reproducibility. It is important to exercise caution when identifying changes in optic nerve or RNFL structure. Most studies of reproducibility have excluded poor-quality scans with low signal strength; they have analyzed short-term (rather than long-term) reproducibility. In clinical practice, patients are followed up over the course of many years, and long-term variability may be considerably greater than short-term variability. Many OCT devices now include some form of glaucoma progression analysis software based on age-adjusted measurements; some devices also include diverse racial demographics in their normative databases.

Clinical Pearl Detecting disease progression essentially depends on the ability to differentiate among disease-induced change, inherent test–retest variability, and changes attributable to normal aging.

In addition to the identification of progression in eyes with existing damage, OCT-based assessments of longitudinal changes are important in the detection of changes in eyes with suspected disease; these findings can help to confirm a diagnosis of glaucoma. Because there is a wide range of normative values, substantial changes in RNFL thickness or other parameters may be observed well before the measurements reach the "outside normal limits" range (Fig 5-14).

Considering the relative stability of the BMO as a point of reference for repeated scans, it might be reasonable to assume that, compared with conventional structural measurements, measurements taken relative to the BMO would be more useful for detecting glaucoma progression. However, it may be more difficult to detect changes using BMO-MRW and rim area measurements because of a relatively low longitudinal signal-to-noise ratio, compared with peripapillary RNFL thickness. This observation may result from changes in BMO location over time, possibly related to fluctuations in intraocular pressure or to connective tissue remodeling that occurs during glaucoma progression.

Regardless of the optimal measurement parameter, there is now extensive evidence that changes measured with OCT are clinically relevant. Faster rates of RNFL loss, visualized by OCT, are also associated with a higher risk of future visual field defects. Progressive structural changes can precede loss of visual function, which is what patients are most concerned about. In addition, patients who demonstrate a faster rate of change on OCT are at increased risk for progressive vision loss; as a result of this OCT finding, these patients have the opportunity to escalate treatment at an earlier stage, which may preserve more visual function. The ability to assess glaucoma progression is likely to be further enhanced by novel approaches that incorporate information from OCT and visual fields, thereby reducing the noise inherent in both tests. For further discussion, see Chapter 6.

Tatham AJ, Medeiros FA. Detecting structural progression in glaucoma with optical coherence tomography. *Ophthalmology*. 2017;124(12S):S57–S65.

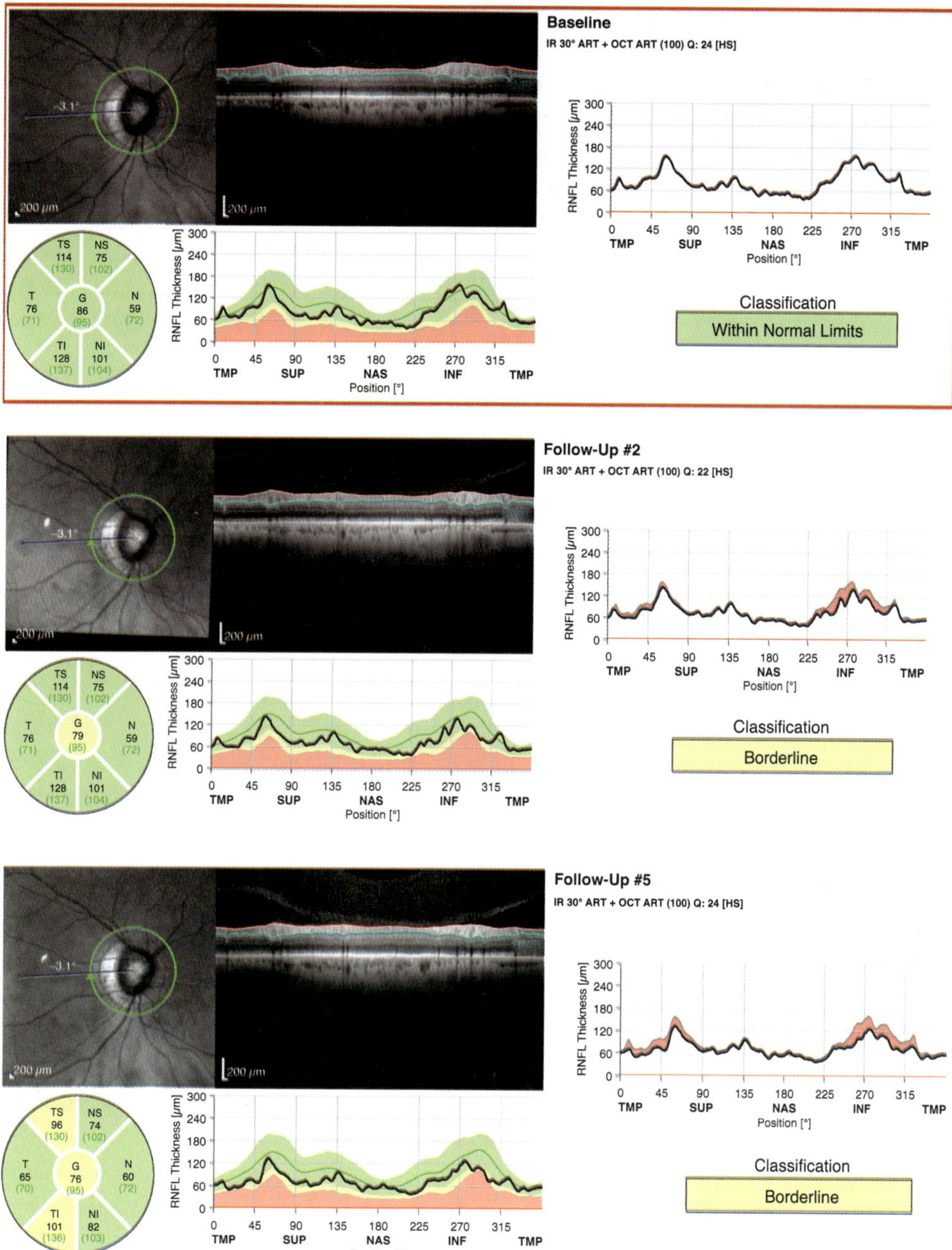

Figure 5-14 Series of OCT RNFL scans of a patient over 4 years of follow-up. Glaucoma was suspected because of the ONH morphology. Note that the initial scan does not show any obvious abnormalities, and all parameters are within normal limits. Progressive RNFL loss begins in the inferior region and gradually affects the superior region. Note that the global and sectoral RNFL thickness parameters only become clearly abnormal *(flagged in red)* after 4 years. *(Courtesy of Felipe A. Medeiros, MD, PhD.)*

(Continued)

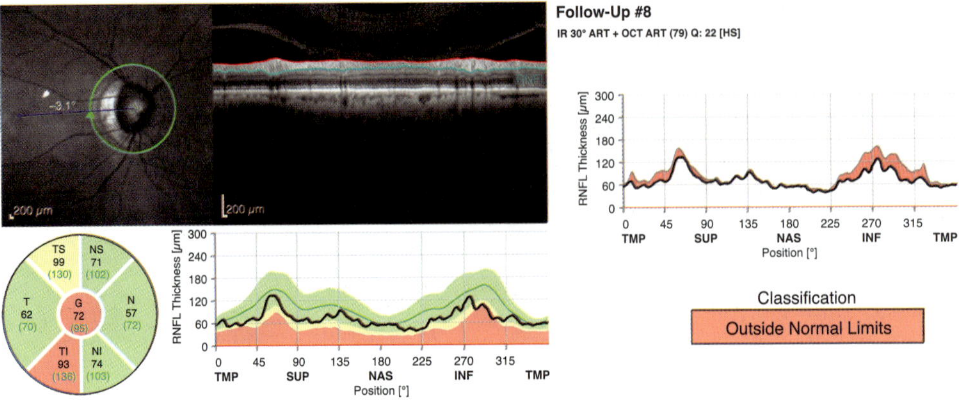

Figure 5-14 *(continued)*

Imaging of the Lamina Cribrosa

The lamina cribrosa is important to the pathophysiology of glaucoma (see Chapter 1), as it is recognized as the site of retinal ganglion cell axonal injury in this disease. Although histologic examination has shown that early glaucomatous cupping begins with structural damage to the lamina cribrosa, until recently, the use of imaging to evaluate the lamina cribrosa was challenging because of its location deep within the ONH. However, advances in OCT technologies such as enhanced depth imaging (EDI) and swept-source OCT (SS-OCT) have allowed imaging of deeper ocular structures, including the lamina cribrosa. In EDI-OCT, the most tightly focused illumination is located more posteriorly, at the level of the choroid and inner sclera.

The wavelength of light used in an OCT system affects image resolution; when penetration depth increases, image resolution and signal strength decrease. Commonly used OCT systems utilize wavelengths in the range of 840–880 nm. However, SS-OCT devices use wavelengths around 1000 nm, allowing greater penetration with less light absorption and dispersion by the vitreous; these characteristics improve the visualization of deeper ONH structures. Figure 5-15 shows EDI-OCT and SS-OCT images of the right eye of a patient with glaucoma who had a clinically visible lamina cribrosa defect, along with images of a healthy eye.

Imaging has enabled the identification of general and localized configurational changes in the lamina cribrosa of glaucomatous eyes, including posterior laminar displacement, altered laminar thickness, and focal laminar defects that have spatial associations with conventional structural and functional losses. In addition to changes in lamina cribrosa depth and thickness, focal lamina cribrosa defects may be important structural features in glaucoma; they could potentially be predictors of glaucomatous visual field loss. There is increasing evidence of an association between lamina cribrosa structure and other measures of glaucoma, indicating that evaluation of the lamina cribrosa may be useful (in combination with clinical imaging tools) for the detection of glaucoma and monitoring of glaucoma progression. The temporal relationship between the lamina cribrosa and neural changes remains unclear.

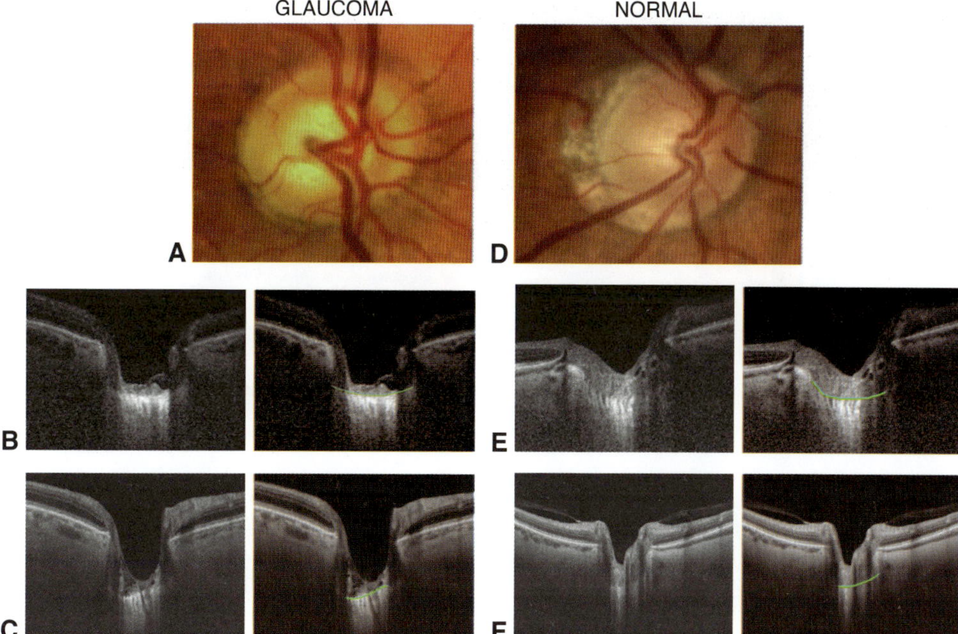

Figure 5-15 Images of the optic nerve in patients with and without glaucoma. The anterior border of the lamina cribrosa is highlighted with a *green line* in parts **B, C, E,** and **F. A,** Photograph of the ONH, right eye, in a patient with glaucoma. **B,** Enhanced depth imaging (EDI) OCT scan of the optic nerve, right eye, of a patient with glaucoma. **C,** Swept-source (SS) OCT scan, right eye, of a patient with glaucoma. **D,** Photograph of the ONH, right eye, in a patient without glaucoma. **E,** EDI-OCT image of a normal eye's right optic nerve. **F,** SS-OCT scan of a normal eye's right optic nerve. *(Courtesy of Teresa C. Chen, MD, and Ashley Kim.)*

Optical Coherence Tomography Angiography

The potential roles of microvasculature and blood flow in glaucoma pathophysiology have been extensively investigated and debated. Studies have demonstrated reduced ocular blood flow in the ONH, retina, choroid, and retrobulbar circulation in eyes with glaucoma. These changes may simply be a consequence of glaucomatous damage to retinal ganglion cells and may have no predictive value. Previously, the lack of a reproducible and relevant in vivo quantitative assessment method hindered analyses of pathophysiology related to ocular perfusion and microvascular networks as potential causes and predictors of future vision loss. OCT angiography (OCTA) is a relatively new imaging modality that can be used to characterize vasculature in various retinal layers, allowing quantitative assessment of the microcirculation in the ONH, peripapillary region, and macula.

The theory underlying OCTA imaging is that blood vessels can be distinguished from static tissue by assessing changes in the OCT signal caused by flowing blood cells. OCTA constructs a blood flow map by comparing differences in backscattered OCT signal intensity or amplitude between sequential OCT scans acquired at identical tissue depth. After the removal of patient movement–related artifacts, sites of motion between repeated OCT scans are assumed to represent erythrocytes in retinal blood vessels.

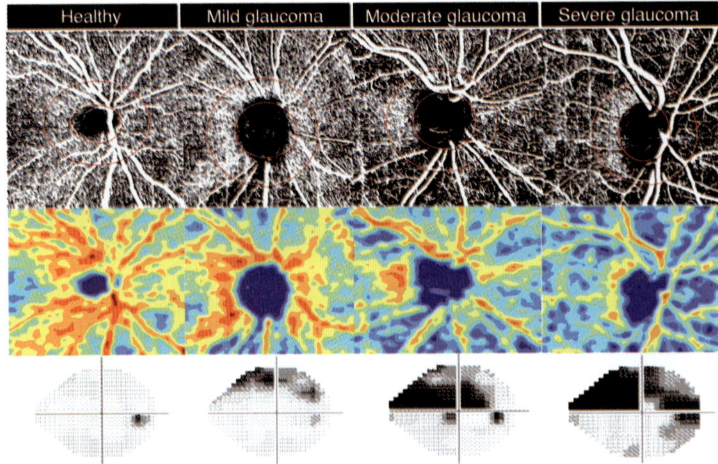

Figure 5-16 Optical coherence tomography angiography (OCTA) scans of a healthy eye and eyes with mild, moderate, and severe glaucomatous damage. OCTA scans show a dense peripapillary vessel network in the healthy eye, illustrated in red and yellow in the color-coded map. Eyes with glaucoma show decreased vessel density and replacement of the red/yellow areas with blue, indicating absence of vessels or no flow. *(Reproduced from Yarmohammadi A, Zangwill LM, Diniz-Filho A, et al. Relationship between optical coherence tomography angiography vessel density and severity of visual field loss in glaucoma.* Ophthalmology. *2016;123(12):2498–2508. With permission from Elsevier.)*

Available OCTA parameters include vessel density, which corresponds to the percentage of detected vessel area within the imaged area, and flow index, which is a dimensionless parameter (ranging from 0 to 1) that represents the average signal. Importantly, these indices are surrogate measures; their validity in blood flow measurement has not been fully determined. Studies have shown that vessel density and flow index within the peripapillary and macular regions significantly differ between patients with glaucoma and healthy individuals. In addition, these indices exhibit significant associations with measures of visual field loss. Figure 5-16 shows OCTA scans of a healthy eye and the eyes of patients with glaucoma who display different degrees of glaucomatous damage.

Motion artifacts and projection artifacts are common in OCTA images. It remains unclear whether OCTA will be able to provide sufficient information to facilitate diagnosis of glaucoma and monitoring of glaucoma progression beyond the current capabilities achieved using OCT-based measurements of the nerve fiber layer relative to the vasculature.

WuDunn D, Takusagawa HL, Sit AJ, et al. OCT angiography for the diagnosis of glaucoma: a report by the American Academy of Ophthalmology. *Ophthalmology.* 2021;128(8):1222–1235.

CHAPTER 6

Perimetry

Highlights

- Standard ("white-on-white") automated perimetry remains the most used method for functional evaluation in glaucoma.
- A high false-positive rate (>15%) is detrimental to a visual field test, as it indicates that the test is likely unreliable and not representative of the patient's visual function.
- When assessing an abnormality on a visual field test, the clinician should determine whether the defect is repeatable and present in approximately the same location on subsequent testing and also verify that the abnormality is not due to an artifact.
- When the visual field is assessed for disease progression, it is important to (a) confirm that a new defect or expansion of a preexisting defect is repeatable on subsequent examinations; and (b) compare the current test results with the results obtained at baseline (often a pair of baseline visual field tests).
- Estimating the rate of visual field change by trend-based analysis is helpful for predicting the risk of functional impairment and determining how aggressive treatment should be.

Introduction

For many years, the standard method of measuring the visual dysfunction that occurs with glaucomatous injury has been assessment of the visual field with *perimetry,* which measures differential light sensitivity, or an individual's ability to detect a stimulus on a uniformly illuminated background.

Perimetry serves 2 major purposes in the management of glaucoma:

- identification and quantification of abnormalities in the visual field
- longitudinal assessment to detect disease worsening and measure the rate of change

Quantitation of visual sensitivity enables detection of visual field defects by comparison of the patient's perimetric results with results from age-matched normal subjects. Regular visual field testing in patients with known disease provides valuable information that can help differentiate between stability and progressive loss.

The current standard method for assessing visual function in glaucoma is automated static perimetry. With this method, sensitivity measurements are performed at a number of test locations using white stimuli on a white background ("white on white"); this is known as *standard automated perimetry (SAP).* One obvious advantage of automated perimetry compared with manual perimetry is that in the former, both stimulus presentation and the recording of patient responses can be standardized, which leads to results with better reproducibility. Manual perimetry introduces the variability of the person performing the test in addition to the variability of the patient. Consequently, manual kinetic perimetry is now rarely performed for visual field assessment in glaucoma. However, kinetic perimetry may be useful in monitoring visual fields in patients who are unable to perform the automated test. Some perimeters can perform automated kinetic perimetry, although its value for assessing visual field loss in glaucoma is not established.

Basic Principles of Automated Perimetry

In SAP, the sensitivity of a patient's central and peripheral vision is quantified by using computerized algorithms to accurately ascertain the retina's sensitivity to light at multiple locations in the field of vision. At each location, stimuli of varying intensities are presented in a systematic sequence of ascending and descending brightness. The patient's responses are then used to calculate the sensitivity to light at each location.

Modern perimeters use stimulus sizes numbered with roman numerals I through V. Each stimulus covers a 4-fold-greater area, ranging from 0.25 mm^2 for a Size I stimulus to 64 mm^2 for a Size V stimulus. The most commonly used stimulus size for the Humphrey Field Analyzer (HFA; Carl Zeiss Meditec AG) is stimulus Size III, which has an area of 4 mm^2.

Full-threshold strategies start by testing a single location in the field of view. If the stimulus is seen, subsequent stimuli at that location are dimmed a fixed amount at a time until the stimulus is no longer seen. If the initial stimulus is not seen, subsequent presentations are made brighter in steps until the patient responds. This process can be repeated at the same location with reversal of the steps to confirm that the threshold of sensitivity has been accurately ascertained. The process of mapping a threshold for each test location requires prohibitively long test sessions, leading to patient fatigue. More efficient approaches have thus been developed to expedite testing (discussed in the section Testing Strategies).

The HFA tests light intensities over 5 orders of magnitude, from 10,000 apostilbs (asb) to 0.1 asb. Every log unit (10×) change in light intensity corresponds to 10 dB; the machine can measure sensitivities over a 50-dB range. Test locations at which a stimulus of 10,000 asb is not detected are assigned a value of <0 dB. Of note, this applies to the specific stimulus size being used. For example, a <0 dB location when testing with stimulus Size III means that the stimulus with maximum intensity of 10,000 asb and Size III was not seen. However, this does not imply that the location is totally blind. A larger stimulus in the same location, such as stimulus Size V, may be visible and detected by the patient. The threshold values reported for each location reflect the extent to which light can be dimmed (by a series of neutral density filters used in the perimeter) and still detected. For example, a value of 30 dB indicates that the stimulus can be dimmed 1000-fold, from

10,000 to 10 asb, and still be seen. The biological significance of this logarithmic test is that small changes in the output (dB scale) correspond to much larger changes in the number of lost retinal ganglion cells (RGCs).

The state of light adaptation of the eye during the visual field test influences luminance sensitivities. The HFA uses background lighting of 31.5 asb to saturate rod photoreceptors, producing photopic conditions in which cones are primarily tested.

Quigley HA, Dunkelberger GR, Green WR. Retinal ganglion cell atrophy correlated with automated perimetry in human eyes with glaucoma. *Am J Ophthalmol.* 1989;107(5): 453–464. doi:10.1016/0002-9394(89)90488-1

Testing Strategies

The standard method for threshold measurement used by the HFA is currently the family of Swedish Interactive Threshold Algorithms (SITAs). SITA is a Bayesian test strategy that uses information from a database of healthy individuals and persons with disease to generate a probability distribution function (PDF) representing the probabilities that the visual field sensitivity will be of a particular value at a particular visual field location. As the test progresses, the distribution adjusts according to how the person being tested responded to prior stimulus presentations. This continues until the probability distribution is within a small range, at which point the mean of the distribution is selected as the threshold sensitivity estimate. The initial PDFs are adjusted for the age of the individual, the visual field location tested, the sensitivity values of neighboring test locations, and the results of previous stimulus presentations. Compared with the full-threshold strategy, SITA has been shown to have equal or lower test–retest variability, and testing can often be done in half the time.

The SITA strategy is available in the Humphrey perimeters as SITA Standard and SITA Fast. As the name implies, SITA Fast is a faster testing method than SITA Standard and thus reduces the likelihood of test fatigue. The accuracy and reliability of SITA Fast are similar to those of SITA Standard. SITA Fast may be a more difficult test for some patients because the test stimuli tend to be closer to the patient's threshold, thus creating a less positive experience for the patient. Any patient struggling with perimetry may benefit from careful instruction by the perimetrist, closer surveillance, and positive feedback during the test.

SITA Faster is a newer strategy with testing times approximately 30% shorter than those of SITA Fast and 50% shorter than those of SITA Standard. The reduction in testing time is achieved by several modifications, including changes in the starting stimulus intensity and in the number of reversals needed to confirm the threshold, as well as elimination of false-negative and fixation-loss catch trials (see the section Test Reliability). Although initial studies indicate that SITA Faster may offer results comparable to those of SITA Standard, there may be a trade-off in terms of reliability.

Like the SITA testing strategy for the HFA, the *tendency-oriented perimetry (TOP)* algorithm, available on the Octopus perimeter (Haag-Streit), was developed as an alternative to the lengthy staircase threshold procedures. TOP differs from SITA in that only 1 stimulus is shown at a single location in the visual field. Therefore, in order to estimate the threshold sensitivity at a particular location, TOP supplements this single data point per test location with information obtained at adjoining test locations.

Phu J, Khuu SK, Agar A, Kalloniatis M. Clinical evaluation of Swedish Interactive Thresholding Algorithm-Faster compared with Swedish Interactive Thresholding Algorithm-Standard in normal subjects, glaucoma suspects, and patients with glaucoma. *Am J Ophthalmol.* 2019;208:251–264.

Patterns of Test Points

For glaucoma diagnosis and management, the most common patterns used for assessing visual function test the central 48°–60° (diameter) of the retina and visual field (Fig 6-1), as for example, the 32 and G1 patterns of the Octopus perimeter and the 24-2 and 30-2 patterns of the Humphrey perimeter. The 24-2 and 30-2 patterns test the central visual field using a 6° grid, with the "24" referring to the radius of the test (in degrees). The "-2" designation indicates that test points are offset from the midlines by 3°, thereby facilitating diagnosis of glaucomatous and neurologic defects that respect horizontal and vertical midlines, respectively. A 24-2 pattern test performed with the SITA Standard strategy for obtaining threshold estimates is then usually referred to as *SITA Standard 24-2.*

For patients with advanced visual field loss or with paracentral defects, testing of the central visual field with the 10-2 or C8 pattern is appropriate (Fig 6-2). The 10-2 pattern evaluates the central 20° (diameter) of vision, testing points every 2°, with test points offset from the midlines by 1°. Alternatively, a larger stimulus (Size V) can be used in patients with advanced disease or reduced visual acuity. For patients with the most advanced disease, stimulus size V testing can be combined with the 10-2 pattern. For patients with visual acuity worse than 20/200, testing with automated perimetry becomes challenging. Although a strategy that tests the visual field between 30° and 60° is available on most static threshold perimeters, it is rarely used because the variability is very high in these more peripheral regions.

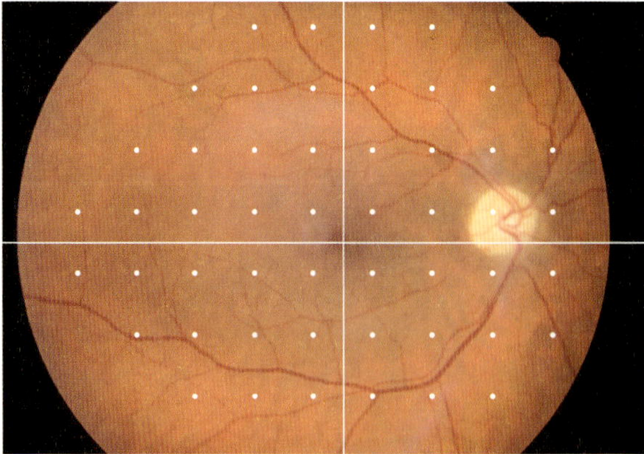

Figure 6-1 The 24-2 test pattern, right eye, showing the relationship to the fundus. *(Courtesy of Michael V. Boland, MD, PhD. Grid drawn by Cyndie C. H. Wooley.)*

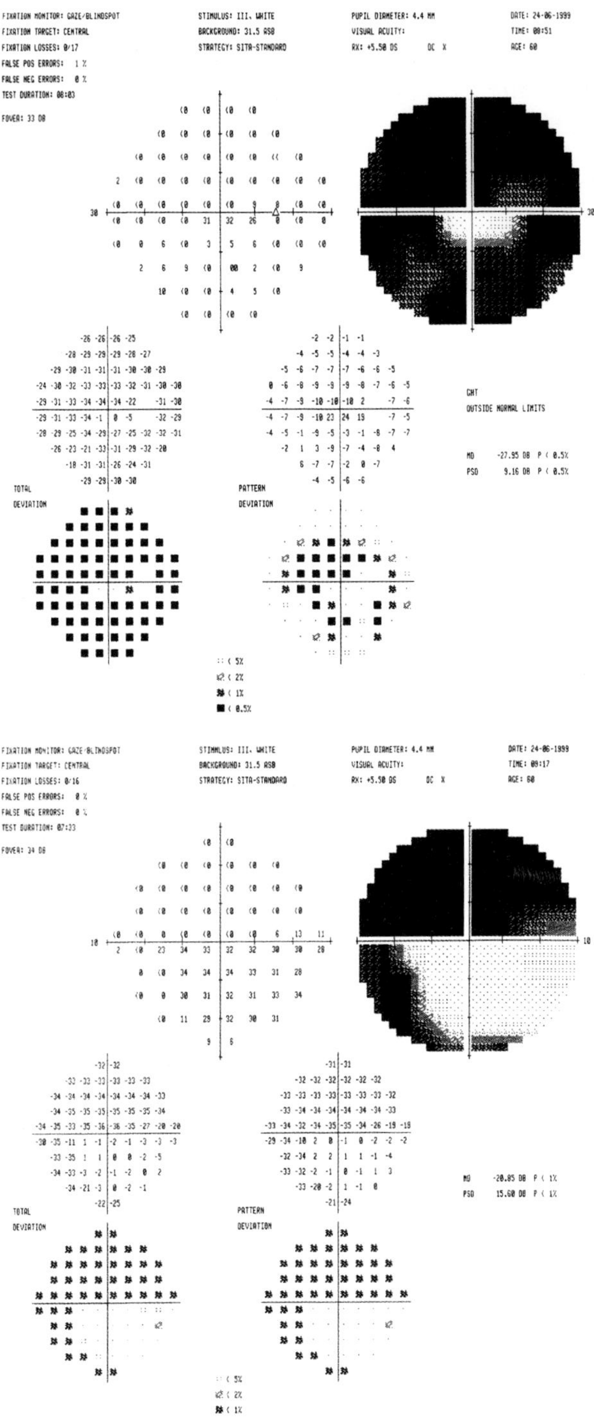

Figure 6-2 Results of a visual field test in a patient with advanced glaucomatous visual field loss. The test with the 30-2 pattern *(top)* evaluates only a few points in the central visual field. The 10-2 pattern *(bottom)* evaluates more points in the central visual field, allowing better evaluation of potential progression over time in this case. *(Courtesy of Felipe A. Medeiros, MD, PhD.)*

Factors Affecting Perimetry Results

Perimetry is a psychophysical test, and many factors can affect the results obtained with it, including the patient's level of attentiveness, the perimetrist's administration of the test, and refractive error. The interaction between the perimetrist and the patient is fundamental to improving the likelihood of successful visual field testing.

Patient

Individuals vary in their attentiveness and response time from moment to moment and from day to day. Longer tests are more likely to cause fatigue and to diminish the patient's ability to attend to the test. The use of perimetry in patients with cognitive issues can be challenging. Finally, although children can be tested, the normative databases used by the perimeter algorithms do not include data for children; thus, the definition of abnormal results in these patients is provided by the standard analyses.

Perimetrist

Although the perimetrist has less influence on the results of automated perimetry than on those of manual perimetry, this technician still plays an essential role in the outcome of the test. It is important for the perimetrist to instruct the patient on various aspects of the test, such as the following: what to expect (eg, how long the test will take); when to blink; what the stimulus will look like; where the stimulus might appear; and how to pause the test if necessary. Also, it is helpful to inform patients that the stimuli are likely to be barely visible throughout the test and that more than half of the stimuli presented may not be visible. This knowledge can decrease a patient's anxiety and improve cooperation during the test. The patient should be monitored during the test to ensure proper positioning and fixation, and the perimetrist should be available to intervene if necessary to ensure proper testing conditions.

Other Factors

Other factors that may affect perimetry results include the patient's refractive error and pupil size. Uncorrected refractive error causes retinal blurring and decreases stimuli visibility. Thus, proper neutralization of refractive error is essential for accurate perimetry. In addition, presbyopic patients must be given a refractive correction that focuses on the perimeter bowl. Care needs to be taken to position the patient close to the instrument's corrective lens to avoid a lens rim artifact, in which the rim blocks peripheral stimuli.

A small pupil (<2.5 mm) may cause artifacts on perimetry by reducing the amount of light entering the eye. However, such artifacts are now rare because the use of miotics (eg, pilocarpine) is less common.

Evaluation and Interpretation of Visual Field Results

The clinician should exercise caution when interpreting perimetry results. Even with improved strategies, these remain subjective tests. Therefore, confirmation of a new defect or worsening of an existing defect is usually necessary to validate the clinical implication of the visual field result in conjunction with all other pertinent data. Evaluation of visual field results involves (1) assessing the reliability of the visual field test, (2) determining whether the test results are normal or abnormal, and (3) identifying artifacts.

Test Reliability

The first step in the evaluation of visual field results is assessing the reliability of the test. Reliability indices include the percentage of fixation losses, false-positives, and false-negatives, as well as test duration. The false-positive rate measures the patient's tendency to press the response button even when no stimulus has been presented. With the SITA strategies, patient responses made at impossible or unlikely times (eg, responses made before, during, or too soon after a stimulus presentation) are used to estimate the false-positive response rate. Of the reliability indices, a high percentage of false-positives is most detrimental to a visual field test. Visual field tests with a false-positive rate greater than 15% are more likely to appear "better" than the patient's true visual function.

The percentage of fixation losses measures the patient's gaze stability during the test. If a patient does not maintain correct fixation during the test, the assessment of peripheral vision will be unreliable. Fixation losses can be estimated by periodically presenting stimuli within the physiologic blind spot. Patients who see these stimuli are presumed to be looking away from the fixation target. However, this method can sometimes fail in detecting fixation losses when the location of the blind spot has not been appropriately identified at the beginning of the test. Modern perimeters possess a gaze tracker that monitors pupil location throughout the test. A record of gaze stability is shown at the bottom of the report. Lines extending upward indicate gaze error, while lines downward indicate that the tracker was not able to successfully track the gaze direction, for example, during blinks. Of the reliability indices, a high fixation loss rate is least detrimental to a visual field test.

The false-negative rate, which was originally devised to assess inattention during the test, indicates lack of response to stimuli that should have been seen based on prior responses at that location. Although a high false-negative rate could indicate an inattentive patient, damaged areas of the visual field show increased variability, which can lead to a high false-negative rate. Thus, false-negative response rates can be elevated in abnormal visual fields regardless of patient attentiveness, and visual field tests should not necessarily be disregarded because of high false-negative rates. Accordingly, newer testing algorithms no longer measure this parameter.

Yohannan J, Wang J, Brown J, et al. Evidence-based criteria for assessment of visual field reliability. *Ophthalmology.* 2017;124(11):1612–1620.

Normality or Abnormality of the Visual Field

The next step in the evaluation of visual field results is determining whether the results are normal or abnormal. A normal visual field demonstrates the greatest sensitivity centrally, with sensitivity falling steadily toward the periphery. Figure 6-3 shows a single field analysis of a test obtained with the HFA. The results are presented as a series of numerical plots, probability maps, and a corresponding grayscale map of sensitivity (see

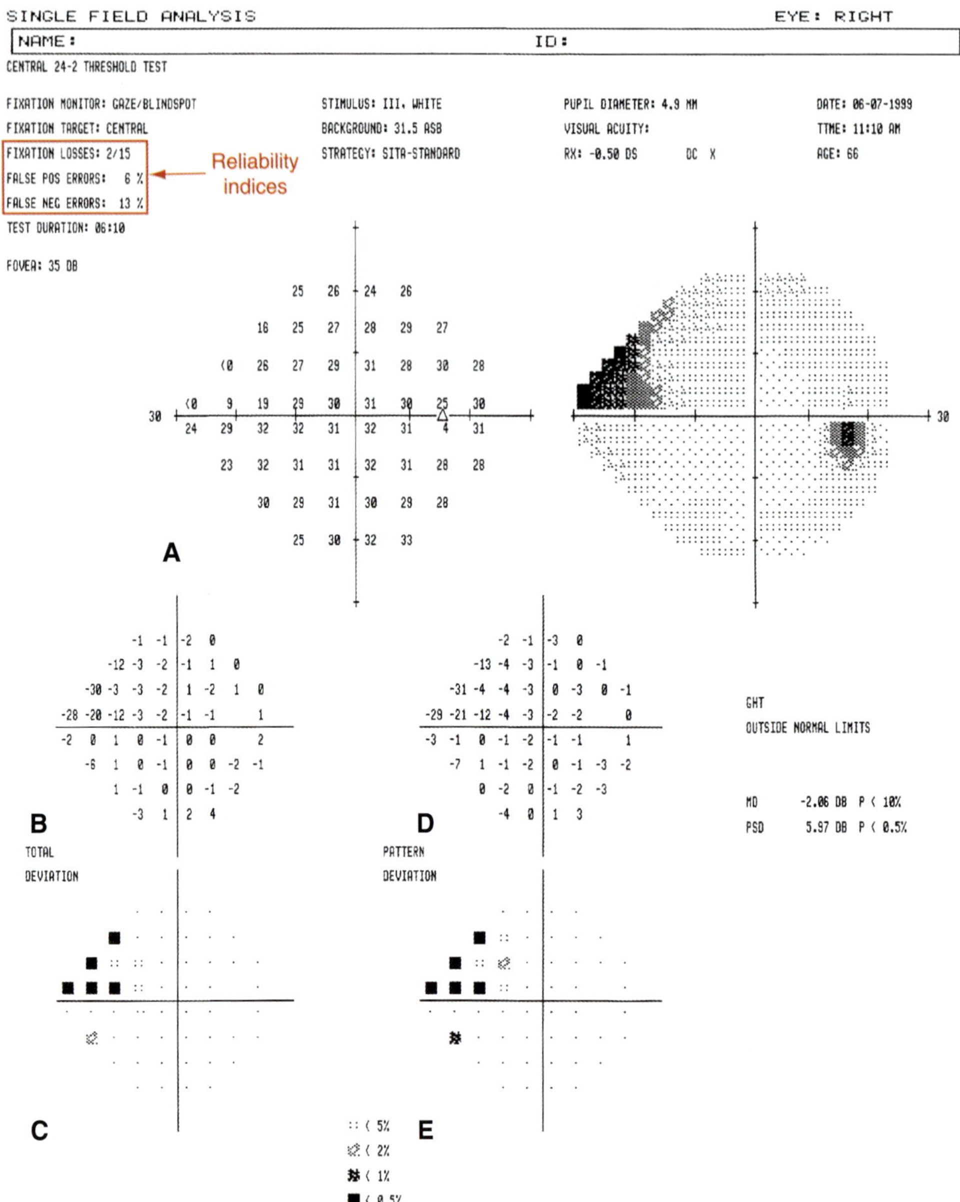

Figure 6-3 Report from a visual field test obtained with a Humphrey Field Analyzer (HFA) using the Swedish Interactive Threshold Algorithm (SITA) Standard 24-2 test strategy. **A,** Raw visual sensitivity threshold values *(left)* and corresponding interpolated grayscale plot *(right)*. **B,** Total deviation values, calculated as the difference between the patient's sensitivity and the age-corrected normal value at each test point. **C,** Probability of abnormality for the total deviation values. See the scale below the plot for the corresponding probability values that a given point is normal. **D,** Pattern deviation values, calculated from the total deviation values by subtracting the "average" defect. **E,** Probability of abnormality for the pattern deviation values (same scale as for part C).

Fig 6-3A). The total deviation plot displays deviations from age-corrected normal sensitivities (see Fig 6-3B), and the corresponding total deviation probability map shows deviations that fall outside the statistical range of normal (see Fig 6-3C). The pattern deviation map shows the localized loss after correcting for any overall decrease in sensitivity (see Fig 6-3D) and, again, a pattern deviation probability map shows the statistical abnormality at each point (see Fig 6-3E).

The HFA also provides a series of summary indices, including the following:

- *Mean deviation (MD).* This is a weighted average of the total deviation values. Zero equates to no deviation from normal, 0 dB to −2 dB is typical for normal results, and more-negative values indicate more advanced loss.
- *Pattern standard deviation (PSD).* The PSD is a summary index of visual field spatial variability (local abnormality) that worsens until an MD of approximately −12 dB, at which it begins to "improve" as the field becomes more uniformly abnormal (and hence less spatially variable).
- *Glaucoma Hemifield Test (GHT).* This index categorizes eyes as "within normal limits," "borderline," or "outside normal limits" based on a comparison of visual field sensitivities at corresponding areas of the superior and inferior hemifields. Because glaucoma frequently causes asymmetric damage to the superior and inferior hemifields, the GHT is a sensitive (but not specific) tool for identification of glaucomatous visual field defects (Fig 6-4).

Several criteria have been proposed for defining a visual field as abnormal. The system employed by the Ocular Hypertension Treatment Study (OHTS) is simple and widely accepted. In the OHTS, an abnormal visual field was defined by the presence of a PSD value found in fewer than 5% of normal participants or the presence of a GHT with a result outside normal limits. The abnormality had to be present in 3 consecutive visual field tests. In the analysis of a visual field report, it is also important to evaluate the probability

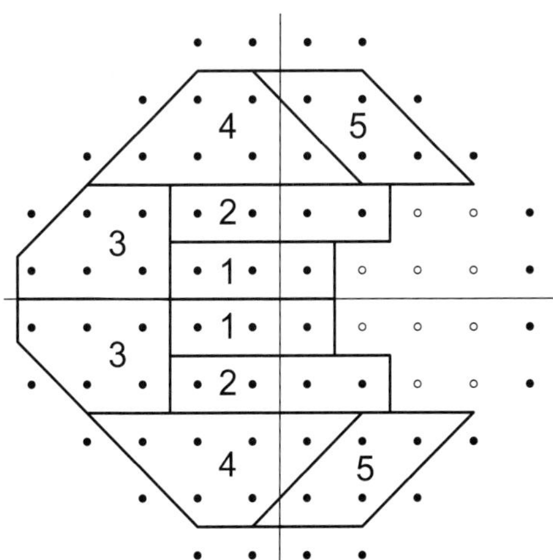

Figure 6-4 The Glaucoma Hemifield Test (GHT) compares pattern deviation probability values in 5 predetermined zones in the superior hemifield with corresponding zones in the inferior hemifield. *(Courtesy of Michael V. Boland, MD, PhD.)*

maps, especially the pattern deviation probability plot. The presence of a cluster of at least 3 abnormal points ($P < 5\%$) on the pattern deviation plot, with at least 1 of those points with $P < 1\%$, is also commonly used to define a visual field as abnormal.

It is important that the clinician carefully review the visual field report to (1) determine whether any defects are repeatable and present in approximately the same location on subsequent tests; and (2) verify that the abnormalities are not due to the presence of artifacts. Although the points that are abnormal will not be exactly the same in all confirmatory tests, the area of visual field abnormality should be similar among the tests.

Artifacts

Identifying artifacts is another step in the evaluation of visual field results. Common artifacts seen on automated perimetry include the following:

- *Lens rim.* If the machine's corrective lens is decentered or set too far from the eye, the lens rim may block peripheral stimuli, often causing an absolute defect (complete attenuation of light) (Fig 6-5).
- *Inappropriate corrective lens.* If an inappropriate corrective lens is used, the resulting visual field may show generalized depression. This commonly occurs, for example, in young pseudophakic patients or in a patient wearing a contact lens that is not considered when the corrective lens power is selected.
- *Eyelid artifact.* Partial eyelid ptosis may lead to a superior visual field defect.
- *Cloverleaf visual field.* If a patient stops paying attention and ceases to respond partway through the test, a distinctive visual field pattern may develop. Figure 6-6 shows a cloverleaf visual field, the result of the testing order of the Humphrey perimeter, which begins testing with the points circled in this figure and proceeds outward. This pattern may also be seen when a patient is malingering.

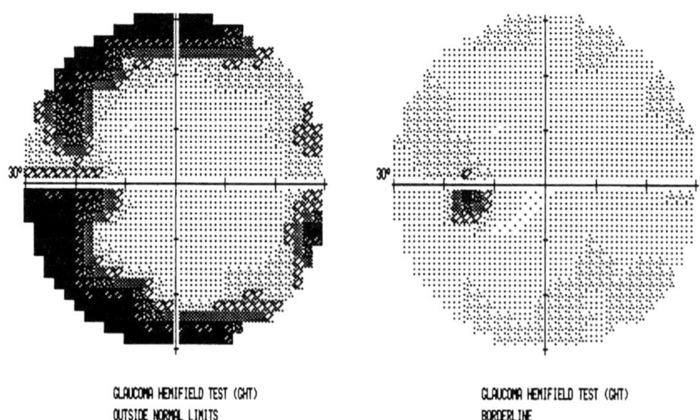

Figure 6-5 Visual fields with and without a lens rim artifact. The 2 visual fields shown were obtained 9 days apart. *Left,* A typical lens rim artifact due to inappropriate position of the corrective lens. *Right,* The corrective lens was positioned appropriately so no artifact is present (Humphrey 30-2 pattern).

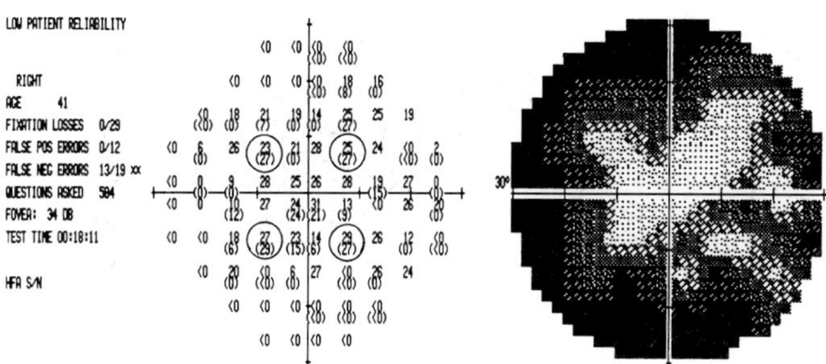

Figure 6-6 Cloverleaf visual field. The HFA begins testing with the 4 circled points, from which testing in each quadrant proceeds outward. If the patient stops responding after only a few points have been tested, the result is some variation of the cloverleaf visual field shown at right (full-threshold strategy and 30-2 pattern).

- *High false-positive rate.* When a patient responds at a time when no test stimulus is presented, a false-positive response is recorded. As previously mentioned, false-positive rates greater than 15% suggest an unreliable test that can mask or minimize an actual scotoma and can, in extreme cases, result in a visual field with impossibly high threshold values (Fig 6-7). Carefully instructing patients to press the response button only when they are sure they see the stimulus may sometimes resolve this artifact.
- *Pattern reversal.* The HFA algorithm used to correct for generalized visual sensitivity loss can lead to more points being abnormal on the pattern deviation plot (corrected for age and generalized depression of sensitivity) than on the total deviation plot (corrected only for age). This typically occurs in tests with a high percentage of false-positives where the total deviation values are artificially inflated. Although pattern reversal may indicate artifactual loss, some data suggest that it could also be an early sign of true paracentral loss.

Chang AC, Camp AS, Patella VM, Weinreb RN. Association of visual field pattern reversal with paracentral visual field loss. *Ophthalmol Glaucoma.* 2022;5(3):353–358.

Patterns of Visual Field Loss in Glaucoma

Damage to RGC axons at the optic nerve head leads to RGC death in the retina and loss of visual information processing and transmission. Hence, there is a correspondence between regions of optic nerve head rim thinning and regions of visual field loss. Typical patterns of loss include

- arcuate (Bjerrum) scotoma (Fig 6-8)
- nasal step (Fig 6-9)
- paracentral scotoma (Fig 6-10)
- altitudinal defect (Fig 6-11)
- generalized depression (rare in glaucoma in the absence of localized loss)
- temporal wedge (rare)

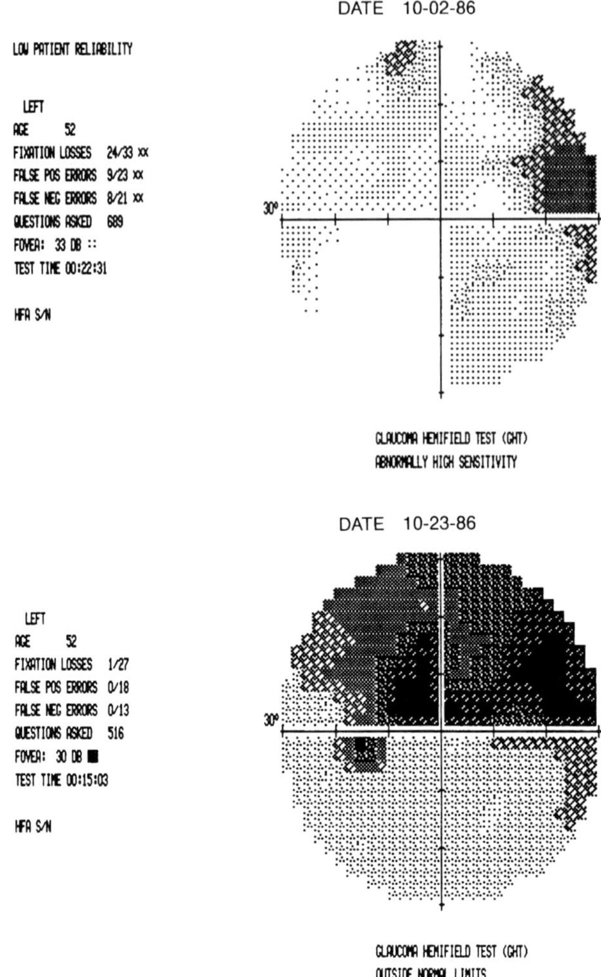

Figure 6-7 High false-positive rate. The top visual field contains characteristic "white scotomas," which represent areas of impossibly high retinal sensitivity. On the return visit 3 weeks later, the patient was carefully instructed to respond only when she saw the light, resulting in the bottom visual field, which shows good reliability and demonstrates the patient's dense superior visual field loss (30-2 pattern).

The common names for the classic visual field defects are derived from the defect appearance as plotted using a kinetic perimeter. In static perimetry, however, the sample points are in a grid pattern, and the representation of visual field defects on a static perimetry chart generally lacks the smooth contours suggested by such terms as *arcuate.*

The superior and inferior poles of the optic nerve are most susceptible to glaucomatous damage. However, damage to small, scattered bundles of optic nerve axons commonly produces a generalized decrease in sensitivity, which is harder to recognize than focal defects. Combinations of superior and inferior visual field loss, such as double arcuate scotomas, may occur, resulting in profound peripheral vision loss. Typically, the

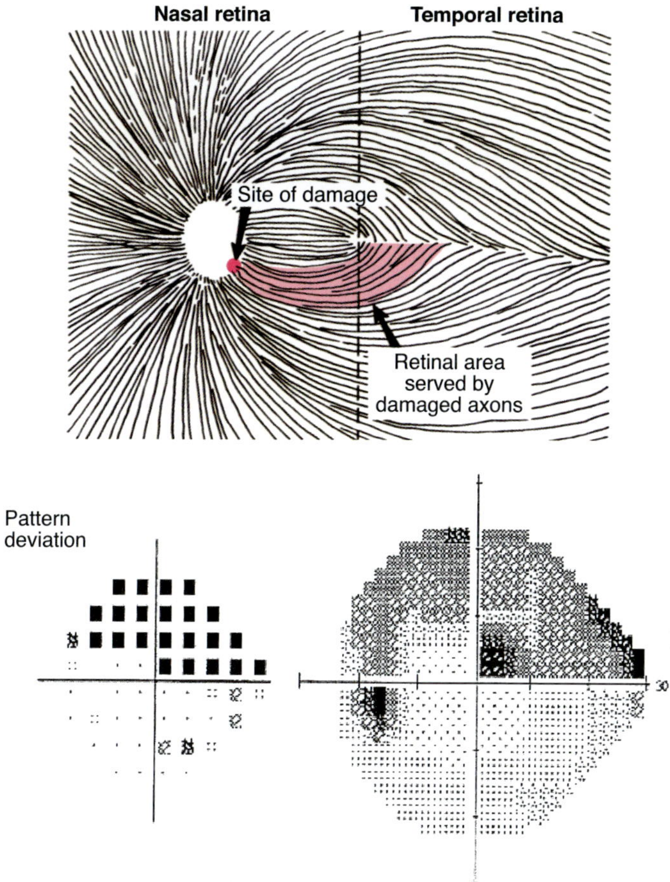

Figure 6-8 An *arcuate scotoma* occurs in the area 10°–20° from fixation. Glaucomatous damage to a nerve fiber bundle containing axons from both the inferonasal and inferotemporal retina resulted in the arcuate defect shown. The scotoma often begins as a single area of relative loss, which then becomes larger, deeper, and multifocal. In its full form, an arcuate scotoma arches from the blind spot and ends at the nasal raphe, becoming wider and closer to fixation on the nasal side (24-2 pattern). *(Visual field courtesy of G. A. Cioffi, MD.)*

central island of vision and the inferotemporal visual field are retained until late in the course of glaucomatous optic nerve damage (see Fig 6-2).

Interpretation of a Series of Visual Field Tests and Detection of Visual Field Progression

Interpretation of serial visual field tests should meet 2 goals:

- separating real change from ordinary variation in responses
- determining the likelihood that a change is related to glaucoma as opposed to other ophthalmic diseases

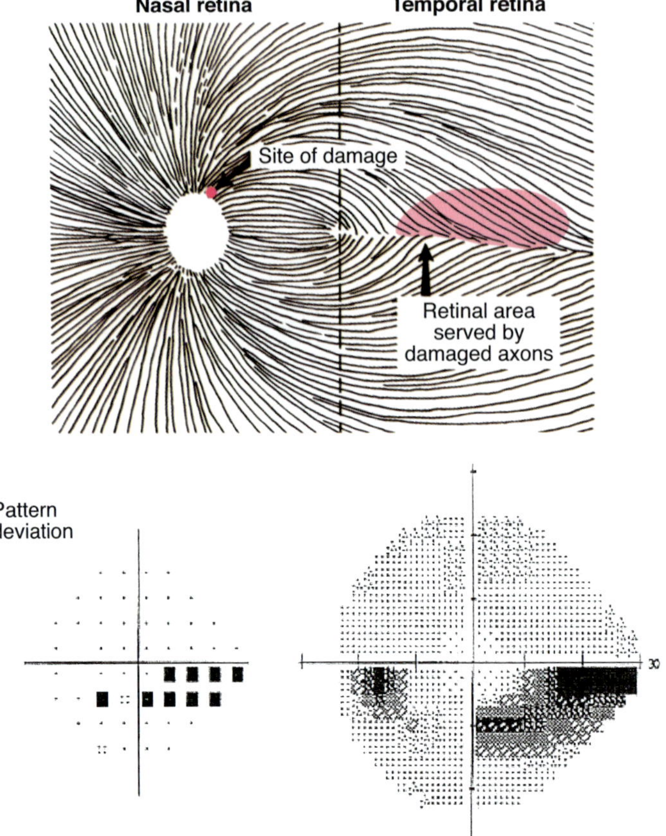

Figure 6-9 A *nasal step* is a relative depression of 1 horizontal hemifield compared with the other. Damage to superior nerve fibers serving the superotemporal retina beyond the paracentral area resulted in this nasal step. In kinetic perimetry, the nasal step is defined as a discontinuity or depression in 1 or more nasal isopters near the horizontal raphe (24-2 pattern). *(Visual field courtesy of G. A. Cioffi, MD.)*

Visual field testing is a subjective examination, and different responses may be obtained each time the test is performed or even during the same test. This fluctuation can greatly confound the detection of disease progression. In order to detect true visual field progression, the clinician needs to evaluate whether the observed change exceeds the expected variability for a particular point or area.

In general, there are 2 main approaches to analyzing visual field progression: event-based analysis and trend-based analysis. In *event-based analysis,* the results of the current test (or a few recent tests for confirmation) are compared with the results obtained at baseline (often a pair of baseline visual field tests). If the results of the follow-up examination(s) are statistically worse than baseline, progression is said to have occurred. This approach defines progression based on incremental deterioration compared with baseline.

In *trend-based analysis,* instead of comparing the current test result with a baseline test result, the clinician or algorithm determines a rate of change in visual field points

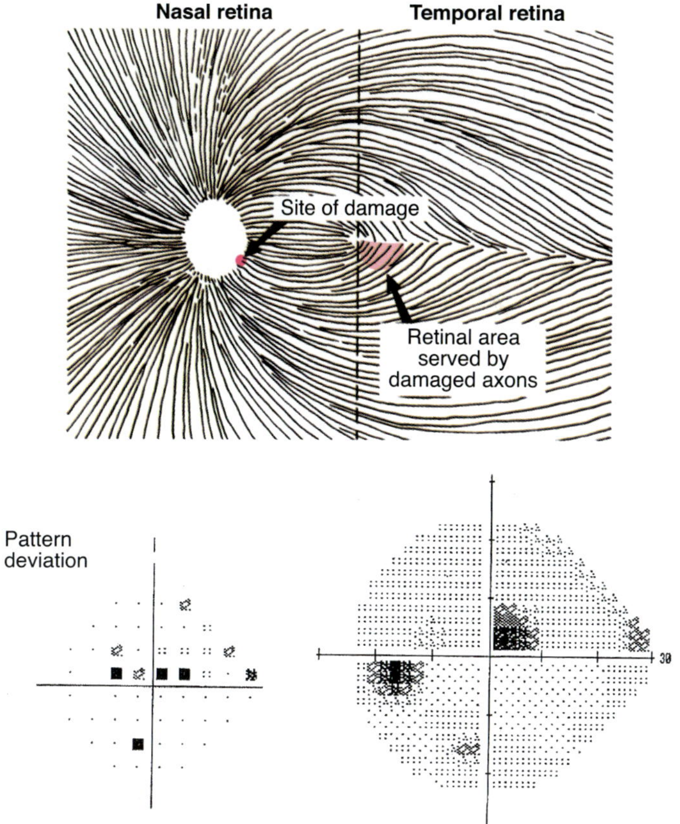

Figure 6-10 A *paracentral scotoma* is an island of relative or absolute vision loss within 10° of fixation. Loss of nerve fibers from the inferior pole, originating from the inferotemporal retina, resulted in the superonasal scotoma shown. Paracentral scotomas may be single, as in this case, or multiple. They may occur as isolated findings or may be associated with other early defects (24-2 pattern). *(Visual field courtesy of G. A. Cioffi, MD.)*

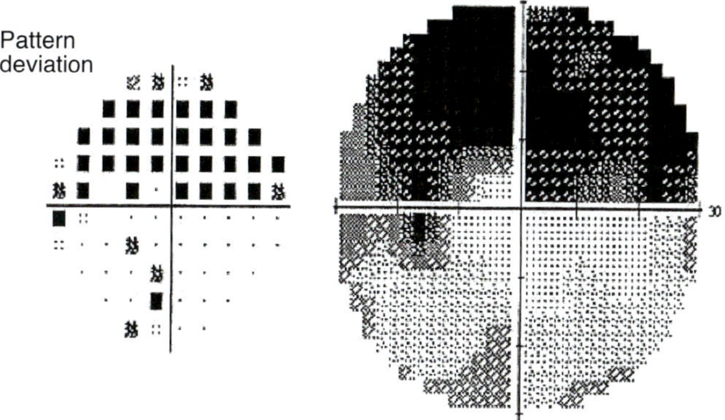

Figure 6-11 Altitudinal defect with nearly complete loss of the superior visual field, characteristic of moderate to advanced glaucomatous optic neuropathy (left eye). *(Visual field courtesy of G. A. Cioffi, MD.)*

or summary statistics for all tests available in a specific period. Change is observed as a statistically significant rate of change in the values over time. In addition to evaluating whether progression has occurred, trend-based analysis provides an estimate of the rate of progression. It is well known that some patients decline faster than others; estimating each patient's rate of progression is helpful for predicting the risk of functional impairment and determining how aggressive treatment should be, especially when viewed in light of the patient's life expectancy.

A variety of tools are available to assist clinicians in identifying visual field progression, and there is no consensus about the best method for detecting change. The simplest and most general method uses the MD index analyzed against time. A statistically significant decline would indicate disease worsening. Deterioration of the MD index may represent glaucomatous progression or progression of cataract or other media opacities. Conversely, in a glaucoma patient who has undergone cataract surgery, true underlying progression of glaucoma may be masked by this method.

The variability inherent in visual field testing is a major impediment to interpretation, leading to both false-negatives and false-positives. In the OHTS, participants flagged as progressing on 2 consecutive reliable visual field tests still had a 66% chance of having normal results on subsequent testing. In contrast, participants with abnormal results on 3 consecutive visual field tests had only a 12% chance of reversion, emphasizing the need for multiple tests to confirm progression. Moreover, the use of multiple tests as a baseline is important to counter the inherent variability as patients learn to take the test.

The HFA provides Guided Progression Analysis (GPA) software to assist in detecting visual field progression (Fig 6-12). This software presents an event-based method that is based on the pattern deviation plot and, therefore, adjusts for the potential confounding effects of diffuse loss of sensitivity from media opacities. New or worsening visual field defects are identified by comparison of follow-up tests with a pair of baseline tests; thus, it is critical to have reliable baseline examinations. Often, the patient experiences a learning effect, and the second visual field may show substantial improvement over the first. To address this phenomenon, at least 2 visual field tests should be performed as early as possible in the course of a patient's disease. If the results are quite different, a third test should be performed. The GPA algorithm automatically selects the first 2 available examinations as the baseline tests. However, this selection can be easily overridden to a more suitable time point (eg, change in therapy after progression) or to avoid initial learning effects (which could reduce the sensitivity to detect progression). The algorithm then compares each follow-up test to the average of the baseline tests (Fig 6-13). It identifies points that show change greater than the expected variability (at the 95% significance level), as determined by previous studies involving patients with stable glaucoma. If statistically significant change is detected in at least 3 points and repeated for the same points in 2 consecutive follow-up tests, the algorithm will flag the last examination as *Possible Progression.* If a significant change is detected and repeated for the same 3 or more points in 3 consecutive follow-up tests, the GPA algorithm will flag the last examination as *Likely Progression.* Using both real and simulated data, studies have shown that *Possible Progression* and *Likely Progression* designations have a false-positive rate between 19% and 34% and 3% and 7%, respectively.

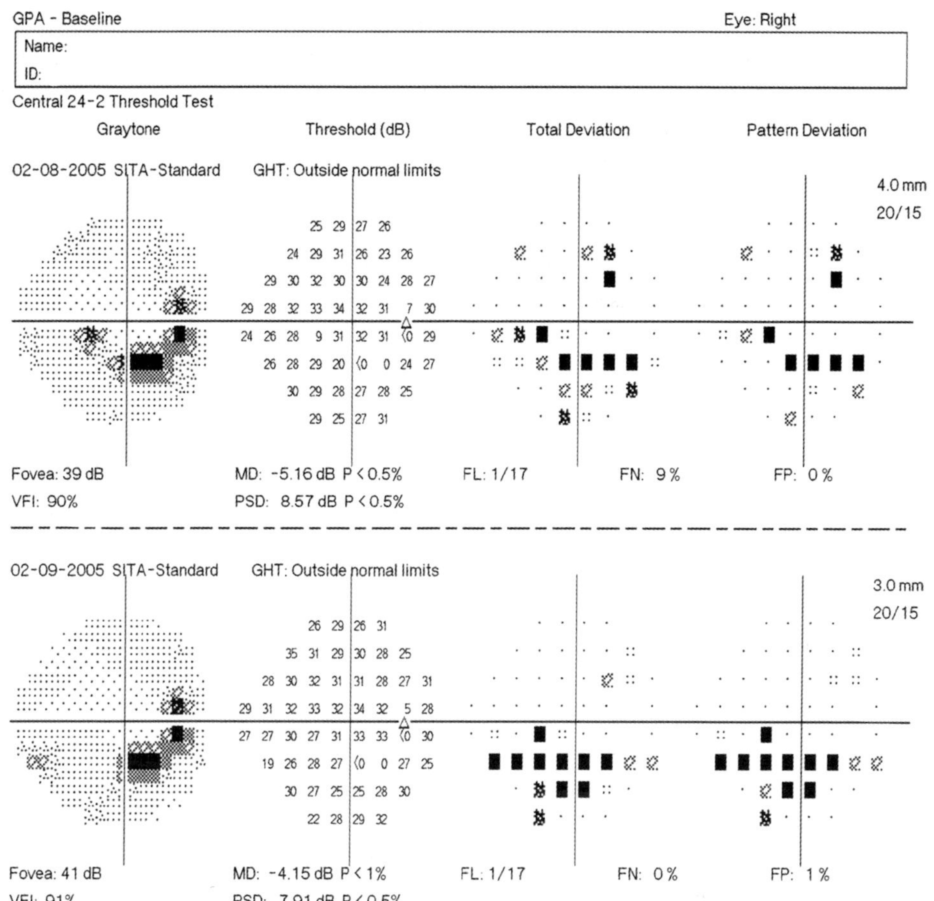

Figure 6-12 Analysis of visual field progression using the Guided Progression Analysis software of the HFA. These visual field tests were selected as the baseline. Results of each follow-up visual field test (see Fig 6-13) are compared with the average of the 2 baseline tests. *(Courtesy of Felipe A. Medeiros, MD, PhD.)*

The HFA also provides the Visual Field Index (VFI) (Fig 6-14), which is calculated as the percentage of normal visual field, weighted more heavily for central vision and adjusted for age. Therefore, a VFI of 100% represents a completely normal visual field, while a VFI of 0% represents a perimetrically blind visual field. The VFI is shown on the HFA report as a percentage value for each examination. A trend-based analysis of VFI as a function of the patient's age is presented with a future projection that predicts the VFI, assuming the same estimated rate of decline, 5 years in the future. Whereas the MD is based only on the total deviation values, and is thus affected by cataract, the VFI is based both on the pattern deviation probability values, for the identification of possibly progressing points, and on the total deviation values, used for the actual calculation of change of the total deviation value. In addition, the algorithm applies different weights to different locations, giving more weight to central points, which have greater impact on the patient's quality of vision. The final VFI score is the mean of all weighted scores.

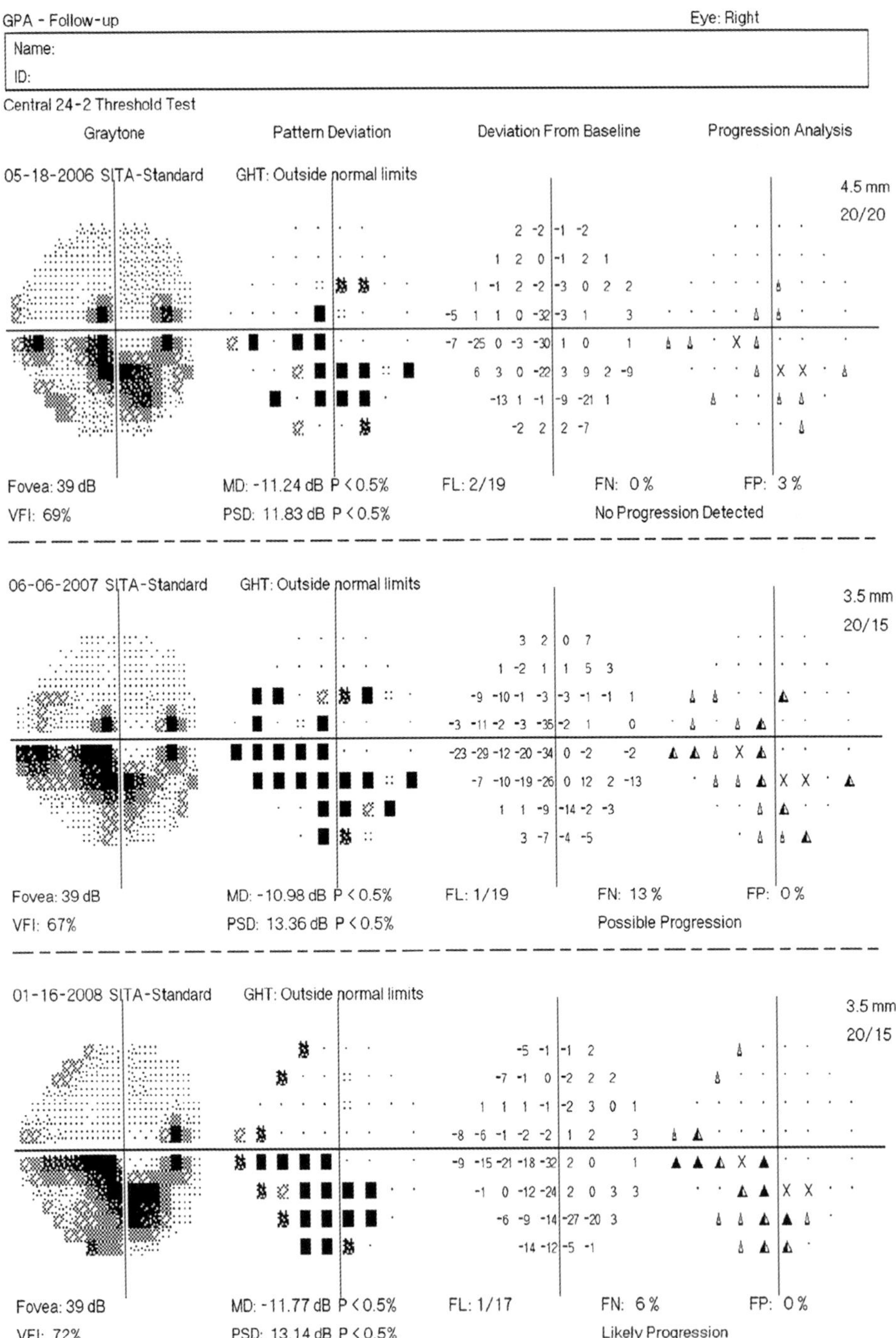

Figure 6-13 Visual fields from consecutive follow-up examinations (see Figure 6-12 for baseline visual field tests for this patient). Several points are flagged as showing significant deterioration. A number of points in the inferonasal region show repeatable significant change *(black-filled triangles)*. The last visual field is then flagged as Likely Progression. *(Courtesy of Felipe A. Medeiros, MD, PhD.)*

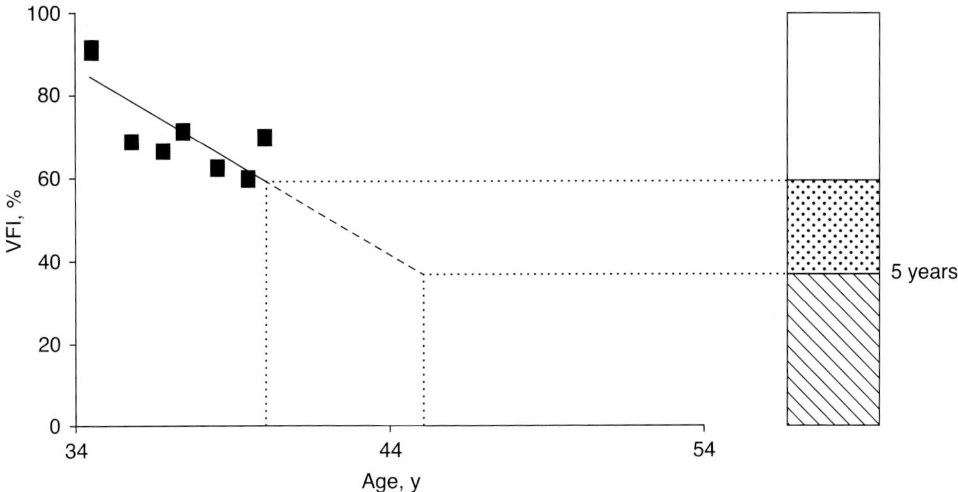

Rate of progression: –4.5 ± 3.3%/year (95% CI)
Slope significant at $P < 5\%$

Figure 6-14 Visual Field Index (VFI) plot corresponding to the visual fields shown in Figures 6-12 and 6-13. The slope of change was significant and estimated at –4.5% per year. CI = confidence interval. *(Courtesy of Felipe A. Medeiros, MD, PhD.)*

The Octopus perimeter also provides a comprehensive statistical package (EyeSuite) for evaluation of visual field progression. The software calculates rates of progression in terms of mean defect change per year (in dB/year), similar to the MD index from Humphrey perimetry. In addition, the software provides an analysis of progression by individual test points (pointwise linear regression) and by clusters, where test locations are combined according to nerve fiber bundle patterns.

Artes PH, O'Leary N, Nicolela MT, Chauhan BC, Crabb DP. Visual field progression in glaucoma: what is the specificity of the Guided Progression Analysis? *Ophthalmology.* 2014;121(10):2023–2027.

Crabb DP, Garway-Heath DF. Intervals between visual field tests when monitoring the glaucomatous patient: wait-and-see approach. *Invest Ophthalmol Vis Sci.* 2012;53(6): 2770–2776. doi:https://doi.org/10.1167/iovs.12-9476

Keltner JL, Johnson CA, Levine RA, et al. Normal visual field test results following glaucomatous visual field end points in the Ocular Hypertension Treatment Study. *Arch Ophthalmol.* 2005;123(9):1201–1206.

Wu Z, Medeiros FA. Comparison of visual field point-wise event-based and global trend-based analysis for detecting glaucomatous progression. *Transl Vis Sci Technol.* 2018;7(4):20. doi:https://doi.org/10.1167/tvst.7.4.20

Frequency of Testing

Accurate and timely detection of progressive changes can be difficult because of the inherent variability of visual field testing. The time required to detect new visual field loss depends on the frequency of testing and follow-up scheme used. The recommended testing frequency varies depending on patient characteristics such as age, disease severity, presence of risk factors for progression, concomitant clinical findings, and risk for functional impairment. To precisely estimate a rate of progression, many tests are needed over time. Studies have shown that the strategy of acquiring only 1 visual field test per year is insufficient in a large number of cases, resulting in delayed detection of disease progression and imprecise estimation of rates of change. Although the optimal testing strategy will vary, obtaining at least 2 or 3 tests per year during the first 2 years of follow-up is recommended to exclude the possibility of fast progression. Thereafter, a testing strategy consisting of 2 tests per year may be sufficient in most cases.

Wu Z, Saunders LJ, Daga FB, Diniz-Filho A, Medeiros FA. Frequency of testing to detect visual field progression derived using a longitudinal cohort of glaucoma patients. *Ophthalmology.* 2017;124(6):786–792.

Structure and Function Relationship

It is important to correlate changes in the visual field (function) with those in the optic nerve (structure). If such correlation is lacking, the ophthalmologist should consider other causes of vision loss, such as ischemic optic neuropathy, demyelinating or other neurologic disease, or pituitary tumor. This consideration is especially important in the following situations:

- The patient's optic nerve head seems less cupped than would be expected for the degree of visual field loss.
- The pallor of the optic nerve head is more impressive than the cupping.
- The rate of visual field loss seems too rapid for a patient with treated glaucoma.
- The pattern of visual field loss is uncharacteristic for glaucoma—for example, it respects the vertical midline.
- The location of the cupping or thinning of the neural rim does not correspond to the location of the visual field defect.

However, it should be noted that progressive visual field loss may sometimes be seen in the absence of optic nerve head changes and vice versa. In cases of early disease, progressive structural changes of the optic nerve and retinal nerve fiber layer can frequently be seen despite lack of apparent visual field progression. Conversely, in cases of more severe disease, progressive visual field losses tend to occur despite a lack of detectable structural change. This apparent disagreement may be explained by the different characteristics of the tests, including scaling, variability, and presence of floor/ceiling effects. Therefore, follow-up of patients with glaucoma should be performed using both structural and functional assessments.

Recent studies have suggested that early glaucomatous visual field defects may sometimes be seen in the macular area and detected with central 10-2 testing in the absence of defects detected with the 24-2 pattern. This has led to the suggestion that central tests be incorporated into the regular management scheme of patients with glaucoma or in those suspected of having the disease. However, the benefit of adding more 10-2 pattern tests in these cases needs to be weighed against the increased patient burden and the missed opportunity of obtaining another 24-2 pattern test to better assess progression. Moreover, there is some evidence that the 10-2 test does not outperform the 24-2 test. Finally, a hybrid option is available on the HFA, the 24-2C pattern, which adds 10 test points within the central 10°; however, its role in clinical use remains to be determined.

De Moraes CG, Hood DC, Thenappan A, et al. 24-2 visual fields miss central defects shown on 10-2 tests in glaucoma suspects, ocular hypertensives, and early glaucoma. *Ophthalmology.* 2017;124(10):1449–1456.

Medeiros FA, Zangwill LM, Bowd C, Mansouri K, Weinreb RN. The structure and function relationship in glaucoma: implications for detection of progression and measurement of rates of change. *Invest Ophthalmol Vis Sci.* 2012;53(11):6939–6946.

Orbach A, Ang GS, Camp AS, et al. Qualitative evaluation of the 10-2 and 24-2 visual field tests for detecting central visual field abnormalities in glaucoma. *Am J Ophthalmol.* 2021;229:26–33.

Other Perimetric Tests

Many psychophysical tests of visual function have been developed for detecting early glaucomatous vision loss. Among these are frequency-doubling technology (FDT), short-wavelength automated perimetry (SWAP), and flicker-defined form (FDF) perimetry (see Figure 6-15 on the next page). These tests aim to target subpopulations of RGCs by evaluating specific aspects of visual function (eg, motion perception, contrast sensitivity, color vision) and thereby reduce the ability of the visual system to use other pathways to compensate. It has been hypothesized that in its early stages, glaucoma may damage predominantly magnocellular RGCs, which project to the magnocellular layers of the lateral geniculate nucleus (ie, the magnocellular [M] pathway); however, whether such preferential loss indeed occurs remains unclear.

Although psychophysical tests such as FDT, SWAP, and FDF perimetry attempt to minimize potential input from other pathways, it is unlikely that any stimulus can be 100% specific for a single visual pathway or a single subset of RGCs. Furthermore, it is unlikely that a single ganglion cell type is always affected first in glaucoma. As previously mentioned, perimetric tests are also subjective examinations, so responses may vary on repeated testing or during the same test; this reduces the ability to confidently detect true early abnormalities.

Other tests that measure the integrity of the visual field include contrast sensitivity perimetry, flicker sensitivity, microperimetry, visual evoked potential, and multifocal electroretinography. These tests are not commonly used in the evaluation of patients with glaucoma. See BCSC Section 5, *Neuro-Ophthalmology,* and Section 12, *Retina and Vitreous,* for discussion of visual evoked potentials and multifocal electroretinography.

Meira-Freitas D, Tatham AJ, Lisboa R, et al. Predicting progression of glaucoma from rates of frequency doubling technology perimetry change. *Ophthalmology.* 2014;121(2): 498–507.

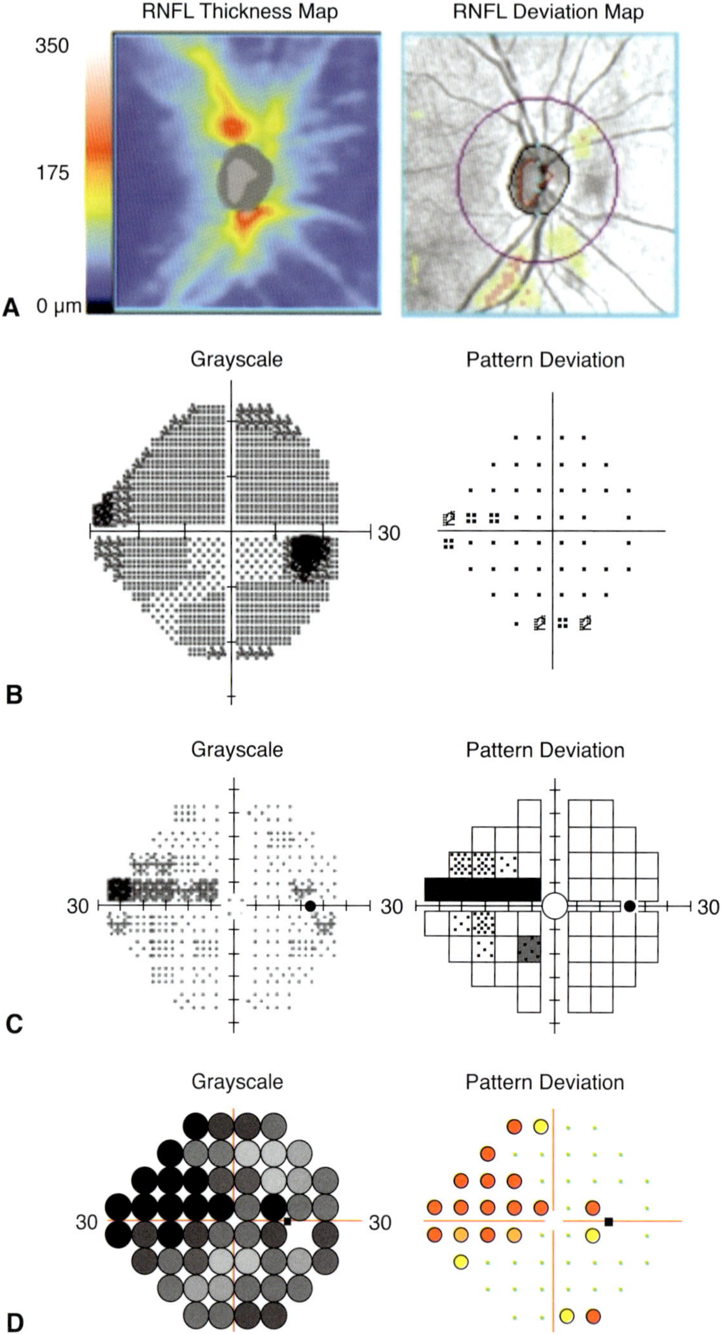

Figure 6-15 Findings from a right eye with glaucoma. **A,** Inferior retinal nerve fiber layer (RNFL) thinning is visible on optical coherence tomography. **B,** Standard automated perimetry shows a small corresponding superonasal visual field defect that is more pronounced on frequency-doubling technology perimetry **(C)** and flicker-defined form perimetry **(D).** *(Courtesy of Felipe A. Medeiros, MD, PhD.)*

CHAPTER 7

Primary Open-Angle Glaucoma

Highlights

- Important risk factors for primary open-angle glaucoma include age, race and ethnicity, family history, central corneal thickness, myopia, and intraocular pressure (IOP).
- The relationship between blood pressure and open-angle glaucoma is complex, but there is convincing evidence that lower ocular perfusion pressure (defined as diastolic blood pressure + 1/3 systolic blood pressure − IOP) is a risk factor for glaucoma development.
- Open-angle glaucoma can develop at any pressure level within the range of IOPs observed in the general population.
- Lowering IOP with medication, laser surgery, incisional surgery, or a combination of these is currently the only means of treating open-angle glaucoma.
- Treatment of ocular hypertension reduces the risk of progression to glaucoma.

Primary Open-Angle Glaucoma

Primary open-angle glaucoma (POAG) is typically a chronic, slowly progressive optic neuropathy with characteristic patterns of optic nerve damage and visual field loss. Numerous factors affect an individual's susceptibility to POAG, which is a multifactorial disease process. These factors include intraocular pressure (IOP), age, race or ethnicity, central corneal thickness, myopia, and family history of glaucoma. Factors that may contribute to disease susceptibility include low corneal hysteresis, low ocular perfusion pressure, low cerebrospinal fluid pressure, abnormalities of axonal or ganglion cell metabolism, and disorders of the extracellular matrix of the lamina cribrosa. Unfortunately, we do not yet fully understand the interplay of the multiple factors involved in the development of POAG. Secondary OAG differs from POAG in that identifiable factors contribute to its development, such as the dispersed pigment in pigmentary glaucoma and the pseudoexfoliative material of pseudoexfoliation syndrome. Secondary OAG is discussed in Chapter 8.

Clinical Features

Primary open-angle glaucoma is typically insidious in onset, slowly progressive, and painless. It is usually bilateral but can be asymmetric. Patients may be asymptomatic until the later stages of the disease, when central vision is affected. POAG is diagnosed primarily on the basis of findings from the assessment of the optic nerve and nerve fiber layer and the results of visual field testing.

Gonioscopic findings

The diagnosis of POAG requires verification that the anterior chamber angle is open. Gonioscopy (discussed in Chapter 4) is indicated for all patients evaluated for glaucoma. In patients with established OAG, gonioscopy should be repeated periodically to monitor for progressive angle closure caused by lens-induced changes, particularly in patients with hyperopia. Repeated gonioscopy is also indicated when the anterior chamber becomes shallow, when strong miotics are prescribed, after argon laser trabeculoplasty or laser peripheral iridotomy has been performed, and when IOP increases.

Optic nerve head appearance and visual fields

Although elevated IOP is an important risk factor for OAG, it is not required for diagnosis of this disease; rather, the diagnosis is based primarily on the appearance of the optic nerve head (also called *optic disc*) and on the results of visual field testing. See Chapters 5 and 6 for detailed discussions of the optic nerve head and visual fields, respectively. Careful periodic evaluation of the optic nerve and visual field testing are essential in the management of glaucoma. Stereophotographic documentation of the optic nerve or computerized imaging of the optic nerve, retinal nerve fiber layer, and macula facilitates the detection of subtle changes over time. Visual field loss typically correlates with the appearance of the optic nerve head; significant discrepancies between the pattern of visual field loss and optic nerve head appearance warrant additional investigation.

Gedde SJ, Vinod K, Wright MM, et al; American Academy of Ophthalmology Preferred Practice Pattern Glaucoma Panel. Primary Open-Angle Glaucoma Preferred Practice Pattern. *Ophthalmology.* 2021;128(1):P71–P150. doi:10.1016/j.ophtha.2020.10.022

Jonas JB, Budde WM, Panda-Jonas S. Ophthalmoscopic evaluation of the optic nerve head. *Surv Ophthalmol.* 1999;43(4):293–320.

Atypical Findings

In patients who present at a young age or with atypical findings that cannot be explained by the clinical circumstances—for example, unilateral disease, decreased central vision, dyschromatopsia, presence of a relative afferent pupillary defect, neuroretinal rim pallor, or visual field loss inconsistent with optic nerve appearance—additional medical and neurologic evaluation should be considered. This evaluation may include assessment for a compressive etiology, carotid artery insufficiency, anemia, syphilis, certain vitamin deficiencies, giant cell arteritis or other causes of systemic vasculitis, and exposure to a toxic substance. Noninvasive tests of carotid circulation (eg, carotid Doppler ultrasonography) may be helpful. For patients with optic nerve pallor or visual field loss suggestive of a neurologic defect, evaluation of the anterior visual pathway, including the optic chiasm, with magnetic resonance imaging or computed tomography may be warranted. See also BCSC Section 5, *Neuro-Ophthalmology.*

Risk Factors

Intraocular pressure

As previously stated, elevated IOP is an important risk factor for glaucoma but is not required for a POAG diagnosis. Large population-based studies suggest a mean IOP of 15.5 mm Hg (standard deviation [SD] ±2.6 mm Hg) in European-derived populations, but the normal distribution of IOP varies across racial and ethnic groups. This finding led to the definition of "normal" IOP as 2 SDs above and below the mean IOP or a range between 10 and 21 mm Hg. IOP higher than 21 mm Hg was thus traditionally defined as "abnormal," but this definition has shortcomings.

It is known that IOP in the general population is not represented by a normal distribution but rather is skewed toward higher pressures (see Chapter 2, Fig 2-4). Thus, IOPs of 22 mm Hg and above may not necessarily be abnormal from a statistical standpoint. More importantly, IOP distribution curves for glaucomatous and nonglaucomatous eyes show a great deal of overlap. Several studies indicate that as many as 30%–50% of individuals in the general population with glaucomatous optic neuropathy and/or visual field loss have initial IOP measurements below 22 mm Hg. IOP, across its entire range observed in a population, is a continuous risk factor for POAG.

IOP may vary considerably over a 24-hour period, and IOP elevations may occur only intermittently in some glaucomatous eyes (see Chapter 2). Thus, a single IOP measurement taken during office hours does not provide an accurate assessment of IOP variability over time, and glaucoma can be present in a patient with low IOP. Of note, large diurnal (daytime) fluctuation in IOP has been identified as an independent risk factor for glaucoma progression in some studies, but not in others. Physiologic diurnal variation in IOP is one reason that high IOP may be undetected. Other reasons include undiagnosed angle closure or uveitis, use of systemic medications that lower (eg, β-blockers) or raise (eg, corticosteroids) IOP, variable glaucoma medication adherence, and inaccurate IOP measurement.

Bengtsson B, Leske MC, Hyman L, Heijl A; Early Manifest Glaucoma Trial Group. Fluctuation of intraocular pressure and glaucoma progression in the early manifest glaucoma trial. *Ophthalmology.* 2007;114(2):205–209.

Liu JH, Kripke DF, Twa MD, et al. Twenty-four-hour pattern of intraocular pressure in the aging population. *Invest Ophthalmol Vis Sci.* 1999;40(12):2912–2917.

Intraocular pressure and central corneal thickness As discussed in Chapter 2, central corneal thickness (CCT) affects the measurement of IOP. Thicker corneas resist the deformation inherent in most methods of tonometry, resulting in an overestimation of IOP. In contrast, tonometry in eyes with thin corneas underestimates the IOP. The average CCT in adult eyes, determined by ultrasonic pachymetry, ranges between approximately 525 and 550 µm and varies with race and ethnicity. For example, mean CCT is lower in persons of African ancestry than in those of European ancestry. Attempts at adjusting IOP measurements for the effect of CCT have not provided a clear benefit in terms of predicting glaucoma progression.

Bhan A, Browning AC, Shah S, Hamilton R, Dave D, Dua HS. Effect of corneal thickness on intraocular pressure measurements with the pneumotonometer, Goldmann applanation tonometer, and Tono-Pen. *Invest Ophthalmol Vis Sci.* 2002;43(5):1389–1392.

Brandt JD, Beiser JA, Kass MA, Gordon MO. Central corneal thickness in the Ocular Hypertension Treatment Study (OHTS). *Ophthalmology.* 2001;108(10):1779–1788.

Brandt JD, Gordon MO, Gao F, Besider JA, Miller JP, Kass MA; Ocular Hypertension Treatment Study. Adjusting intraocular pressure for central corneal thickness does not improve prediction models for primary open-angle glaucoma. *Ophthalmology.* 2012;119(3):437–442.

Older age

The Baltimore Eye Survey found that the prevalence of glaucoma increases dramatically with age, particularly among Black individuals, in whom prevalence exceeded 11% among those 80 years and older. In the Collaborative Initial Glaucoma Treatment Study (CIGTS; see Clinical Trial 7-1 at the end of this chapter), visual field defects were 7 times more likely to progress in patients 60 years or older than in those younger than 40 years. The Ocular Hypertension Treatment Study (OHTS; see Clinical Trial 7-2) found an increased risk of progression to OAG with age (per decade): 43% in the univariate analysis and 22% in the multivariate analysis. Older age is an independent risk factor for both the development and the progression of glaucoma.

Race and ethnicity

Although race and ethnicity are, in part, social constructs, they do represent crude markers of genetic heritage, and many studies have identified race and ethnicity (as defined in the studies) to be a risk factor for glaucoma. They may also serve as markers of social determinants of health, such as access to health care and socioeconomic status. The prevalence of POAG in the United States is 3–4 times higher in individuals of African descent or Hispanic ethnicity than in primarily European-derived populations. Blindness due to glaucoma is at least 4 times more common in Black individuals than in White individuals. In addition, Black patients are more likely to be diagnosed with glaucoma at a younger age and at a more advanced stage than are White patients.

In a univariate analysis, the OHTS found that glaucoma was 59% more likely to develop in Black/African American patients with ocular hypertension (defined in this study as IOP ≥24 mm Hg in the absence of optic nerve or visual field abnormalities) than in White patients with ocular hypertension. This relationship was not present after controlling for corneal thickness and baseline vertical cup–disc ratio in a multivariate analysis, suggesting a genetic basis for these physiologic parameters. However, the 20-year cumulative incidence of POAG was higher among Black/African American participants compared with that among participants of European descent. The difference in POAG prevalence noted over the 10 years during which "standard therapy" was offered to all participants suggests an effect of social determinants of health on race-related health disparities. For more information on social determinants of health, see BCSC Section 1 *Update on General Medicine.*

Kass MA, Heuer DK, Higginbotham EJ, et al; Ocular Hypertension Study Group. Assessment of cumulative incidence and severity of primary open-angle glaucoma among participants in the Ocular Hypertension Treatment Study after 20 years of follow-up. *JAMA Ophthalmol.* 2021;139(5):1–9.

Thin central cornea and low corneal hysteresis

A thinner cornea is an important risk factor for disease progression in individuals with POAG (who have higher baseline IOPs) and for the development of glaucoma in individuals with ocular hypertension. This risk may not be entirely due to the underestimation of IOP measured by Goldmann tonometry in patients with thin corneas. Thin corneas may be a biomarker for disease susceptibility. As mentioned previously, Black patients have thinner corneas on average than White patients. Studies of corneal biomechanics, particularly hysteresis, have shown a relationship between these measurements and glaucoma progression (see Chapter 2).

Family history

In the Baltimore Eye Survey, the relative risk of POAG increased approximately 3.7-fold for individuals who had a sibling with POAG. The increased risk of glaucoma within families is likely genetic, although simple mendelian inheritance of glaucoma is not common (see Chapter 1).

Myopia

Population-based data support an association between POAG and myopia. In the Beaver Dam Eye Study (United States), myopia of greater than 1 diopter (D) spherical equivalent was significantly associated with a diagnosis of glaucoma. In the Rotterdam (Netherlands) follow-up study, high myopia of greater than 4 D was associated with a hazard ratio (HR) of 2.3 for developing glaucoma over 10 years. Myopia was also shown to be a risk factor in the Beijing Eye Study, in which high myopia (>6 D spherical equivalent) conferred an odds ratio of 8 for having glaucoma compared with emmetropia. The Blue Mountains Eye Study (Australia) found an odds ratio of 3.3 for participants with myopia of greater than 3 D. However, in the OHTS, no association between myopia and progression to glaucoma was observed.

The concurrence of POAG and myopia may complicate diagnosis and management in several ways. Evaluation of the optic nerve head is particularly challenging in highly myopic eyes that have tilted discs or posterior staphylomas. Also, the myopic refractive error may cause optical minification of the optic nerve, further complicating accurate optic nerve assessment. Myopia-related retinal degeneration or anomalies can cause visual field abnormalities that are difficult to distinguish from those caused by glaucoma (for more on myopia and pathologic myopia, see BCSC Section 12, *Retina and Vitreous*). In addition, patients who are highly myopic may have difficulty performing visual field tests, making interpretation of visual field abnormalities more challenging.

Mitchell P, Hourihan F, Sandbach J, Wang JJ. The relationship between glaucoma and myopia: the Blue Mountains Eye Study. *Ophthalmology.* 1999;106(10):2010–2015.

Varma R, Ying-Lai M, Francis BA, et al; Los Angeles Latino Eye Study Group. Prevalence of open-angle glaucoma and ocular hypertension in Latinos: the Los Angeles Latino Eye Study. *Ophthalmology.* 2004;111(8):1439–1448.

Wong TY, Klein BE, Klein R, Knudtson M, Lee KE. Refractive errors, intraocular pressure, and glaucoma in a white population. *Ophthalmology.* 2003;110(1):211–217.

Xu L, Wang Y, Wang S, Wang Y, Jonas JB. High myopia and glaucoma susceptibility: the Beijing Eye Study. *Ophthalmology.* 2007;114(2):216–220.

Association With Systemic Conditions

Diabetes

The evidence related to diabetes as a risk factor for glaucoma is difficult to interpret. The Beaver Dam Eye Study, the Blue Mountains Eye Study, and the Los Angeles Latino Eye Study found an increased risk of OAG in participants with diabetes. However, the Framingham Study, the Baltimore Eye Survey, the Barbados Eye Study, and a revised analysis of the Rotterdam Study did not find an association. Furthermore, the Rotterdam Study and the Barbados Eye Study, which were large longitudinal population-based studies, did not identify diabetes as a risk factor for the incident development of glaucoma. In the OHTS, depending on how the analysis was performed, diabetes was either associated with a reduced risk of developing glaucoma or not associated with glaucoma. One possible explanation for these results is that the cohort of patients with diabetes was skewed in the OHTS because the presence of retinopathy was an exclusion criterion.

de Voogd S, Ikram MK, Wolfs RC, et al. Is diabetes mellitus a risk factor for open-angle glaucoma? The Rotterdam Study. *Ophthalmology.* 2006;113(10):1827–1831.

Hypertension

The Baltimore Eye Survey found that systemic hypertension was associated with a lower risk of glaucoma in younger (<65 years) patients and a higher risk of glaucoma in older patients. The hypothesis is that younger individuals with high blood pressure may have better optic nerve perfusion, but as these patients age, their chronic hypertension may have adverse effects on the microcirculation of the optic nerve that increase the nerve's susceptibility to glaucomatous damage. Conversely, in the Barbados Eye Study, the relative risk of developing glaucoma among study participants with systemic hypertension was less than 1 in all age groups, including those aged 70 years and older.

Lower ocular perfusion pressure

There is compelling evidence that lower ocular perfusion pressure (OPP; defined as diastolic blood pressure + 1/3 systolic blood pressure − IOP) is a risk factor for the development of glaucoma. The Baltimore Eye Survey found a sixfold increase in the prevalence of glaucoma in those patients with the lowest OPP levels. Low systolic perfusion pressure was also a risk factor for glaucoma progression in the Early Manifest Glaucoma Trial (HR 1.42 for systolic perfusion pressure ≤160 mm Hg). Although the concept of OPP oversimplifies actual ocular blood flow, several factors, including autoregulatory mechanisms in central nervous system perfusion, make the association between OPP and glaucoma intriguing. The overtreatment of systemic hypertension may contribute to glaucoma progression and should be considered in some cases (eg, worsening of seemingly well-treated glaucoma).

Costa VP, Harris A, Anderson D, et al. Ocular perfusion pressure in glaucoma. *Acta Ophthalmol.* 2014;92(4):e252–e266.

Other associated conditions

Sleep apnea, thyroid disorders, hypercholesterolemia, migraine, low cerebrospinal fluid pressure, and Raynaud phenomenon have been identified in 1 or more studies as potential risk factors for the development of glaucoma. Further research is required in order to clarify the significance of these conditions in patients with POAG and their relationship to glaucoma, if any.

Prognosis and Therapy

Most patients with POAG retain useful vision for their entire lives. The patients at greatest risk of blindness are those who present with visual field loss at the time of diagnosis. In a single-institution study, the cumulative risk of unilateral and bilateral blindness in patients with OAG was 7.4% and 3.4%, respectively, within 10 years of diagnosis, and 13.5% and 4.3%, respectively, within 20 years of diagnosis.

Treatment with topical medication, laser surgery, incisional surgery, or a combination of these to lower IOP has been shown to significantly reduce the risk of glaucomatous progression (see the Clinical Trials at the end of this chapter). Patients with symptomatically decreased visual function (eg, visual acuity worse than 20/40, severe visual field damage, decreased contrast sensitivity) can be referred to a vision rehabilitation specialist. These specialists can help improve visual function by optimizing lighting, enhancing contrast, reducing glare, and providing adaptations to facilitate activities of daily living. Orientation and mobility specialists can be consulted and vision substitution strategies (eg, talking books and watches) used to improve daily function and quality of life for these patients. The American Academy of Ophthalmology's Initiative in Vision Rehabilitation page on the ONE Network (aao.org/education/low-vision-and-vision-rehab) provides resources for low vision management, including patient handouts and information about additional vision rehabilitation opportunities beyond those provided by the ophthalmologist. See also BCSC Section 3, *Clinical Optics and Vision Rehabilitation,* for in-depth discussion of low vision aids.

Boland MV, Ervin AM, Friedman DS, et al. Comparative effectiveness of treatments for open-angle glaucoma: a systematic review for the US Preventive Services Task Force. *Ann Intern Med.* 2013;158(4):271–279.

Jackson ML, Virgili G, Shepherd JD, et al; American Academy of Ophthalmology Preferred Practice Pattern Vision Rehabilitation Committee. Vision Rehabilitation Preferred Practice Pattern. *Ophthalmology.* 2023;130(3):P271–P335. doi:10.1016/j.ophtha.2022.10.033

Malihi M, Moura Filho ER, Hodge DO, Sit AJ. Long-term trends in glaucoma-related blindness in Olmsted County, Minnesota. *Ophthalmology.* 2014;121(1):134–141.

The Glaucoma Suspect

A *glaucoma suspect* is defined as an individual who has 1 or more of the following characteristics:

- an optic nerve or nerve fiber layer appearance suggestive of glaucoma in the absence of a visual field defect
- a visual field defect suggestive of glaucoma in the absence of a corresponding glaucomatous optic nerve abnormality
- a family history of glaucoma in a first-degree relative
- elevated IOP without evidence of optic nerve damage (see the section Ocular Hypertension)

Patients with such findings or a family history of glaucoma are typically monitored for the development of glaucoma with periodic evaluation of the optic nerve, retinal nerve fiber layer, and visual field. For patients with an absence of visual field defects on standard perimetry (see Chapter 6), the use of frequency-doubling technology perimetry, short-wavelength automated perimetry, and pattern electroretinography have all been proposed, although the role of each is not well supported by available evidence. If signs of optic nerve damage are present, the diagnosis of early POAG and initiation of treatment should be considered. In uncertain cases, close monitoring of the patient without treatment is reasonable in order to better establish a diagnosis (ie, confirm initial findings or detect progressive changes) before initiation of therapy. In glaucoma suspects with elevated IOP and structural or functional findings that are not clearly due to glaucoma, diagnosis may be difficult.

Ocular Hypertension

In this book, *ocular hypertension* is defined as a condition in which IOP is elevated above an arbitrary cutoff value, typically 21 mm Hg, in the absence of optic nerve, retinal nerve fiber layer, or visual field abnormalities. This condition is discussed separately given the availability of high-quality clinical trial data that are not available for other categories of glaucoma suspects. Estimates of the prevalence of ocular hypertension in the United States vary considerably and may be as high as 8 times that of diagnosed POAG. Studies of individuals with elevated IOP for various lengths of time suggest that a higher baseline IOP is associated with an increased risk of developing glaucoma. However, for most individuals with elevated IOP, the risk of developing glaucoma is low.

Distinguishing between ocular hypertension and early POAG is often difficult. The ophthalmologist must look carefully for signs of early optic nerve damage, such as focal notching, asymmetry of cupping, optic disc hemorrhage, nerve fiber layer defects, or subtle visual field defects.

There is no clear consensus about whether elevated IOP should be treated in the absence of signs of early optic nerve damage. Some clinicians, after assessing all risk factors, treat those patients thought to be at greatest risk of developing glaucoma. In the OHTS, patients 40–80 years of age with IOP between 24 and 32 mm Hg were randomized to either observation or treatment with topical ocular hypotensive medications (see Clinical Trial 7-2). During a 5-year period, 4.4% of participants in the treatment group versus 9.5% of participants in the observation group progressed to glaucoma as determined by optic nerve or visual field changes. Thus, this study showed that topical medications reduce the risk of progression to glaucoma in patients with ocular hypertension. However, it should be noted that most untreated participants did not progress over a 5-year period. In the OHTS, the risk of developing glaucoma was increased by 10% for every 1 mm Hg increase in IOP over the mean study IOP; the risk was increased by 32% for each 0.1 increment in vertical cup–disc ratio.

Results from the OHTS suggest that older age, higher IOP, thinner corneas, larger baseline cup–disc ratio, and higher pattern SD on standard automated perimetry are important risk factors for the development of POAG. However, the increased risk of developing glaucoma attributed to thinner corneas in this study was not fully explained by the estimated artifactual error in measured IOP. As previously noted, thinner corneas may be a biomarker for glaucoma susceptibility based on factors other than IOP. The increased risk of progression to glaucoma in Black participants (in univariate but not multivariate analyses) may be attributed to thinner corneas and greater cup–disc ratios. Other potential risk factors, such as myopia, diabetes, migraine, and high or low blood pressure, were not confirmed in the OHTS as significant risk factors for the development of glaucoma.

A follow-up study of the OHTS participants found that delayed initiation of treatment still resulted in a decrease in the rate of developing glaucoma, as it did earlier in the course. This suggests that careful observation without initial treatment may be appropriate for some patients. The decision of whether to treat a patient with ocular hypertension may be based on a combination of the results from the OHTS, findings from the clinical examination, and discussions with the patient. The clinician and patient should consider whether the risk of developing glaucoma outweighs the inconvenience, cost, and potential side effects of therapy for the patient. Additional factors to consider include the patient's age and likely life span; for patients with no glaucomatous damage and a relatively short life expectancy, it may be reasonable to observe rather than treat. Data from the OHTS and the European Glaucoma Prevention Study were combined to create a risk calculation model (https://ohts.wustl.edu/risk) to help clinicians predict the 5-year risk of conversion from ocular hypertension to glaucoma, based on risk factors in the 2 studies (ie, older age, higher IOP, thinner corneas, larger baseline cup–disc ratio, higher pattern SD on standard automated perimetry).

Brandt JD, Beiser JA, Kass MA, Gordon MO; Ocular Hypertension Treatment Study (OHTS) Group. Central corneal thickness in the Ocular Hypertension Treatment Study (OHTS). *Ophthalmology.* 2020;127(4S):S72–S81.

Kass MA, Gordon MO, Gao F, et al. Delaying treatment of ocular hypertension: The Ocular Hypertension Treatment Study. *Arch Ophthalmol.* 2010;128(3):276–287.

Kass MA, Heuer DK, Higginbotham EJ, et al. The Ocular Hypertension Treatment Study: a randomized trial determines that topical ocular hypotensive medication delays or prevents the onset of primary open-angle glaucoma. *Arch Ophthalmol.* 2002;120(6):701–713; discussion 829–830.

Retinal vein occlusion

Glaucoma and ocular hypertension are risk factors for the development of central retinal vein occlusion (CRVO). In patients with a history of partial or complete CRVO, consideration may be given to treating elevated IOP in order to reduce the risk of a vein occlusion in the fellow eye.

Open-Angle Glaucoma Without Elevated IOP

Controversy remains as to whether normal-tension glaucoma (NTG; also called *low-tension glaucoma*) represents a distinct disease entity or whether it is simply POAG developing in individuals with IOP within the statistically normal range. As stated previously, glaucoma can develop at any IOP level within the range of pressures observed in the general population, and IOP is a continuous risk factor for glaucoma; any cutoff between "normal" and "abnormal" IOP is arbitrary. Accordingly, many authorities believe the terms *normal-tension glaucoma* and *low-tension glaucoma* should be abandoned.

Risk Factors and Clinical Features

As previously emphasized, glaucoma is a multifactorial disease process for which elevated IOP is just 1 of several risk factors. Studies of Japanese populations, which have found that a particularly high proportion of patients with OAG have IOPs in the statistically normal range, illustrate that other risk factors may play a greater role in individuals with NTG than in those who have POAG with higher IOPs. One hypothesis is that local vascular factors may have a substantial role in the development of NTG. Some studies suggest that patients with NTG have a higher incidence of vasospastic conditions or diseases (eg, migraine and Raynaud phenomenon), ischemic vascular disease, autoimmune disease, sleep apnea, systemic hypotension, and coagulopathies than patients with high-tension POAG. However, these findings have not been consistent.

As in POAG, NTG is characteristically bilateral but often asymmetric. In glaucomatous eyes with IOPs that are within the statistically normal range but asymmetric, worse damage typically occurs in the eye with the higher IOP. Optic disc hemorrhage may be more common among patients with NTG than among those with high-tension POAG (Fig 7-1).

The visual field defects in NTG tend to be more focal, deeper, and closer to fixation, especially with early disease, than the defects commonly seen in high-tension POAG. Also, a dense paracentral scotoma encroaching near fixation is not an unusual initial finding

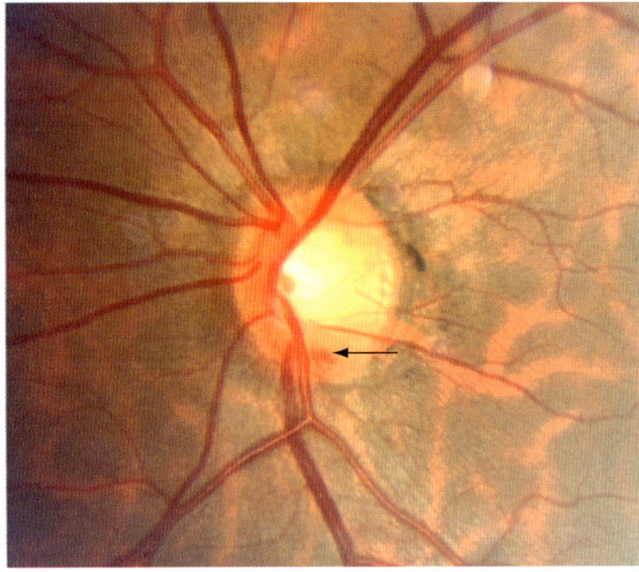

Figure 7-1 Subtle optic disc hemorrhage *(arrow)* in a patient with open-angle glaucoma. See Chapter 5, Figure 5-6 for an example of a flame-shaped optic disc hemorrhage in a patient with open-angle glaucoma. *(Courtesy of Wallace L. M. Alward, MD. ©The University of Iowa.)*

on the visual field tests of patients with NTG. However, these differences may be due to detection bias, given that patients experiencing visual disturbance are more likely to seek care. Further, differences in optic nerve appearance and visual field defects between patients with NTG and those with high-tension POAG have not been uniformly confirmed in studies. Thus, for any individual patient, there is no characteristic optic nerve or visual field abnormality that distinguishes NTG from high-tension POAG. Rates of glaucoma progression for patients with NTG are highly variable.

Cartwright MJ, Anderson DR. Correlation of asymmetric damage with asymmetric intraocular pressure in normal-tension glaucoma (low-tension glaucoma). *Arch Ophthalmol.* 1988;106(7):898–900.

Sommer A. Ocular hypertension and normal-tension glaucoma: time for banishment and burial. *Arch Ophthalmol.* 2011;129(6):785–787.

Differential Diagnosis

Normal-tension glaucoma can be mimicked by conditions other than glaucoma. It is therefore essential to distinguish glaucoma from other optic neuropathies (eg, optic disc drusen, ischemic optic neuropathy) because appropriate therapy will differ (Table 7-1). Visual field defects in some of these conditions may appear similar to those seen with NTG and can be progressive.

Patients with "normal" IOP in clinic may have higher pressures outside clinic hours. While diurnal IOP measurement may help in the determination of target IOPs by identifying peak pressures and IOP fluctuation, it does not capture nocturnal IOP patterns. Also, as previously mentioned, elevated IOP can be obscured in patients taking systemic medication, particularly systemic β-blockers. In addition, some patients with apparent NTG may have artifactually low tonometry readings because of altered corneoscleral biomechanics, 1 marker of which may be a thin central cornea. Similarly, decreased corneal thickness in patients who have undergone refractive surgery may result in underestimation of true IOP.

Diagnostic Evaluation

The clinical assessment of patients with NTG should mirror that of patients with any other OAG (see Chapters 3–5). In addition, the clinician must carefully review the patient's medical history for conditions that cause an optic nerve appearance and/or visual

Table 7-1 Differential Diagnosis for Glaucomatous Optic Neuropathy

Differential Diagnosis for Glaucomatous Optic Neuropathy
Congenital anomalies (eg, coloboma, optic nerve pit, myopic optic nerve head)
Physiologic cupping due to a large scleral canal
Optic disc drusen
Compressive lesions of the optic nerve and chiasm
Arteritic anterior ischemic optic neuropathy
Posterior ischemic optic neuropathy
Toxic (eg, methanol exposure) or nutritional (eg, vitamin B_{12} deficiency) optic neuropathy

field defects similar to those seen in NTG. These conditions include significant systemic hemorrhage causing low blood pressure, myocardial infarction, or shock.

Prognosis and Therapy

The initial goal of therapy is often to achieve a near 30% reduction in IOP from a carefully determined baseline IOP. Once the target pressure is established, routine evaluations with appropriate individualized adjustments are recommended. In making these adjustments, the clinician should consider baseline severity of optic nerve damage and visual field loss, potential risks of therapy, comorbid conditions, life expectancy of the patient, and other relevant factors. The target pressure may be reassessed and adjusted as needed during follow-up visits in order to maintain visual function.

In a secondary analysis of the Collaborative Normal-Tension Glaucoma Study (CNTGS; see Clinical Trial 7-3), lowering IOP by at least 30% reduced the 5-year risk of visual field progression from 35% to 12%, supporting the role of IOP in NTG. Of note, the protective effect of IOP reduction was evident only after adjusting for the effect of cataracts, which were more frequent in the treatment group. In light of the findings of the CNTGS, treatment of NTG is generally recommended unless the optic neuropathy is determined to be stable. Interestingly, approximately half of the patients who did not receive treatment in this study showed no progression over the study duration, whereas in 12% of patients in the treatment group, worsening of their glaucomatous visual field damage occurred despite a 30% reduction of IOP. Factors in addition to IOP are likely important in patients with NTG. In those who worsened, the rate of visual field progression was highly variable yet slow in most but not all patients. In addition, this study showed a lower treatment benefit among patients with a baseline history of optic disc hemorrhage.

Treatment of NTG differs little from that of other OAGs. Some glaucoma specialists are wary of treating NTG with topical β-blocker medications because of their association with low OPP (see the subsection "Lower ocular perfusion pressure"). The Low-Pressure Glaucoma Treatment Study showed that patients with low-pressure glaucoma treated with timolol had a high rate of glaucomatous progression. However, there was a significant loss of follow-up in this study, and its results must be interpreted with that in mind. In the Early Manifest Glaucoma Trial (EMGT; see Clinical Trial 7-4), IOP lowering with the combination of betaxolol and argon laser trabeculoplasty was minimal in eyes with baseline IOPs of 15 mm Hg or lower. This finding suggests that patients with a lower baseline IOP who are progressing may need incisional surgery or medications other than β-blockers to stabilize their disease. Tailoring treatment to each patient is relevant to all forms of glaucoma. See Chapter 13 for further discussion of indications for surgery.

Bhandari A, Crabb DP, Poinoosawmy D, Fitzke FW, Hitchings RA, Noureddin BN. Effect of surgery on visual field progression in normal-tension glaucoma. *Ophthalmology.* 1997;104(7):1131–1137.

Collaborative Normal-Tension Glaucoma Study Group. Comparison of glaucomatous progression between untreated patients with normal-tension glaucoma and patients with therapeutically reduced intraocular pressures. *Am J Ophthalmol.* 1998;126(4):487–497.

Collaborative Normal-Tension Glaucoma Study Group. The effectiveness of intraocular pressure reduction in the treatment of normal-tension glaucoma. *Am J Ophthalmol.* 1998;126(4):498–505.

CLINICAL TRIAL 7-1

Collaborative Initial Glaucoma Treatment Study (CIGTS) Essentials

Purpose: To determine whether patients with newly diagnosed open-angle glaucoma (OAG) are better treated by initial treatment with medications or by immediate filtering surgery.

Study design: Multicenter randomized controlled clinical trial comparing initial medical therapy with initial surgical therapy for OAG.

Participants: A total of 607 patients with OAG (primary, pigmentary, or pseudoexfoliation).

Results: Although intraocular pressure (IOP) was lower in the group initially treated with trabeculectomy, initial medical and initial surgical therapy resulted in similar visual field outcomes after up to 9 years of follow-up. Early visual acuity loss was greater in the surgery group, but the differences between groups converged over time. Also, cataracts were more common in the surgery group. At the 8-year follow-up examination, substantial worsening (≥3 dB) of visual field mean deviation from baseline was found in 21.3% of the initial surgery group and 25.5% of the initial medical therapy group. Patients with worse baseline visual fields were less likely to progress if treated with trabeculectomy first. Patients with diabetes were more likely to progress if treated initially with surgery.

The quality of life (QOL) reported by the 2 treatment groups was similar. The most persistent QOL finding was a greater number of symptoms reported at a higher frequency by the surgery group.

The overall rate of progression of OAG was lower in CIGTS than in many clinical trials, possibly because of more aggressive IOP-lowering goals and the disease stage. Individualized target IOPs were determined according to a formula that accounted for baseline IOP and visual field loss. Over the course of follow-up, IOP in the medical therapy group averaged 17–18 mm Hg (IOP reduction of approximately 38%), whereas IOP in the surgery group averaged 14–15 mm Hg (IOP reduction of approximately 46%). IOP fluctuation was a risk factor for progression in the medically treated group but not the surgically treated group. The rate of cataract removal was greater in the surgically treated group.

CLINICAL TRIAL 7-2

Ocular Hypertension Treatment Study (OHTS) Essentials

Purpose: To evaluate the safety and efficacy of topical ocular hypotensive medications in preventing or delaying the onset of visual field loss and/or optic nerve damage in participants with ocular hypertension.

Study design: Multicenter randomized controlled clinical trial comparing observation and medical therapy for ocular hypertension.

(Continued on next page)

(continued)

Participants: A total of 1637 patients with ocular hypertension recruited between 1994 and 1996.

Results 2002: Topical ocular hypotensive medication was effective in delaying or preventing the onset of primary open-angle glaucoma (POAG). The incidence of glaucoma was lower in the medication group than in the observation group (4.4% vs 9.5%, respectively) at 60 months' follow-up. No increase in adverse events was detected in the medication group.

The 5-year risk of developing POAG was associated with the following baseline factors: older age (22% increase in relative risk [RR] per decade), larger vertical and horizontal cup–disc ratios (32% and 27% increases in RR per 0.1 increase, respectively), higher pattern standard deviation (22% increase in RR per 0.2 dB increase), and higher baseline IOP (10% increase in RR per 1-mm-Hg increase). Central corneal thickness (CCT) was found to be a powerful predictor for the development of POAG (81% increase in RR for every 40 μm thinner). The corneas in OHTS participants were thicker than those in the general population, and Black/African American participants had thinner corneas than others in the study.

Results 2010: Topical ocular hypotensive medication was initiated in the original observation group after 7.5 years (median) without medication, and medication was continued for 5.5 years thereafter. Participants in the original medication group continued topical ocular hypotensive medications for a median of 13 years. The proportion of participants who developed POAG was 0.22 in the original observation group and 0.16 in the original medication group. The primary purpose of the follow-up study was to determine whether delaying treatment resulted in a persistently increased risk of conversion to glaucoma, even after the initiation of therapy. It was found that delayed initiation of treatment still resulted in a decrease in the rate of developing glaucoma, as it did earlier in the course.

Results 2021: Over 20 years of follow-up, the cumulative incidence of POAG was 55.2% (95% CI, 47.9%–61.5%) among Black/African American participants and 42.7% (95% CI, 38.9%–46.3%) among participants of other races. Approximately one-fourth of all participants experienced visual field loss at 20 years.

CLINICAL TRIAL 7-3

Collaborative Normal-Tension Glaucoma Study (CNTGS) Essentials

Purpose: To determine whether the optic nerve damage seen in eyes without statistically elevated IOP was IOP dependent or IOP independent.

Study design: Multicenter randomized controlled clinical trial comparing observation and treatment for normal-tension glaucoma (NTG).

Randomization to treatment (30% reduction in IOP after treatment with medications, laser trabeculoplasty, or incisional surgery) or observation occurred at enrollment only if there was clear evidence of glaucoma worsening before enrollment. Otherwise, eyes were observed and then randomized after they showed worsening of glaucoma, determined primarily by using a study-specific analysis of visual fields. Determination of worsening could also be made by observation of optic nerve head changes.

Participants: From 24 centers, 230 eyes of 230 participants were enrolled, meeting the following criteria:

- the presence of glaucoma in 1 or both eyes (as determined by the investigators)
- age between 20 and 90 years
- recorded IOPs never above 24 mm Hg

In addition to meeting these criteria, each participant underwent 10 IOP readings after medication washout in order to determine baseline IOP. The median IOP had to be 20 mm Hg or lower, with none of the readings above 24 mm Hg. Each participant completed 3 reliable visual field tests within 1 month. Exclusion criteria were use of systemic β-blockers or clonidine, comorbid ocular disease, prior intraocular surgery, narrow angles, visual acuity worse than 20/30, and severe visual field loss.

Results: Seventy-nine eyes were randomized to observation; 66, to treatment. The remaining 85 eyes never showed evidence of worsening. In the intention-to-treat analysis, visual field worsening occurred in 31 eyes (39%) in the observation group and 22 (33%) in the treatment group; this difference was not statistically significant. When the data were reevaluated by censoring results obtained after the development of visually significant cataract, visual field worsening was more likely in the observation group (27%) than in the treatment group (12%). The difference in the 2 analyses was attributed to the higher rate of cataract in the group that underwent filtration surgery.

In a secondary analysis of participants who met the treatment target, 28 (35%) of the observation eyes and 7 (12%) of the treated eyes worsened after randomization. Visually significant cataract developed in 11 eyes (14%) in the observation group and 23 (38%) in the treatment group. In a secondary analysis of the 160 participants in the untreated group, half demonstrated a detectable change in visual field after 7 years.

CLINICAL TRIAL 7-4

Early Manifest Glaucoma Trial (EMGT) Essentials

Purpose: To evaluate the effectiveness of lowering IOP in patients with early, newly detected OAG.

(Continued on next page)

(continued)

Study design: Multicenter randomized controlled clinical trial comparing observation and treatment with betaxolol and argon laser trabeculoplasty for OAG.

Participants: Patients 50 to 80 years of age with newly diagnosed OAG and early glaucomatous visual field loss were identified mainly through a population-based screening of more than 44,000 residents of Malmö and Helsingborg, Sweden. Exclusion criteria were as follows: advanced visual field loss; mean IOP greater than 30 mm Hg or any IOP greater than 35 mm Hg; and visual acuity less than 0.5 (20/40). Between 1993 and 1997, 255 patients were randomized.

Results: At 6 years, 62% of untreated patients showed progression, whereas 45% of treated patients progressed. On average, treatment reduced IOP by 25%. In a univariate analysis, risk factors for progression included no IOP-lowering treatment, older age, higher IOP, pseudoexfoliation syndrome, more advanced visual field loss, and bilateral glaucoma. In multivariate analyses, the risk of progression with IOP-lowering treatment was reduced by half (HR = 0.50; 95% CI, 0.35–0.71). Each millimeter of mercury of IOP lowering decreased the risk of glaucomatous progression by 10%. Risk factors for progression in multivariate analyses included higher baseline IOP, older age, pseudoexfoliation syndrome, bilateral disease, worse mean deviation, and frequent optic disc hemorrhages. IOP fluctuation was not found to be a significant risk factor.

In the observation group, the rate of visual field progression was most rapid in the subgroup of patients with pseudoexfoliation syndrome and slowest in patients with baseline IOPs within the normal range.

CLINICAL TRIAL 7-5

Advanced Glaucoma Intervention Study (AGIS) Essentials

Purpose: To compare the clinical outcomes of 2 treatment sequences: argon laser trabeculoplasty–trabeculectomy–trabeculectomy (ATT) and trabeculectomy–argon laser trabeculoplasty–trabeculectomy (TAT).

Study design: Multicenter randomized controlled clinical trial comparing 2 treatment sequences (ATT and TAT) for patients with OAG uncontrolled with medical therapy.

Participants: A total of 789 eyes of 591 patients with medically uncontrolled OAG recruited from 1988 to 1992.

Results:

AGIS 4 and AGIS 13: Black patients treated with the ATT sequence had a lower combined visual acuity and visual field loss than those treated with the TAT sequence. White patients had a lower combined visual acuity and visual field loss at 7 years if initially treated with the TAT sequence.

In the initial follow-up period, White patients in the TAT group had greater visual acuity loss than those in the ATT group; by 7 years, this loss was similar.

AGIS 5: The mean IOP at the 4-week postoperative visit was higher in eyes with encapsulated blebs than in those without; with resumption of medical therapy, eyes with and without encapsulated blebs had similar IOPs after 1 year.

AGIS 6: Visual function scores improved after cataract surgery. Adjustment for cataract did not alter the findings of previous AGIS studies.

AGIS 7: Lower IOP was associated with less visual field progression. Less visual field progression was observed in eyes with an average IOP of 14 mm Hg or less during the first 18 months after the first surgical intervention, and for eyes with IOP of 18 mm Hg or less for all study visits.

AGIS 8: Approximately half of the study patients developed cataract in the first 5 years of follow-up. Trabeculectomy increased the relative risk of cataract formation by 78%.

AGIS 9: The treatment protocol with initial trabeculectomy slows the progression of glaucoma more effectively in White patients than in Black patients. The treatment protocol with initial argon laser trabeculoplasty (ALT) was slightly more effective in Black participants than in White participants.

AGIS 10: Assessment of optic nerve findings showed good intraobserver but poor interobserver agreement.

AGIS 11: Reduced effectiveness of ALT was associated with younger age and higher IOP. The ineffectiveness of trabeculectomy was associated with younger age, higher IOP, diabetes mellitus, and postoperative complications (markedly elevated IOP and inflammation).

AGIS 12: Risk factors for sustained decrease of the visual field included better baseline visual fields, male sex, worse baseline visual acuity, and diabetes mellitus. Risk factors for sustained decrease in visual acuity included better baseline visual acuity, older age, and less formal education.

AGIS 14: In patients with visual field progression, a single 6-month confirmatory visual field test had a 72% probability of verifying a persistent defect. When the number of confirmatory visual field tests was increased from 1 to 2, the percentage of eyes that showed a persistent defect increased to 84%.

2009 AGIS Report: IOP fluctuation was an independent predictor of OAG progression in eyes with lower baseline IOPs but not in those with higher baseline IOPs.

Most of the relevant findings from AGIS that reflect clinical practice are from post hoc analysis; thus, they may not fully take into account unmeasurable confounding factors and enrollment bias.

CLINICAL TRIAL 7-6

The United Kingdom Glaucoma Treatment Study (UKGTS) Essentials

Purpose: To determine the change in the frequency of visual field deterioration in treatment-naïve patients treated with latanoprost compared with those treated with placebo.

Study design: Participants were randomized 1:1 to treatment with latanoprost 0.005% or to placebo and monitored with frequent visual field tests and optic nerve imaging during 11 visits within 2 years. Visual field worsening was determined with the guided progression analysis (GPA) available on the Humphrey Field Analyzer. The optic nerve was imaged with confocal scanning laser ophthalmoscopy, scanning laser polarimetry, time-domain optical coherence tomography, and monoscopic disc photography. IOP was measured with Goldmann tonometry, dynamic contour tonometry, and the ocular response analyzer. Study endpoints were visual field worsening determined by GPA, IOP greater than 35 mm Hg on 2 visits, and decline of corrected distance visual acuity to worse than 20/60. The UKGTS was designed with a short observation period, achieved by a novel arrangement of the visual field tests in which they were clustered at the beginning and end of the study period.

Participants: From 10 centers, 516 patients with newly diagnosed mild to moderate OAG were enrolled. Exclusion criteria were as follows:

- mean deviation worse than −10 dB in the better eye or −16 dB in the worse eye
- IOP above 35 mm Hg on 2 visits or IOP that averaged more than 30 mm Hg on 2 visits
- unreliable performance on visual field tests
- poor-quality optic nerve imaging with confocal scanning laser ophthalmoscopy
- presence of significant cataract
- previous intraocular surgery other than cataract extraction
- diabetic retinopathy

Results: The UKGTS is important because it is the first randomized, placebo-controlled study of the effect of topical glaucoma medications and because of its novel design of testing intervals and clustering, which allowed the investigators to identify differences in visual field worsening in a relatively short time. Over 24 months, 59 participants in the placebo group had worsening of their visual field compared with 35 in the latanoprost group. The mean change in visual field mean deviation in those who worsened was −1.6 dB.

CLINICAL TRIAL 7-7

Laser in Glaucoma and Ocular Hypertension (LiGHT) Trial Essentials

Purpose: To compare selective laser trabeculoplasty (SLT) and topical ocular hypotensive therapy (eyedrops) as first-line treatment for OAG and ocular hypertension.

Study design: Multicenter, observer-masked randomized controlled trial in the United Kingdom. The target IOP was determined according to glaucoma severity. The primary outcome was QOL; secondary outcomes were related to target IOP, need for additional surgery, and cost.

Participants: A total of 718 previously untreated adults with ocular hypertension or OAG and no ocular comorbidities were recruited at 6 centers between 2012 and 2014.

Results: Of 718 patients enrolled, 356 were randomized to receive SLT and 362 to receive eyedrops. Following randomization, there was no significant difference in scores on the QOL instrument between the two groups. At 36 months, 74.2% (95% CI, 69.3–78. 6) of participants in the SLT group required no eyedrops to maintain IOP at target. Eyes of participants in the SLT group were within target IOP at more visits (93.0%) than those in the eyedrops group (91.3%). Glaucoma surgery was required for 11 eyes in the eyedrops group and none in the SLT group. The cost analysis favored SLT. In an analysis of an extended 6-year cohort study, participants in the SLT arm had less visual field progression and were less likely to require trabeculectomy than participants in the medication arm.

CHAPTER 8

Secondary Open-Angle Glaucoma

This chapter includes a case study. Go to aao.org/bcsccasestudy_section10 or scan the QR code in the text to access this content.

Highlights

- Pseudoexfoliation syndrome is the most common cause of secondary open-angle glaucoma (OAG).
- The lens can cause secondary OAG through a variety of inflammatory mechanisms.
- Ocular inflammatory syndromes may be linked to OAG through both inflammation and the eye's physiologic response to corticosteroids.
- Nonpenetrating ocular trauma may cause a variety of anterior segment conditions that can lead to secondary glaucoma.
- Repeated intravitreous injections of anti–vascular endothelial growth factor agents may result in sustained intraocular pressure elevation.

Secondary Open-Angle Glaucoma

Pseudoexfoliation Syndrome

The most common cause of secondary open-angle glaucoma (OAG) is *pseudoexfoliation syndrome,* which is characterized by the extracellular deposition of a distinctive fibrillar material in the anterior segment of the eye. On histologic examination, this material has been found in and on the lens epithelium and capsule, pupillary margin, ciliary epithelium, iris pigment epithelium, iris stroma, iris blood vessels, and subconjunctival tissue. The material has also been identified in other parts of the body, including the skin, lungs, heart, and liver. Pathogenic variants in a single gene, lysyl oxidase like 1 *(LOXL1),* are present in nearly all cases of pseudoexfoliation syndrome and pseudoexfoliation glaucoma. However, these disease-associated variations are also common in populations without pseudoexfoliation syndrome, and other genes have also been implicated in genome-wide association studies, suggesting a multifactorial etiology for this disease. The exact relationship between genetic and environmental factors in pseudoexfoliation syndrome remains unclear.

Pseudoexfoliation syndrome is typically asymmetric and often presents unilaterally, although the uninvolved eye may manifest signs of the disease at a later time. Strongly age-related, this syndrome is rarely seen in persons younger than 50 years and occurs most commonly in individuals older than 70 years.

The classic characteristic of pseudoexfoliation syndrome is the deposition of fibrillar material in a “bull's-eye” pattern on the anterior lens capsule, best viewed after pupillary dilation. This pattern is presumably caused by iris movement that scrapes the pseudoexfoliative material from the lens, resulting in an intermediate clear area between a central zone and a peripheral zone of the material (Fig 8-1). Clinically, this fibrillar extracellular material can be seen on the pupillary margin, zonular fibers of the lens, ciliary processes, inferior anterior chamber angle, corneal endothelium, and anterior vitreous (Figs 8-2, 8-3).

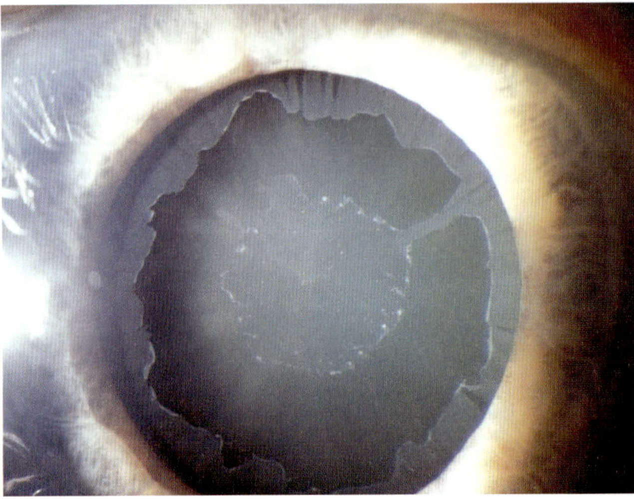

Figure 8-1 Pseudoexfoliation syndrome. Pseudoexfoliative material deposited on the anterior lens capsule in a classic "bull's-eye" pattern, viewed in a dilated eye. *(Courtesy of Wallace L. M. Alward, MD. From the* Iowa Glaucoma Curriculum *[curriculum.iowaglaucoma.org]. © The University of Iowa.)*

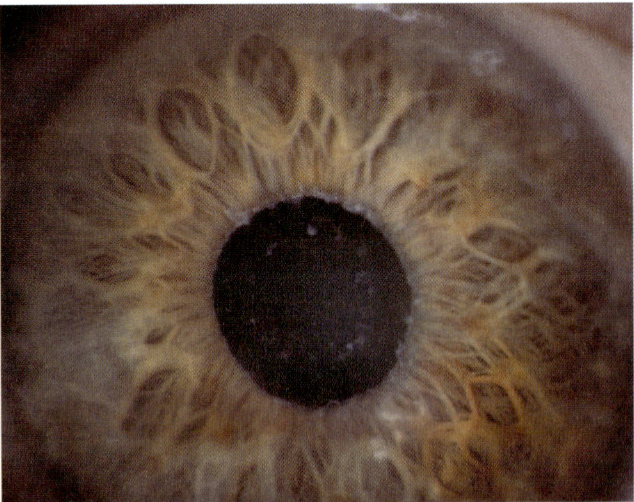

Figure 8-2 Pseudoexfoliative material deposited on the pupillary margin and anterior lens capsule, viewed in an undilated eye. *(Courtesy of Wallace L. M. Alward, MD. From the* Iowa Glaucoma Curriculum *[curriculum.iowaglaucoma.org]. © The University of Iowa.)*

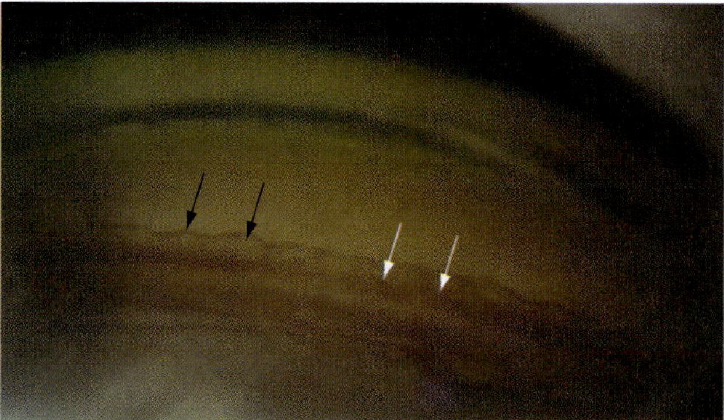

Figure 8-3 Goniophotograph of the anterior chamber angle in an eye with pseudoexfoliation syndrome. Note the Sampaolesi line *(black arrows)*. *White arrows* indicate the anterior border of the pigmented trabecular meshwork. *(Courtesy of Angelo P. Tanna, MD.)*

Individuals with pseudoexfoliation syndrome may also have peripupillary atrophy with transillumination defects. In these patients, the pupil often dilates poorly, probably because of infiltration of fibrillar material into the iris stroma. Phacodonesis results from the weak zonular fibers. Thus, great care must be taken during cataract surgery to reduce the risk of zonular dehiscence, vitreous loss, lens dislocation, and other complications (see also BCSC Section 11, *Lens and Cataract*). Iris angiography has shown abnormalities of the iris vessels with leakage of fluorescein.

On gonioscopy, the trabecular meshwork is typically heavily pigmented, sometimes in a variegated fashion. Pigment deposition anterior to the Schwalbe line, known as the *Sampaolesi line,* is commonly seen (see Fig 8-3). Anterior migration of the lens due to zonular laxity may lead to secondary angle closure.

The intraocular pressure (IOP) elevation associated with pseudoexfoliation syndrome is likely attributable to deposits of fibrillar material in the conventional (trabecular meshwork) and uveoscleral outflow pathways that impede the outflow of aqueous humor. In addition, because elastin is an important component of the lamina cribrosa, pseudoexfoliation syndrome may increase the susceptibility of the optic nerve to injury. This increased susceptibility may, in turn, contribute to the increased risk of development and progression of glaucoma in these patients, as was found in the Early Manifest Glaucoma Trial (see Chapter 7, Clinical Trial 7-4).

Individuals with pseudoexfoliation syndrome with elevated IOP that results in optic nerve damage or visual field loss are described as having *pseudoexfoliation glaucoma.* Pseudoexfoliation syndrome is associated with OAG in all populations, but the prevalence varies considerably. In Scandinavian countries, pseudoexfoliation syndrome accounts for more than 50% of OAG cases. The risk of progression to glaucoma also varies widely and can be as high as 40% of patients in a 10-year period. Patients with pseudoexfoliation syndrome often have higher IOP, with greater diurnal IOP fluctuations, than do patients with primary open-angle glaucoma (POAG). The overall prognosis for glaucoma is worse for patients with pseudoexfoliation glaucoma than for those with POAG. Laser trabeculoplasty can be very effective, but the duration of the response may be shorter in pseudoexfoliation glaucoma than in POAG.

Aboobakar IF, Johnson WM, Stamer WD, Hauser MA, Allingham RR. Major review: exfoliation syndrome; advances in disease genetics, molecular biology, and epidemiology. *Exp Eye Res.* 2017;154:88–103.

Thorleifsson G, Magnusson KP, Sulem P, et al. Common sequence variants in the *LOXL1* gene confer susceptibility to exfoliation glaucoma. *Science.* 2007;317(5843):1397–1400.

Pigment Dispersion Syndrome

In pigment dispersion syndrome, the zonular fibers rub the posterior iris pigment epithelium, resulting in the release of pigment granules into the anterior segment. Posterior bowing of the iris caused by the so-called reverse pupillary block configuration is present in many eyes with pigment dispersion syndrome. This concave iris configuration results in greater contact with the zonular fibers, causing increased release of pigment granules.

Pigment dispersion syndrome characteristically presents with pigment deposits on the corneal endothelium, trabecular meshwork, and lens periphery, as well as with midperipheral iris transillumination defects in a spokelike pattern. The pigment is typically deposited on the corneal endothelium in a vertical spindle pattern, referred to as a *Krukenberg spindle* (Fig 8-4); the pattern of corneal pigment deposition is the result of aqueous convection currents and subsequent phagocytosis of pigment by the corneal endothelium. The presence of a Krukenberg spindle is not necessary for a diagnosis of pigment dispersion syndrome. Moreover, this sign may be present in other diseases, such as pseudoexfoliation syndrome. The midperipheral iris transillumination defects are a result of contact between the zonular fibers and the posterior iris pigment epithelium (Fig 8-5). On gonioscopy, the trabecular meshwork commonly appears as homogeneous and densely pigmented, with speckled pigment at or anterior to the Schwalbe line (Fig 8-6), forming a Sampaolesi line. When the eye is dilated, pigment deposits may be seen on the zonular fibers, on the anterior hyaloid, and in the equatorial region of the lens capsule (*Zentmayer line/ring,* or *Scheie stripe;* Fig 8-7).

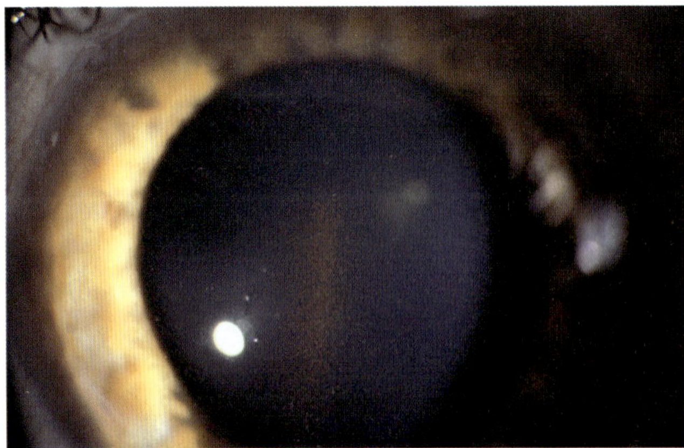

Figure 8-4 Krukenberg spindle in a patient with pigmentary glaucoma. *(Reproduced from Alward WLM, Longmuir RA.* Color Atlas of Gonioscopy. *2nd ed. American Academy of Ophthalmology; 2008:75. Fig 9-1.)*

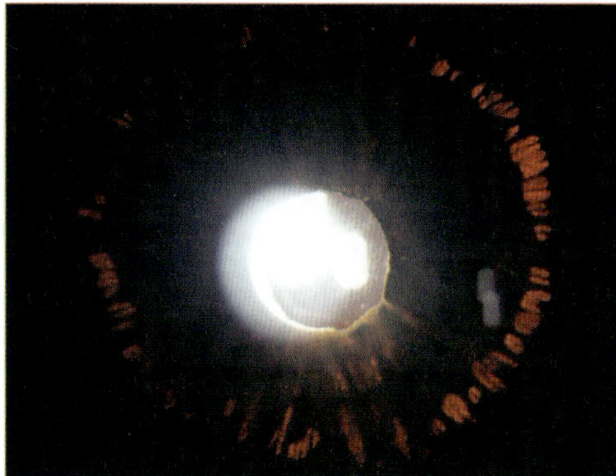

Figure 8-5 The classic spokelike iris transillumination defects of pigment dispersion syndrome. *(Courtesy of Angelo P. Tanna, MD.)*

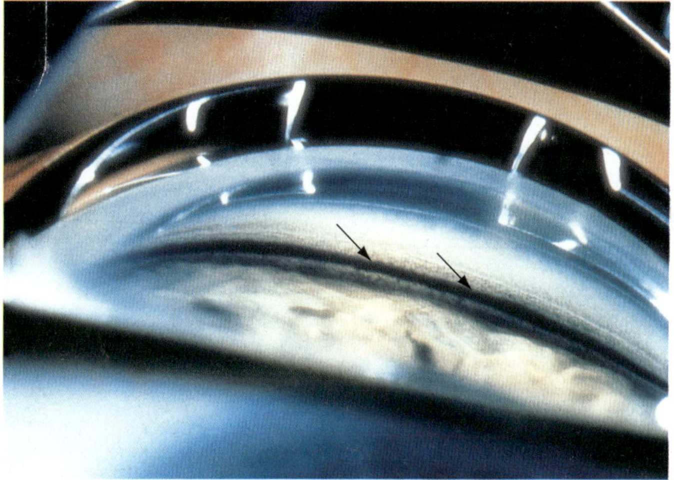

Figure 8-6 Characteristic heavy, uniform pigmentation of the trabecular meshwork *(arrows)* that occurs in pigment dispersion syndrome and pigmentary glaucoma. *(Courtesy of M. Roy Wilson, MD.)*

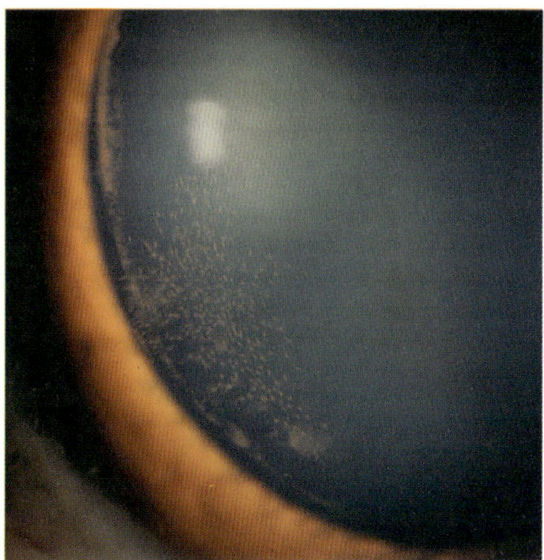

Figure 8-7 Pigment dispersion syndrome. Pigment deposits are visible in the equatorial region of the lens capsule (Zentmayer line or ring; also called *Scheie stripe*) and on the zonular fibers. *(Courtesy of Angelo P. Tanna, MD.)*

With increasing age, the signs of pigment dispersion may decrease as a result of normal growth of the lens, inducing a physiologic pupillary block and anterior movement of the iris. Loss of accommodation may also occur. As pigment dispersion is reduced, the deposited pigment may fade from the corneal endothelium, trabecular meshwork, or anterior surface of the iris.

Approximately 15% of cases of pigment dispersion syndrome progress to glaucoma or elevated IOP that requires treatment. *Pigmentary glaucoma* is 3 times more common in men than in women, particularly men who are young or middle-aged (20–50 years) and myopic. The presumed mechanism of elevated IOP is obstruction of the trabecular meshwork by pigment granules. Pigmentary glaucoma is characterized by wide fluctuations in IOP, which can exceed 50 mm Hg in untreated eyes. Affected patients may have extreme elevations in IOP after exercise or pupillary dilation because of an excessive liberation of pigment. Symptoms associated with such elevated IOPs may include halos, intermittent blurry vision, and ocular pain.

Medical treatment is often successful in reducing elevated IOP. Most patients respond reasonably well to laser trabeculoplasty, although its effect may be short-lived. Studies have shown paradoxical IOP elevations after laser trabeculoplasty in eyes with heavy trabecular meshwork pigmentation, including pigmentary glaucoma; thus, it may be advisable to use lower laser energy in this condition. Filtering surgery is usually successful; however, extra care is warranted in young male patients with myopia, who are at increased risk for hypotony maculopathy. Laser peripheral iridotomy (LPI) has been proposed as a means of minimizing posterior bowing of the iris by alleviating the pressure differential between the anterior chamber and the posterior chamber. However, multiple studies, including randomized trials, have failed to show a benefit of LPI for treatment of this condition.

Niyadurupola N, Broadway DC. Pigment dispersion syndrome and pigmentary glaucoma—a major review. *Clin Exp Ophthalmol.* 2008;36(9):868–882.

Reistad CE, Shields MB, Campbell DG, et al; American Glaucoma Society Pigmentary Glaucoma Iridotomy Study Group. The influence of peripheral iridotomy on the intraocular pressure course in patients with pigmentary glaucoma. *J Glaucoma.* 2005;14(4):255–259.

Siddiqui Y, Ten Hulzen RD, Cameron JD, Hodge DO, Johnson DH. What is the risk of developing pigmentary glaucoma from pigment dispersion syndrome? *Am J Ophthalmol.* 2003;135(6):794–799.

Lens-Induced Glaucoma

The lens can play a role in the development of both open-angle and angle-closure glaucoma. Lens-induced open-angle mechanisms are the cause of 3 clinical entities:

- phacolytic glaucoma
- lens particle glaucoma
- phacoantigenic glaucoma

Lens-induced angle-closure glaucomas include phacomorphic glaucoma and ectopia lentis and are discussed in Chapter 10. See also BCSC Section 9, *Uveitis and Ocular Inflammation,* and Section 11, *Lens and Cataract.*

Phacolytic glaucoma

As the lens ages, its protein composition changes, with an increased concentration of high-molecular-weight proteins. Phacolytic glaucoma is an inflammatory glaucoma caused by the leakage of such proteins through microscopic openings in the lens capsule of a mature or hypermature cataract (Fig 8-8). These proteins, lens-laden macrophages, and other inflammatory debris subsequently obstruct the trabecular meshwork, resulting in elevated IOP.

Individuals with phacolytic glaucoma are usually older patients with a history of poor vision. They have sudden onset of pain, conjunctival hyperemia, and worsening vision. Examination reveals markedly elevated IOP, microcystic corneal edema, prominent cell and flare without keratic precipitates (KPs), an open anterior chamber angle, and a mature or hypermature cataract (Fig 8-9). The lack of KPs helps distinguish phacolytic glaucoma from phacoantigenic glaucoma. Cellular debris may be seen layered in the anterior chamber angle, and a pseudohypopyon may be present. Large white particles (clumps of lens protein) may also be present in the anterior chamber. The anterior lens capsule of the mature, hypermature, or morgagnian cataract may exhibit wrinkling, which represents loss of cortical volume and the release of lens material (see Fig 8-8). Ocular hypotensive medications may be necessary to reduce the IOP; however, definitive therapy requires cataract extraction.

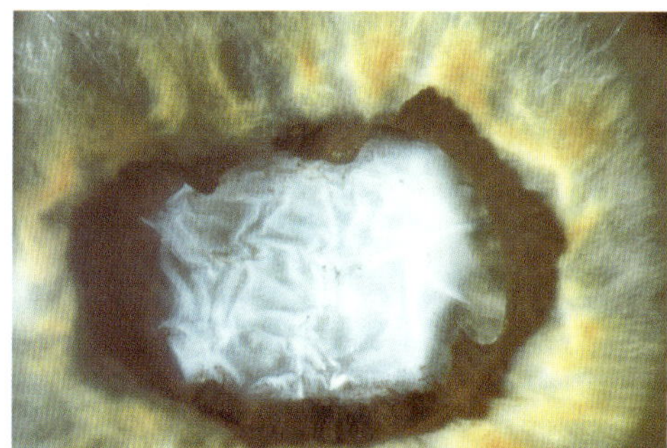

Figure 8-8 Characteristic appearance of a hypermature cataract with wrinkling of the anterior lens capsule, which results from loss of cortical volume. Extensive posterior synechiae are present, which suggests previous inflammation. *(Courtesy of Steven T. Simmons, MD.)*

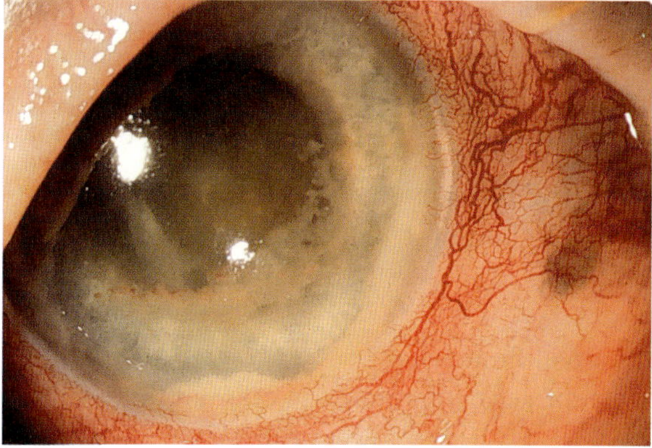

Figure 8-9 Phacolytic glaucoma. The typical presentation of phacolytic glaucoma is conjunctival hyperemia, microcystic corneal edema, mature cataract, and prominent anterior chamber reaction, as shown in this photograph. Note the lens protein deposits on the endothelium and layering in the angle, which create a pseudohypopyon. *(Courtesy of G. A. Cioffi, MD.)*

Lens particle glaucoma

In lens particle glaucoma, retention of lens material in the eye after cataract extraction, capsulotomy, or ocular trauma results in obstruction of the trabecular meshwork. The severity of IOP elevation depends on the quantity of lens material released, the degree of inflammation, the ability of the trabecular meshwork to clear the lens material, and the functional status of the ciliary body, which is often altered after surgery or trauma.

Lens particle glaucoma usually occurs within weeks of the initial surgery or trauma, but it may occur months or years later. Clinical findings include cortical material in the anterior chamber, elevated IOP, moderate anterior chamber reaction, microcystic corneal edema, and with time, posterior synechiae and peripheral anterior synechiae (PAS).

Medical therapy may be needed to reduce the IOP while the residual lens material resorbs. Appropriate therapy includes medications to decrease aqueous formation, mydriatics to inhibit posterior synechiae formation, and topical corticosteroids to reduce inflammation. If the IOP cannot be controlled, surgical removal of the lens material may be necessary.

Phacoantigenic glaucoma

Phacoantigenic glaucoma (formerly, *phacoanaphylaxis*) is a rare condition in which patients become sensitized to their own lens protein after surgery or penetrating trauma, resulting in a granulomatous inflammation. The clinical picture is quite varied, but most patients present with a moderate anterior chamber reaction with KPs on both the corneal endothelium and the anterior lens surface. In addition, a low-grade vitritis, posterior synechiae, PAS, and residual lens material in the anterior chamber may be present. Glaucomatous optic neuropathy may occur, but it is not common in eyes with phacoantigenic glaucoma. Initiation of topical corticosteroids and aqueous suppressants are recommended to reduce inflammation and IOP. The residual lens material will likely need to be removed once the inflammation is controlled.

Glaucoma Secondary to Intraocular Tumors

A variety of tumors can cause unilateral glaucoma. Many of the tumors described in this section are also discussed in BCSC Section 4, *Ophthalmic Pathology and Intraocular Tumors.* Depending on the size, type, and location of the tumor, IOP elevation can result from several different mechanisms, including the following:

- direct tumor invasion of the anterior chamber angle
- angle closure resulting from rotation of the ciliary body or from anterior displacement of the lens–iris interface (see Chapter 10)
- intraocular hemorrhage
- neovascularization of the angle
- deposition of tumor cells, inflammatory cells, and cellular debris within the trabecular meshwork

Choroidal and retinal tumors typically cause a secondary angle-closure glaucoma by the anterior displacement of the lens–iris diaphragm, which results in the closure of the anterior chamber angle. Posterior synechiae may develop as a result of inflammation of necrotic tumors; they exacerbate angle closure through a pupillary block mechanism. Choroidal melanomas, medulloepitheliomas, and retinoblastomas may also cause neovascularization of the angle, which can result in angle closure. Neovascularization of the angle may also occur after radiation therapy for intraocular tumors.

The most common cause of IOP elevation associated with primary or metastatic tumors of the ciliary body is direct invasion of the anterior chamber angle. This can be exacerbated by anterior segment hemorrhage and inflammation, which further obstruct aqueous outflow. Necrotic tumor and tumor-laden macrophages obstruct the trabecular meshwork, resulting in OAG. Tumors causing a secondary glaucoma in adults include uveal melanoma and melanocytoma (Figs 8-10, 8-11), metastatic carcinoma, lymphoma, and leukemia. In children, tumors associated with glaucoma include retinoblastoma, juvenile xanthogranuloma, and medulloepithelioma.

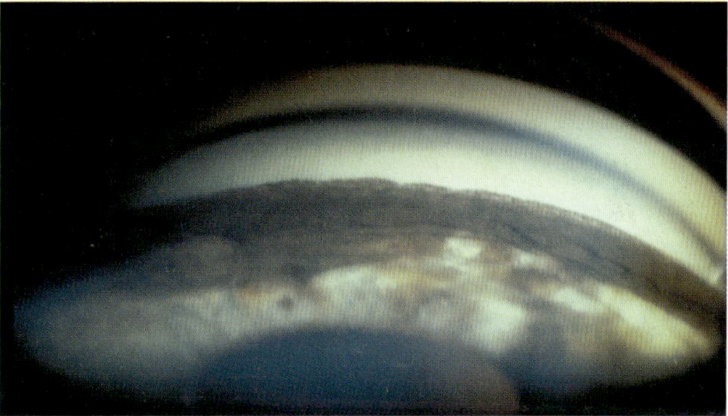

Figure 8-10 Goniophotograph of a ciliary body melanoma in the anterior chamber angle. *(Courtesy of Wallace L. M. Alward, MD. From the* Iowa Glaucoma Curriculum *[curriculum.iowaglaucoma.org]. © The University of Iowa.)*

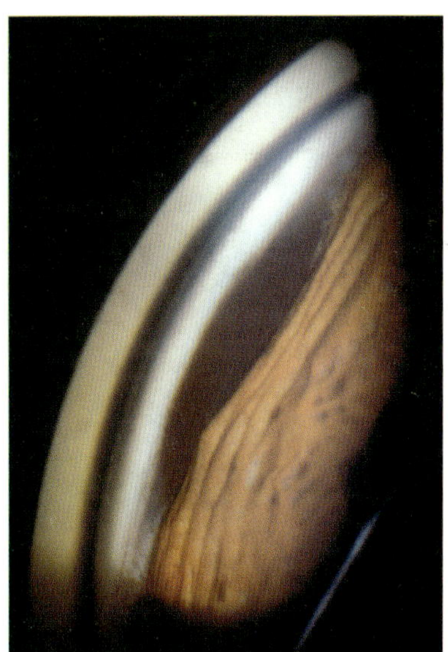

Figure 8-11 Goniophotograph of a ciliary body melanocytoma in the anterior chamber angle. *(Courtesy of Wallace L. M. Alward, MD. From the* Iowa Glaucoma Curriculum *[curriculum.iowaglaucoma.org]. © The University of Iowa.)*

Camp DA, Yadav P, Dalvin LA, Shields CL. Glaucoma secondary to intraocular tumors: mechanisms and management. *Curr Opin Ophthalmol.* 2019;30(2):71–81.

Shields CL, Materin MA, Shields JA, Gershenbaum E, Singh AD, Smith A. Factors associated with elevated intraocular pressure in eyes with iris melanoma. *Br J Ophthalmol.* 2001;85(6):666–669.

Ocular Inflammation and Secondary Glaucoma

Inflammatory, or uveitic, glaucoma is a secondary glaucoma that often combines components of open-angle and angle-closure disease (Case Study 8-1). In individuals with uveitis, elevated IOP may be caused by a variety of mechanisms:

- edema of the trabecular meshwork
- endothelial cell dysfunction of the trabecular meshwork
- fibrin and inflammatory cells blocking outflow through the trabecular meshwork or Schlemm canal
- corticosteroid-induced reduction in outflow through the trabecular meshwork
- PAS blocking outflow
- prostaglandin-mediated breakdown of the blood–aqueous barrier

CASE STUDY 8-1 Uveitic glaucoma.
Courtesy of Alice Choi, MD, and Kelly Walton Muir, MD, MHSc.
Available at: aao.org/bcsccasestudy_section10

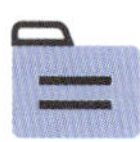

Appropriate therapy depends on the etiology of the uveitis. Most cases of anterior uveitis are idiopathic, but uveitides commonly associated with open-angle inflammatory glaucoma include Fuchs uveitis syndrome, herpes zoster iridocyclitis, herpes simplex keratouveitis, toxoplasmosis, juvenile idiopathic arthritis–associated uveitis, and pars planitis. See also BCSC Section 9, *Uveitis and Ocular Inflammation.*

The presence of KPs suggests anterior uveitis may be the cause of IOP elevation. Gonioscopic evaluation may reveal subtle trabecular meshwork precipitates. Occasionally, PAS or posterior synechiae with iris bombé (forward bulging of the peripheral iris in the setting of annular synechiae) may develop, resulting in angle closure.

The treatment of inflammatory glaucoma is complicated by the fact that corticosteroid therapy may increase IOP, likely by increasing outflow resistance, but also possibly by improving aqueous production, which can be decreased in eyes with intraocular inflammation. Miotic agents are not recommended in patients with anterior uveitis because they may exacerbate the inflammation and result in the formation of central posterior synechiae. Prostaglandin analogues may exacerbate inflammation in some eyes with uveitis and herpetic keratitis; however, this relationship is not clear, and some patients may benefit from their IOP-lowering effects without increased inflammation.

Some patients with uveitis develop low IOP. The etiology is unclear but may be related to a prostaglandin-mediated increase in uveoscleral outflow. Hyposecretion of aqueous humor (particularly if ciliary body detachment is present) has often been assumed to be the etiology for low IOP but has not been confirmed, because aqueous flow currently cannot be measured in the presence of uveitis.

Glaucomatocyclitic crisis

Glaucomatocyclitic crisis (also known as *Posner-Schlossman syndrome*) is an uncommon form of open-angle inflammatory glaucoma characterized by acute, unilateral episodes of markedly elevated IOP accompanied by low-grade anterior chamber inflammation. This condition most frequently affects middle-aged persons, who usually present with unilateral blurred vision and mild ocular pain. The anterior uveitis is mild, with few KPs, which are small, discrete, and round and which usually resolve spontaneously within a few weeks. On gonioscopy, KPs may be seen on the trabecular meshwork, suggesting a "trabeculitis." The elevated IOP may range between 40 and 50 mm Hg, and corneal edema may be present. In between episodes, the IOP usually returns to normal, but with increasing numbers of episodes, chronic secondary glaucoma may develop.

The etiology of this condition is unknown; theories include infections (eg, herpes simplex virus, cytomegalovirus [CMV], *Helicobacter pylori*) and autoimmune disease. Recurrent attacks of acute primary angle closure have been mistaken for this condition. In some cases in which glaucomatocyclitic crisis was initially diagnosed, CMV DNA was subsequently detected in the aqueous humor by polymerase chain reaction (see BCSC Section 9, *Uveitis and Ocular Inflammation,* for more on CMV). Distinguishing glaucomatocyclitic crisis from CMV is important, as specific antiviral therapy for CMV is available.

During a glaucomatocyclitic crisis, treatment should be initiated to control IOP. Topical corticosteroids and topical and/or oral nonsteroidal anti-inflammatory drugs (NSAIDs) may be considered to reduce inflammation. There is no evidence that long-term suppressive therapy with topical NSAIDs or corticosteroids is effective in preventing attacks. In some cases, filtering surgery is performed to prevent IOP spikes in eyes with advanced optic nerve damage or in those undergoing frequent attacks.

Fuchs uveitis syndrome

Fuchs uveitis syndrome (formerly, *Fuchs heterochromic iridocyclitis*) is a relatively rare, insidious, and chronic form of uveitis that is usually unilateral. There is no race or sex predilection, and it often manifests in young to middle adulthood. The syndrome is characterized by iris heterochromia, low-grade anterior chamber inflammation, posterior subcapsular cataracts, and IOP elevation. The heterochromia is caused by loss of iris pigment in the affected eye, which is usually hypochromic in dark irides and hyperchromic in light irides. The low-grade inflammation is often accompanied by small, stellate pancorneal KPs. Despite the low-grade inflammation, patients may be asymptomatic or have minimal symptoms and present with a nonhyperemic eye. Studies have shown an association between Fuchs uveitis syndrome and several infectious agents, including rubella virus, CMV, *Toxoplasma* species, and herpes simplex virus, although these links are difficult to prove given the frequency of those infectious agents in the population.

Secondary OAG occurs in approximately 15% of patients with Fuchs uveitis syndrome. Gonioscopic examination reveals multiple fine vessels that cross the trabecular meshwork (Fig 8-12). These vessels are usually not accompanied by a fibrous membrane and typically do not result in PAS formation or secondary angle closure, although in rare cases the neovascularization may be progressive. The vessels are fragile and may cause an anterior chamber hemorrhage, either spontaneously or as a result of trauma. A classic

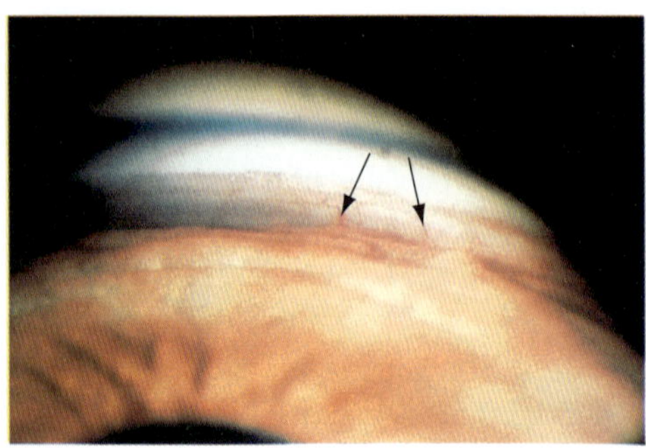

Figure 8-12 Fuchs uveitis syndrome. The goniophotograph shows fine vessels *(arrows)* crossing the trabecular meshwork. This neovascularization is not accompanied by a fibrovascular membrane and does not result in formation of peripheral anterior synechiae or in secondary angle closure. *(Courtesy of Steven T. Simmons, MD.)*

finding is anterior chamber hemorrhage after a paracentesis during intraocular surgery (Amsler sign).

Control of IOP may be difficult, and the IOP does not necessarily correlate with the degree of inflammation. Corticosteroids are generally not effective in treating the low-grade chronic inflammation, and their use can elevate the IOP. See BCSC Section 9, *Uveitis and Ocular Inflammation,* for further discussion.

Birnbaum AD, Tessler HH, Schultz KL, et al. Epidemiologic relationship between Fuchs heterochromic iridocyclitis and the United States rubella vaccination program. *Am J Ophthalmol.* 2007;144(3):424–428.

Elevated Episcleral Venous Pressure

Episcleral venous pressure (EVP) is an important factor in the determination of IOP. Normal EVP ranges between 6 and 9 mm Hg, depending on the measurement technique used. Elevated EVP can be caused by conditions that either obstruct venous outflow or involve vascular malformations (Table 8-1). For example, EVP is often increased in syndromes with facial hemangiomas, such as Sturge-Weber (encephalofacial angiomatosis) (Fig 8-13).

Patients with elevated EVP may note a chronic red eye without ocular discomfort, itching, or discharge. Occasionally, a distant history of substantial head trauma may suggest the cause of a carotid-cavernous sinus (high-flow) fistula or a dural (low-flow) fistula. However, most cases are idiopathic, and some may be familial. Clinically, patients with elevated EVP present with tortuous, dilated episcleral veins (Fig 8-14). These vascular

Table 8-1 Causes of Elevated Episcleral Venous Pressure

Vascular Malformations	Venous Obstruction
Arteriovenous fistula	Retrobulbar tumor
Carotid-cavernous sinus fistula	Superior vena cava syndrome
Dural fistula	Thyroid eye disease
Orbital varix	
Sturge-Weber syndrome (encephalofacial angiomatosis)	

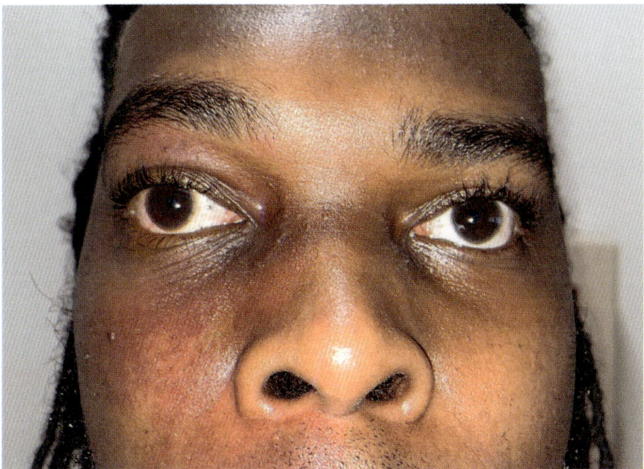

Figure 8-13 Facial hemangioma in a patient with Sturge-Weber syndrome and glaucoma. The hemangioma may be more difficult to recognize in individuals with more darkly pigmented skin. *(Courtesy of Richmond Woodward, MD.)*

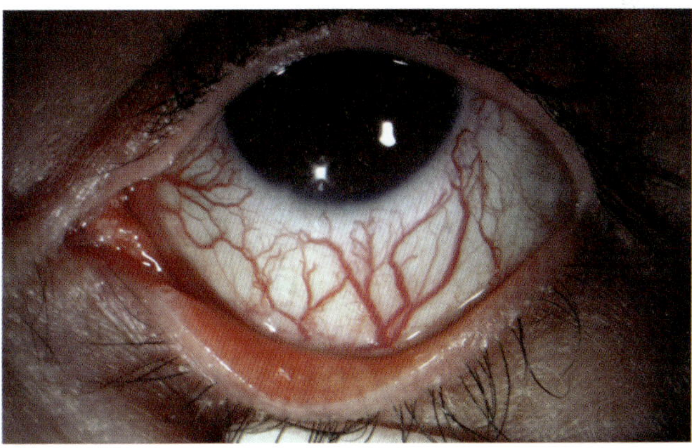

Figure 8-14 Prominent episcleral vessels in a patient with idiopathic elevated episcleral venous pressure. *(Courtesy of Jonathan Eisengart, MD.)*

abnormalities may be unilateral or bilateral. Gonioscopy may reveal blood in the Schlemm canal (see Chapter 4, Fig 4-6). In rare instances, signs of ocular ischemia or venous stasis may be present. Sudden, severe carotid-cavernous fistulas may be accompanied by proptosis and other orbital or neurologic signs. In such cases, magnetic resonance imaging or angiography to rule out a vascular malformation may be appropriate. If these tests fail to show an abnormality and the clinical suspicion is high, traditional angiography with neuroradiologic intervention (eg, coiling of fistula) may be considered when the benefits to the patient outweigh the risks.

Topical ocular hypotensive medications, particularly those that reduce aqueous production, may be effective in some patients. Because of the etiology of the condition, laser trabeculoplasty is not effective. Glaucoma filtering surgery may be indicated. However, given the risk of a ciliochoroidal effusion or suprachoroidal hemorrhage, prophylactic sclerotomies or scleral windows should be considered.

Trauma and Surgery

Nonpenetrating, or blunt, trauma to the eye may cause a variety of anterior segment conditions that can lead to secondary glaucoma, including the following:

- inflammation
- hyphema
- angle recession
- lens subluxation (see the discussion of ectopia lentis in Chapter 10)

These findings, particularly when in combination, often lead to elevated IOP initially after trauma. This elevation tends to be brief but may be protracted and result in glaucoma.

Siderosis or *chalcosis* from a metallic foreign body retained in the eye after a penetrating or perforating injury may lead to IOP elevation and glaucoma.

Chemical injuries, particularly those involving alkali, may cause acute IOP elevation as a result of inflammation, shrinkage of scleral collagen, release of chemical mediators such as prostaglandins, direct damage to the anterior chamber angle, or compromised anterior uveal circulation. Recurrent inflammation or damage to the trabecular meshwork may progress to glaucoma over months or years after a chemical injury.

Traumatic hyphema

The risk of elevated IOP after a traumatic hyphema is increased with recurrent hemorrhage, or rebleeding. The average reported frequency of rebleeding after an initial hyphema is approximately 5%, but it varies significantly with different study populations. Rebleeding usually occurs within 3–7 days of the initial hyphema and may be related to normal clot retraction and lysis. In general, the larger the hyphema, the higher the incidence of increased IOP, although small hemorrhages may also be associated with marked IOP elevation, particularly when the angle is already compromised. Increased IOP occurs as a result of obstruction of the trabecular meshwork with red blood cells (RBCs), inflammatory cells, debris, and fibrin, as well as from direct injury to the trabecular meshwork from the blunt trauma. Gentle gonioscopic examination in individuals with blunt trauma may reveal a subtle hyphema. In addition to glaucomatous damage, prolonged IOP elevation in an eye with a hyphema increases the risk of corneal blood staining (Fig 8-15).

Individuals with sickle cell hemoglobinopathies have an increased risk of elevated IOP following hyphema and are more susceptible to the development of optic neuropathy. Normal RBCs pass through the trabecular meshwork without difficulty. However, in the sickle cell hemoglobinopathies, the low pH of the aqueous humor causes the RBCs to sickle. These more rigid cells become trapped in the trabecular meshwork, and even low numbers of sickle-shaped RBCs may cause marked elevations in IOP. In addition, in sickle cell disease (SCD), the optic nerve is more sensitive to elevated IOP, and affected patients are prone to development of anterior ischemic optic neuropathy and central

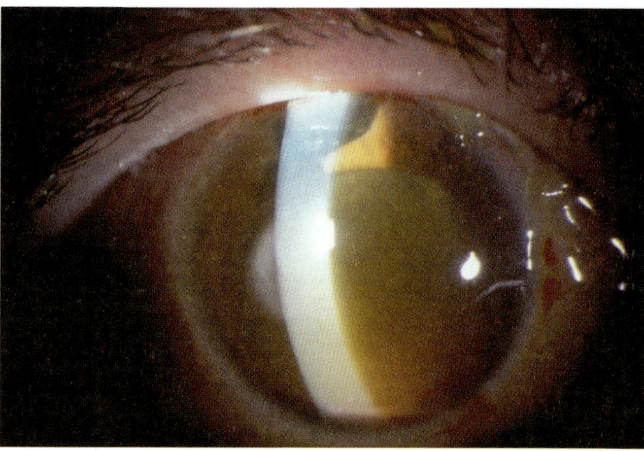

Figure 8-15 Corneal blood staining following trauma. Note the area of layered heme in the inferior angle. *(Courtesy of Wallace L. M. Alward, MD. From the* Iowa Glaucoma Curriculum *[curriculum.iowaglaucoma.org]. © The University of Iowa.)*

retinal artery occlusion as a result of compromised microvascular perfusion. Testing for SCD, which is part of routine newborn screening, may be requested if the diagnosis is unknown.

Management For patients with uncomplicated hyphema, conservative management is generally appropriate and includes wearing an eye shield, limiting physical activity, and elevating the head. Topical and oral corticosteroids may reduce associated inflammation, although their effect on rebleeding is debatable. If substantial ciliary spasm or photophobia occurs, cycloplegic agents may be helpful, but they have no proven benefit for prevention of rebleeding. Oral administration of aminocaproic acid has been shown to reduce rebleeding in some studies. However, this has not been confirmed in all studies, and systemic adverse effects, such as hypotension, syncope, abdominal pain, and nausea, can be considerable. Also, discontinuation of aminocaproic acid may be associated with clot lysis and additional IOP elevation.

Medical treatment of elevated IOP in patients with hyphema includes ocular hypotensive agents, particularly aqueous suppressants, and hyperosmotic agents. It has been suggested that patients with sickle cell hemoglobinopathies avoid carbonic anhydrase inhibitors (CAIs) because these agents may increase the sickling tendency in the anterior chamber by further lowering the pH; however, this relationship has not been firmly established. The use of systemic CAIs and hyperosmotic agents may induce a sickle crisis in susceptible individuals who are significantly dehydrated. Accordingly, systemic CAIs should be avoided in people with SCD and considered with caution in individuals with sickle cell trait. Adrenergic agonists with significant α_1-agonist effects (apraclonidine, dipivefrin, epinephrine) should also be avoided in patients with SCD, because of the potential for anterior segment vasoconstriction with their use. Parasympathomimetic agents may not be appropriate in patients with traumatic hyphema because they may increase inflammation and result in more centrally located posterior synechiae.

Indications for surgical intervention in traumatic hyphema vary (see also BCSC Section 8, *External Disease and Cornea*). For patients with SCD, the threshold for surgical intervention may be lower, given these patients' increased risk of optic neuropathy from elevated IOP. In young children (with or without SCD), obstruction of vision by the hyphema or corneal blood staining may justify early surgical intervention to reduce the risk of amblyopia. If surgery for elevated IOP becomes necessary, anterior chamber irrigation is commonly performed first. If a total hyphema is present, pupillary block may occur; thus, an iridectomy is helpful at the time of the washout. If the IOP remains uncontrolled, filtering surgery may be required. Some surgeons prefer to perform glaucoma filtering surgery with the anterior chamber washout to obtain immediate control of IOP, relieve any pupillary block, and reduce the risk of elevated IOP in the future from damage to the trabecular meshwork.

Campagna JA. Traumatic hyphema: current strategies. *Focal Points: Clinical Modules for Ophthalmologists.* American Academy of Ophthalmology; 2007, module 10.

Gharaibeh A, Savage HI, Scherer RW, Goldberg MF, Lindsley K. Medical interventions for traumatic hyphema. *Cochrane Database Syst Rev.* 2019;1(1):CD005431. https://doi.org/10.1002/14651858.CD005431.pub4

Hemolytic and ghost cell glaucoma

Hemolytic glaucoma, ghost cell glaucoma, or both may develop after a vitreous hemorrhage. In *hemolytic glaucoma,* hemoglobin-laden macrophages block the trabecular meshwork. Red-tinged cells can be seen floating in the anterior chamber, and the trabecular meshwork may appear reddish brown.

Ghost cells are small, degenerated khaki-colored RBCs that have lost their intracellular hemoglobin and become less pliable than normal RBCs (Fig 8-16). RBCs degenerate within 1 to 3 months after a vitreous hemorrhage. They gain access to the anterior chamber through a disrupted hyaloid face, which can occur spontaneously or as a result

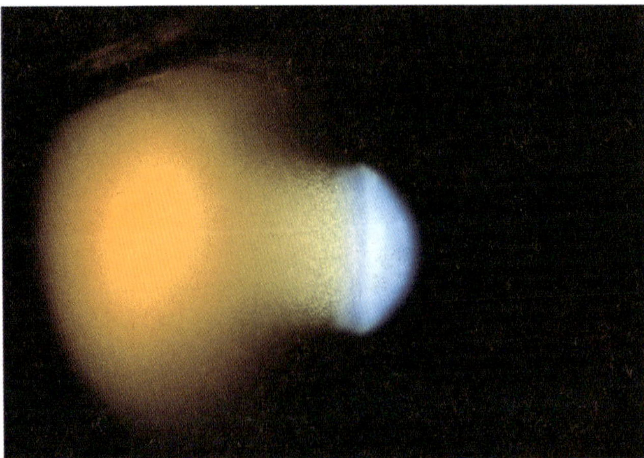

Figure 8-16 Ghost cell glaucoma: the classic appearance of ghost cells in the anterior chamber. These small, khaki-colored cells can become layered, as occurs in a hyphema or hypopyon. *(Courtesy of Ronald L. Gross, MD.)*

of trauma or previous surgery (eg, pars plana vitrectomy, cataract extraction, capsulotomy). The ghost cells obstruct the trabecular meshwork and cause IOP elevation *(ghost cell glaucoma).*

Patients with ghost cell glaucoma typically present with elevated IOP and a history of or current vitreous hemorrhage. On gonioscopy, the angle appears normal except for possible layering of ghost cells in the inferior angle. A long-standing vitreous hemorrhage may be present, with characteristic khaki coloration and clumps of extracellular pigmentation from degenerated hemoglobin.

In both hemolytic glaucoma and ghost cell glaucoma, IOP typically normalizes once the hemorrhage has cleared. Medical therapy with aqueous suppressants is the preferred initial approach. If medical therapy fails to control the IOP, some patients may require anterior chamber irrigation, pars plana vitrectomy, and/or incisional glaucoma surgery. When a collection of RBCs or ghost cells is present in the vitreous, a pars plana vitrectomy is likely necessary for IOP control.

Traumatic, or angle-recession, glaucoma

Angle recession is a common finding after blunt ocular trauma and involves a tear between the longitudinal and circular muscle fibers of the ciliary body. Although angle recession is not necessarily associated with immediate IOP elevation and glaucoma, it is a sign of probable damage to the trabecular meshwork. Traumatic glaucoma is chronic and usually unilateral. It can occur immediately after the ocular trauma or months to years later. Traumatic glaucoma resembles POAG in presentation and clinical course but can be distinguished by its gonioscopic findings (Figs 8-17, 8-18):

- widening of the ciliary body band
- absent or torn iris processes
- white, glistening scleral spur
- irregular and dark pigmentation in the angle
- PAS at the border of the recession

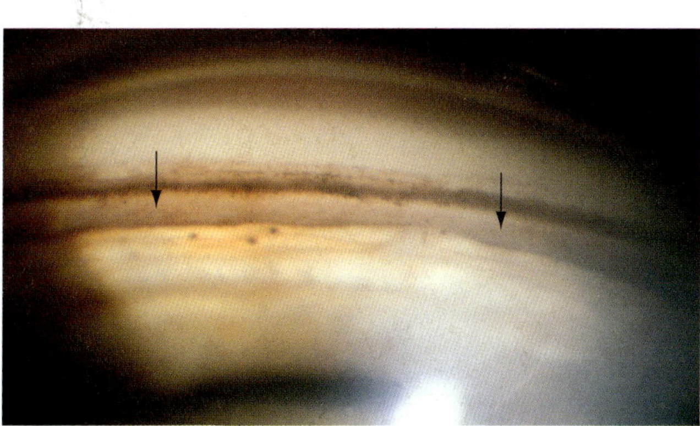

Figure 8-17 Goniophotograph of angle recession. Angle recession occurs when the ciliary body is torn between the longitudinal and circular fibers of the ciliary body, resulting in a deepened angle recess *(arrows).* The dark circular deposits located on the peripheral iris represent old heme. *(Reproduced from Alward WLM, Longmuir RA.* Color Atlas of Gonioscopy. *2nd ed. American Academy of Ophthalmology; 2008:89. Fig 9-50.)*

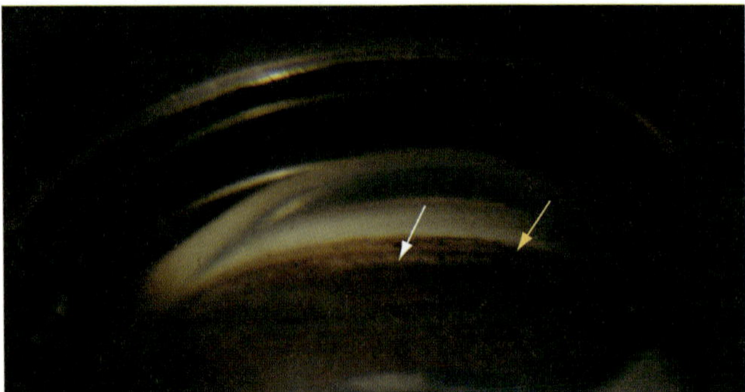

Figure 8-18 Gonioscopic photograph of an eye with angle recession. The recessed angle *(white arrow)* can be more easily appreciated adjacent to the normal portion of the angle *(yellow arrow)*. *(Courtesy of Richard Lee, MD, PhD.)*

Traumatic glaucoma should be considered in a patient with unilateral IOP elevation. The patient's history may reveal the contributing incident, although it may have occurred in the distant past and hence been forgotten. Examination may reveal findings consistent with previous ocular trauma, such as corneal scars, iris injury, angle abnormalities, focal anterior subcapsular cataracts, and phacodonesis. Comparing gonioscopic findings in the affected eye with those in the fellow eye may help the clinician identify areas of recession.

More extensive angle recession is associated with a greater reduction in outflow facility and an increased risk of glaucoma. However, even with substantial angle recession, this risk is not high. Although the risk of developing glaucoma decreases appreciably after several years, it is still present even 25 years or more after injury. In a significant proportion (up to 50%) of fellow eyes, IOP elevation occurs, suggesting that some eyes with trauma that go on to develop glaucoma may have been predisposed to POAG. Alternatively, it is possible that trauma to the fellow eyes occurred in these cases. Because it is not possible to predict which eyes will develop glaucoma, regular monitoring of all eyes with angle recession and their fellow eyes is recommended.

The treatment of traumatic glaucoma is often initiated with aqueous suppressants, prostaglandin analogues, and α_2-adrenergic agonists. Miotics may be useful, but paradoxical responses of increased IOP may occur. The role of laser trabeculoplasty in traumatic glaucoma has not been well studied, but this technique can be considered for these patients. Incisional glaucoma surgery may be required in order to control the IOP in patients not responding to medical therapy.

Surgically induced IOP elevation

Conventional surgical procedures such as cataract extraction are occasionally associated with transient IOP elevation. Similarly, laser surgery—including trabeculoplasty, LPI, and posterior capsulotomy—may be complicated by posttreatment IOP elevation. Although the IOP may rise as high as 50 mm Hg or more, these elevations are usually transient, lasting from a few hours to a few days. Other procedures, including vitrectomy and penetrating keratoplasty, may be followed by a sustained increase in IOP. The exact mechanism of the

IOP elevation is not always known. However, the presence of inflammatory cells, RBCs, and debris; pigment release; mechanical deformation of the trabecular meshwork; oxidative damage; and angle closure may be involved.

Agents used as adjuncts to intraocular surgery or postoperative treatment (eg, corticosteroids) may also cause secondary IOP elevation. For example, the injection of viscoelastic substances into the anterior chamber may result in a transient and possibly severe postoperative increase in IOP. Cohesive viscoelastic agents, especially in higher-molecular-weight forms, may be more likely to cause an IOP increase than dispersive viscoelastics. Silicone oil, used in retinal surgery, can induce glaucoma in several ways: overfill of oil, pupillary block, emulsified oil obstructing the meshwork, and chronic inflammation causing scarring of the outflow track.

Postoperative IOP elevation, even over a short period, can cause considerable damage to the optic nerve in susceptible individuals. Eyes with preexisting glaucoma are particularly at risk of further damage; thus, it is critical to monitor IOP soon after conventional or laser surgery and to consider treatment with IOP-lowering medications at the time of surgery. If a substantial rise in IOP occurs, IOP-lowering therapy may be required, including the use of topical β-blockers, α_2-adrenergic agonists, or CAIs. If postoperative inflammation is present, prostaglandin analogues may be deferred until the inflammation has resolved. Paracentesis with release of aqueous fluid (and possibly viscoelastic) can be used to rapidly lower the IOP if it is substantially high. Persistent IOP elevation may require filtering surgery.

Intraocular lenses The implantation of an intraocular lens (IOL) can lead to a variety of secondary glaucomas, including the following:

- uveitis-glaucoma-hyphema (UGH) syndrome
- secondary pigmentary glaucoma
- pseudophakic pupillary block (see Chapter 10)

UGH syndrome is a secondary inflammatory glaucoma typically caused by chafing of the iris or ciliary body by a malpositioned IOL. It is characterized by 1 or more of the following:

- chronic inflammation
- elevated IOP
- recurrent hyphemas
- cystoid macular edema
- iris neovascularization

Although originally associated with malpositioned anterior chamber IOLs, this syndrome can also occur after implantation of a posterior chamber IOL in the ciliary sulcus or one that is suture-fixated to the iris or sclera. Implantation of single-piece acrylic IOLs in the sulcus is a particular risk factor for UGH syndrome and should be avoided. Gonioscopy and ultrasound biomicroscopy may be helpful in revealing the IOL's exact position in relation to the iris and ciliary body. Persistent or recurrent cases often require IOL repositioning or IOL exchange, which can be technically challenging if synechiae and/or an open posterior capsule is present. UGH syndrome may be mimicked in patients with neovascularization of the internal lip of a corneoscleral wound, which may result in recurrent spontaneous hyphemas and elevated IOP. Laser ablation of the vessels may successfully resolve these cases.

Penetrating keratoplasty Secondary glaucoma is a common complication after penetrating keratoplasty (PKP) and occurs with greater frequency in aphakic and pseudophakic patients and after a second graft. Wound-induced distortion of the trabecular meshwork and progressive angle closure are the most common causes of glaucoma after PKP. Attempts to minimize these changes with different-sized donor grafts, peripheral iridectomies, and surgical repair of the iris sphincter have been only partially successful. Alternative procedures, such as lamellar stromal or endothelial grafts, may be associated with a lower risk of elevated IOP. Long-term use of topical corticosteroids after PKP is another potential cause of elevated IOP and secondary glaucoma. Surgical interventions to treat glaucoma after PKP are associated with an increased risk of graft rejection and failure. See BCSC Section 8, *External Disease and Cornea,* for further discussion of PKP.

Schwartz-Matsuo Syndrome

Individuals with a rhegmatogenous retinal detachment (RRD) typically have lower IOPs, presumably because of increased outflow of fluid through the exposed retinal pigment epithelium. Schwartz was the first to describe elevated IOP associated with an RRD. Matsuo later demonstrated the presence of photoreceptor outer segments in the aqueous humor of patients with RRDs. The postulated mechanism of IOP elevation is the liberation of photoreceptor outer segments, which migrate through the vitreous into the anterior chamber and trabecular meshwork, where they impede aqueous outflow. The IOP tends to normalize after successful surgery to reattach the retina.

Drugs and Glaucoma

Corticosteroid-induced glaucoma is an OAG caused by use of topical, periocular, intravitreous, inhaled, or oral corticosteroids. It mimics POAG in its presentation and clinical course. Approximately one-third of the population without glaucoma demonstrates an IOP increase of between 6 and 15 mm Hg in response to corticosteroids, and only a small percentage (4%–6%) has a significant IOP elevation of more than 15 mm Hg while receiving a short course of corticosteroids. A high percentage (up to 95%) of patients with POAG experience an ocular hypertensive response to topical corticosteroids. The type and potency of the agent, the route and frequency of its administration, and the susceptibility of the patient all affect the timing and extent of the IOP rise. Risk factors for corticosteroid-induced glaucoma include a history of POAG, a first-degree relative with POAG, and very young age (<6 years) or older age. The elevated IOP is a result of increased resistance to aqueous outflow in the trabecular meshwork. See also BCSC Section 9, *Uveitis and Ocular Inflammation,* for further discussion of corticosteroids.

Corticosteroid-induced IOP elevation may develop within weeks, months, or years of use of the drug; thus, regular monitoring of IOP is recommended in patients receiving these agents. In general, the risk of IOP elevation is correlated with the glucocorticoid potency of the drug and its ability to penetrate the ocular surface. For example, some corticosteroid preparations, such as fluorometholone, rimexolone, medrysone, or loteprednol, are less likely to raise IOP than are prednisolone, dexamethasone, or difluprednate (see BCSC Section 2, *Fundamentals and Principles of Ophthalmology*). However, even weaker corticosteroids or lower concentrations of stronger drugs can raise IOP in susceptible individuals. A corticosteroid-induced rise in IOP may cause glaucomatous optic nerve damage in some patients.

The cause of the IOP elevation may be related to an underlying ocular disease, such as anterior uveitis, as opposed to corticosteroid use. After the corticosteroid is discontinued, the IOP usually decreases with a time course similar to or slightly longer than that of the onset of elevation. However, elevated IOP may persist in some cases.

IOP may also become elevated in patients who have excessive levels of endogenous corticosteroids (eg, Cushing syndrome). When the corticosteroid-producing tissue is excised, IOP generally returns to normal.

Periocular injection of a corticosteroid, particularly triamcinolone acetonide, may result in elevated IOP. Medical therapy may lower the IOP, but some patients require excision of the corticosteroid depot or glaucoma surgery.

Intravitreous corticosteroid injection is associated with transient elevations in IOP in more than 50% of patients. Up to 25% of these patients require topical medications to control the IOP, and 1%–2% require incisional glaucoma surgery. In contrast, intravitreous implants that release corticosteroid are frequently associated with elevated IOP, often requiring patients to undergo incisional glaucoma surgery for IOP control. Surgical treatment has a high success rate in lowering IOP in these patients; laser trabeculoplasty may also be of benefit.

Cycloplegic drugs can increase IOP in individuals with narrowed or open angles. Dilation for ophthalmoscopy may increase IOP; people at greater risk include those with POAG, pseudoexfoliation syndrome, or pigment dispersion syndrome, as well as patients receiving miotic therapy.

Intravitreous injection of *anti–vascular endothelial growth factor* (anti-VEGF) agents, which is a common treatment for choroidal neovascularization and macular edema, may result in a transient rise in IOP. Over time, repeated injections may result in sustained IOP elevation. In the Study of Comparative Treatments for Retinal Vein Occlusion 2, of those participants who were not taking glaucoma medications before treatment of the vein occlusion, 8% had IOP elevation more than 10 mm Hg over baseline, and 2% had IOP higher than 35 mm Hg through month 60. The etiology of the elevated IOP is unknown, but theories include increased inflammation and injury to or mechanical blockage of the trabecular meshwork.

Aref AA, Scott IU, VanVeldhuisen PC, et al; Study of Comparative Treatments for Retinal Vein Occlusion 2 (SCORE2) Investigator Group. Intraocular Pressure–Related Events After Anti-Vascular Endothelial Growth Factor Therapy for Macular Edema Due to Central Retinal Vein Occlusion or Hemiretinal Vein Occlusion: SCORE2 Report 16 on a Secondary Analysis of a Randomized Clinical Trial. *JAMA Ophthalmol.* 2021;139(12):1285–1291.

CHAPTER 9

Primary Angle-Closure Disease

This chapter includes related videos. Go to aao.org/bcscvideo_section10 or scan the QR codes in the text to access this content.

This chapter also includes a case study. Go to aao.org/bcsccasestudy_section10 or scan the QR code in the text to access this content.

Highlights

- Primary angle-closure (PAC) disease is a common cause of glaucoma, particularly in Asian populations.
- Although pupillary block is the most common mechanism in the pathogenesis of PAC disease, multiple mechanisms have been recognized, including plateau iris, which is a contributing factor in up to one-third of eyes with PAC.
- Gonioscopy should be performed in all patients in whom glaucoma or narrow angles are suspected, including individuals with hyperopia and older phakic patients.
- Treatment of PAC disease is tailored to the individual patient and may include medical therapy, laser peripheral iridotomy, laser iridoplasty, or lens extraction.

Introduction

Angle closure refers to an anatomical configuration in which there is mechanical blockage of the trabecular meshwork by the peripheral iris. Anatomical alterations in anterior segment structures result in obstruction of the iridocorneal drainage angle either through apposition *(iridotrabecular contact)* or because of the formation of peripheral anterior synechiae (PAS; adhesions of the peripheral iris to the trabecular meshwork).

Angle closure is divided into 2 main categories—primary angle closure and secondary angle closure—based on the etiology of the disease. In *primary angle closure,* no secondary pathologic condition can be identified; there is only an anatomical predisposition to angle closure. In *secondary angle closure,* an identifiable pathologic condition—such as an intumescent lens, iris neovascularization, chronic inflammation, corneal endothelial migration into the angle, or epithelial ingrowth—initiates the angle closure. See Chapter 10 for discussion of secondary angle closure.

The primary form of angle closure is a spectrum of disease and can occur in an acute or chronic form. The term *primary angle-closure disease (PACD)* refers to appositional

Table 9-1 Classification of Primary Angle-Closure Disease

Stage	Definition
Primary angle-closure suspect (PACS)	Iridotrabecular contact ≥180° but no evidence of trabecular meshwork or glaucomatous optic nerve damage
Primary angle closure (PAC)	Iridotrabecular contact ≥180° with statistically elevated IOP or PAS but no glaucomatous optic nerve damage
Primary angle-closure glaucoma (PACG)	PAC but with glaucomatous optic neuropathy

IOP = intraocular pressure; PAS = peripheral anterior synechiae.

or synechial closure of the anterior chamber angle. The current classification categorizes patients with PACD or persons at risk as follows, based on the severity of the condition (Table 9-1):

- *primary angle-closure suspect (PACS),* in which the eye has an anatomical configuration that increases the risk of developing angle-closure disease
- *primary angle closure (PAC),* in which trabecular meshwork damage or dysfunction is already present, characterized by PAS or statistically elevated intraocular pressure (IOP)
- *primary angle-closure glaucoma (PACG),* which is characterized by PAS or statistically elevated IOP (>21 mm Hg) and glaucomatous optic neuropathy (optic nerve cupping, retinal nerve fiber layer loss, and/or visual field loss consistent with glaucoma)

The worldwide prevalence of angle-closure glaucoma (ACG) has been estimated to reach over 23 million in 2020 and over 32 million in 2040. ACG is more common in females and in certain ethnic groups, such as particular Asian populations and the Inuit. Prevalence rates in European and African populations are generally lower than those in Asian populations, but genetic heterogeneity can result in widely varying prevalence within populations of the same region. ACG has been estimated to account for over 90% of blindness due to glaucoma in the Chinese population.

The angle-closure–related disorders are a diverse group of diseases. Although the various forms of angle closure are united by the presence of PAS or iridotrabecular apposition, different mechanisms are responsible for these features. Moreover, the clinical presentation of angle closure varies from the abrupt and dramatic onset of acute angle closure to the insidious and asymptomatic presentation of chronic disease.

To initiate the appropriate therapy, the ophthalmologist must identify the anatomical changes in the angle and the underlying pathophysiology that has precipitated the disease. Early diagnosis and treatment of most forms of angle closure or narrowing can sometimes be curative.

Chan EW, Li X, Tham YC, et al. Glaucoma in Asia: regional prevalence variations and future projections. *Br J Ophthalmol.* 2016;100(1):78–85.

Gedde SJ, Chen PP, Muir KW, et al; American Academy of Ophthalmology Preferred Practice Pattern Glaucoma Panel. Primary Angle-Closure Disease Preferred Practice Pattern. *Ophthalmology.* 2021;128(1):P30–P70. doi:10.1016/j.ophtha.2020.10.021

Tham YC, Li X, Wong TY, Quigley HA, Aung T, Cheng CY. Global prevalence of glaucoma and projections of glaucoma burden through 2040: a systematic review and meta-analysis. *Ophthalmology.* 2014;121(11):2081–2090.

Yip JL, Foster PJ. Ethnic differences in primary angle-closure glaucoma. *Curr Opin Ophthalmol.* 2006;17(2):175–180.

Pathogenesis and Pathophysiology

The hallmark of angle closure is the apposition or adhesion of the peripheral iris to the trabecular meshwork. The portion of the anterior chamber angle affected by such apposition is described as closed, and drainage of aqueous humor through the angle is reduced as a result. Such closure may be transient and intermittent *(appositional)* or permanent *(synechial).* These 2 forms of angle closure can be distinguished by means of dynamic (also called *compression* or *indentation*) gonioscopy. The IOP becomes elevated as a result of reduced aqueous humor outflow through the trabecular meshwork.

In addition to these traditional mechanisms of angle closure, it has been suggested that dynamic changes in iris volume and water content normally occurring in the human eye are dysfunctional in patients with PACD and may play an important role in its pathogenesis. A variety of factors that cause pupillary dilation—certain drugs, pain, emotional upset, and fright, among others—may precipitate acute angle closure.

The major mechanism in the pathogenesis of PACD is pupillary block. However, in up to one-third of eyes with angle closure, plateau iris is a contributing factor.

Aptel F, Denis P. Optical coherence tomography quantitative analysis of iris volume changes after pharmacologic mydriasis. *Ophthalmology.* 2010;117(1):3–10.

Pupillary Block

Pupillary block is the most frequent cause of angle closure. While the pathophysiology of PACD is complex and not completely understood, pupillary block is recognized as a contributing cause in most cases. In eyes with pupillary block, the flow of aqueous humor from the posterior chamber through the pupil is impeded at the level of the lens–iris interface, and this obstruction creates a pressure gradient between the posterior and anterior chambers, causing the peripheral iris to bow forward against the trabecular meshwork (Fig 9-1A). Pupillary block is maximal when the pupil is in the mid-dilated position. In most cases of angle closure, pupillary block results from anatomical factors at the lens–iris interface. Pupillary block may be broken by an unobstructed peripheral iridectomy or iridotomy.

In phakic eyes, the lens plays a critical role in pupillary block. Studies have found that a high lens vault (defined as how far the lens protrudes anterior to the plane of the scleral spur) is a major risk factor for PACD. Iris thickness, area, and volume have also been strongly correlated with a narrower angle and risk for angle closure. Smaller anterior

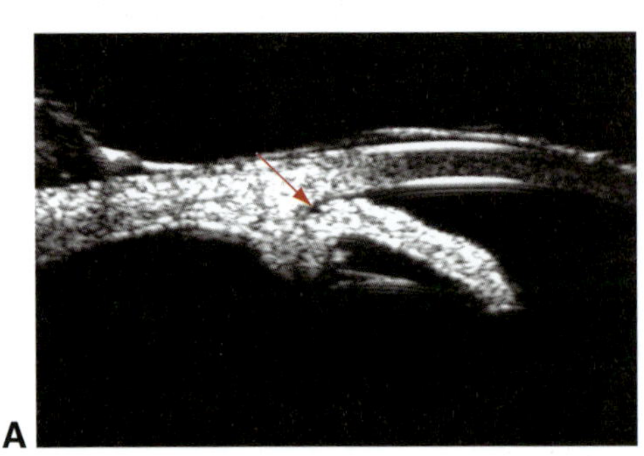

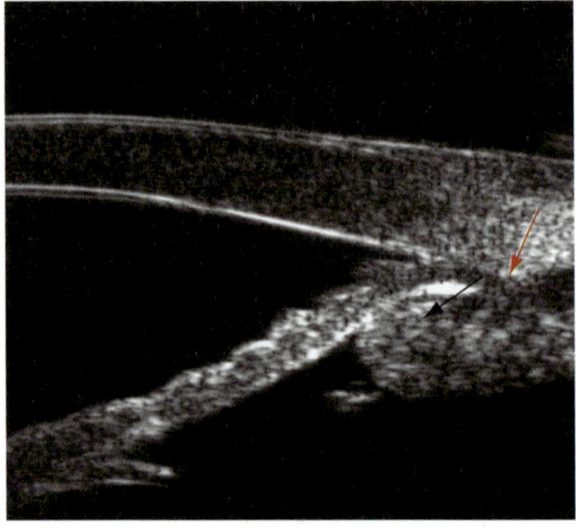

Figure 9-1 Ultrasound biomicroscopy (UBM) imaging. Assessment of UBM images for angle closure begins with identifying the scleral spur (*red arrow* in parts A and B) and determining the degree of angle crowding (see also Chapter 4, Fig 4-11). **A,** Eye with pupillary block. Anterior bowing of the iris occluding the trabecular meshwork is shown. **B,** Eye with plateau iris anatomy. A large, anteriorly rotated ciliary process *(black arrow)* causing appositional angle closure is evident. *(Part A courtesy of Shan C. Lin, MD; part B courtesy of Sunita Radhakrishnan, MD, from the Glaucoma Center of San Francisco archives.)*

chamber dimensions, including anterior chamber depth, width, area, and volume, are also risk factors.

Plateau Iris and Iris-Induced Angle Closure

In plateau iris and iris-induced angle closure, the peripheral iris is apposed to the trabecular meshwork. Iris-induced angle closure can be the result of developmental anomalies such as anterior cleavage abnormalities, in which the iris insertion into the scleral spur or trabecular meshwork is more anterior than normal; a thick peripheral iris, which on dilation "rolls" into the trabecular meshwork; and/or anteriorly displaced ciliary processes (Fig 9-1B), which may secondarily rotate the peripheral iris forward *(plateau iris)* into the trabecular meshwork (see the section Plateau Iris as a Mechanism of Angle Closure). Although it was thought that iris-induced angle closure occurs in aniridia because of rotation of the rudimentary iris leaflets into the angle, evidence suggests that this phenomenon occurs as a result of intraocular surgery rather than spontaneously.

The Role of Medications in Angle Closure

In predisposed eyes with shallow anterior chambers, either mydriatic or miotic agents can precipitate acute angle closure. Mydriatic agents include not only dilating drops but also systemic medications with sympathomimetic or anticholinergic activity that may cause mild pupillary dilation. The effect of miotics is to pull the peripheral iris away from the anterior chamber angle. However, strong miotics may also cause the zonular fibers of the lens to relax, allowing the lens–iris interface to move forward. In addition, use of these agents results in greater iris–lens contact, thus potentially increasing pupillary block. For these reasons, miotics, especially the cholinesterase inhibitors, may induce or worsen angle closure.

In patients with narrow angles, gonioscopy should be repeated soon after miotic drugs are administered.

Systemic drugs with adrenergic (sympathomimetic) or anticholinergic (parasympatholytic) activity have the potential to cause angle closure. They include

- allergy and cold medications
  - adrenergic agents, including ephedrine
  - antihistamines, such as diphenhydramine
- bronchodilator medications (for asthma and chronic obstructive pulmonary disease), such as ipratropium bromide and tiotropium bromide
- antidepressants, anxiolytics, and antipsychotics
  - selective serotonin reuptake inhibitors, such as fluoxetine and paroxetine
  - tricyclic antidepressants, such as amitriptyline and imipramine
  - antihistamine-anxiolytics, such as hydroxyzine
  - phenothiazines, such as chlorpromazine
- urinary antispasmodics, such as tolterodine and oxybutynin
- gastrointestinal drugs
  - antihistamines, including cimetidine
- muscle relaxants, such as orphenadrine and trihexyphenidyl
- antinauseants, including promethazine

Although systemic administration generally does not raise intraocular drug levels as much as topical administration, even slight mydriasis in a patient with a critically narrow angle can induce angle closure. When drugs with adrenergic or anticholinergic activity are administered to patients with potentially occludable angles, it is important to inform the patient of the risk and consider laser peripheral iridotomy.

Risk Factors

Race and Ethnicity

The prevalence of PACG in patients older than 40 years varies greatly, depending on race and ethnicity. For example, it is 0.1%–0.6% in people of African ancestry, 0.1%–0.4% in European-derived populations, 0.3%–2.2% in Japanese individuals, 0.4%–1.7% in Chinese individuals, and 2.1%–4.8% in Inuit persons. Some of this variation in prevalence—for example, between White individuals and Inuit individuals—can be explained by differences in the biometric parameters (anterior chamber depth [ACD], axial length) of these groups. However, the increased prevalence of PACG in Chinese and other East Asian populations cannot be explained by major biometric parameters alone. Anterior segment anatomical studies suggest that other parameters, such as iris thickness and area, dynamic changes in the iris, lens vault, and anterior chamber width (ACW), can be significant contributing factors. Anterior segment optical coherence tomography (AS-OCT) shows that, compared with White persons, Chinese individuals have a shallower ACD, thicker iris, smaller ACW, and increased iris thickness and area when going from light to dark conditions. It has become increasingly clear that the burden of PACG is greater in Asian countries. However, recent increases in the prevalence of myopia (with associated axial elongation) in Asian countries—particularly urban areas—may counterbalance these trends in PACG.

Day AC, Baio G, Gazzard G, et al. The prevalence of primary angle closure glaucoma in European derived populations: a systematic review. *Br J Ophthalmol.* 2012;96(9): 1162–1167.

Quigley HA. Angle-closure glaucoma—simpler answers to complex mechanisms: LXVI Edward Jackson Memorial Lecture. *Am J Ophthalmol.* 2009;148(5):657–669.

Ocular Biometrics

Eyes with PACD tend to have a small, "crowded" anterior segment and short axial length (AL). The most important factors predisposing an eye to angle closure are a shallow anterior chamber, a thick lens, increased anterior curvature of the lens, a short AL, and a small corneal diameter and radius of curvature. Studies using anterior segment imaging have identified additional parameters that are risk factors for angle closure, including increased iris thickness and area and greater lens vault (see the discussion in Chapter 4 on anterior segment imaging). An ACD of <2.5 mm predisposes patients to PAC; in most patients with PAC, the ACD is <2.1 mm. Improvements in ocular biometry techniques have allowed researchers to demonstrate a clear association between ACD and the development of PAS. While primary PAS are uncommon in eyes with ACD >2.4 mm, there is a strong correlation between increasing PAS formation and an ACD of <2.4 mm. However, in some cases, angle closure occurs in eyes with deep anterior chambers, with plateau iris as a cause. Of note, some instruments measure true ACD (endothelium to lens capsule), whereas others (eg, IOLMaster biometer, Carl Zeiss Meditec) measure the distance from the epithelium to the lens capsule. The ACD thresholds noted previously refer to true ACD.

Aung T, Nolan WP, Machin D, et al. Anterior chamber depth and the risk of primary angle closure in 2 East Asian populations. *Arch Ophthalmol.* 2005;123(4):527–532.

Age

The prevalence of angle closure increases with each decade after 40 years of age. This has been explained by the increasing thickness and forward movement of the lens with age and the resultant increase in iridolenticular contact. PACD is rare in persons younger than 40 years, and the etiology of angle closure in young individuals is most often related to structural or developmental anomalies such as plateau iris and retinopathy of prematurity rather than pupillary block.

Ritch R, Chang BM, Liebmann JM. Angle closure in younger patients. *Ophthalmology.* 2003;110(10):1880–1889.

Sex

Primary angle closure is 2–4 times more common in females than in males, irrespective of race. Studies assessing ocular biometry data have found that women tend to have smaller anterior segments and shorter ALs than men. However, these differences do not appear to be large enough to completely explain the sex predilection.

Family History and Genetics

The prevalence of PAC is increased in first-degree relatives of affected individuals. In White individuals, the prevalence of PAC in first-degree relatives has been reported to be between 1% and 12%, whereas results from a survey in a Chinese population showed that the risk was 6 times higher in patients with any family history. Among the Inuit, the relative risk in persons with a family history is increased 3.5 times compared with that in the general Inuit population. These familial associations support a genetic influence in PAC. Recent genome-wide association studies have shown a complex genetic inheritance pattern with variable penetrance of genetic loci.

Rong SS, Tang FY, Chu WK, et al. Genetic associations of primary angle-closure disease: a systematic review and meta-analysis. *Ophthalmology.* 2016;123(6):1211–1221.

Refractive Error

Primary angle-closure disease occurs most commonly in patients with hyperopia, regardless of race. However, angle closure does occur in patients with significant myopia and even in those with simple myopia, particularly in persons of Asian descent. This underscores the importance of performing gonioscopy in all glaucoma patients regardless of their refractive status. Angle closure in a patient with high myopia should prompt the clinician to search for secondary mechanisms such as microspherophakia; plateau iris; or, in eyes with phacomorphic angle closure, nuclear sclerotic cataract. Axial myopia is primarily the result of elongation of the posterior segment of the eye, while the anterior segment sometimes retains properties that predispose to angle closure. Thus, even though myopia and axial elongation are associated with a lower risk for angle closure, there may be some risk in myopic eyes.

Yong KL, Gong T, Nongpiur ME, et al. Myopia in Asian subjects with primary angle closure: implications for glaucoma trends in East Asia. *Ophthalmology.* 2014;121(8):1566–1571.

The Primary Angle-Closure Disease Spectrum

Primary Angle-Closure Suspect

The term *primary angle-closure suspect (PACS)* refers to an eye that has a narrow angle with ≥180° of iridotrabecular contact (often referred to as an *occludable angle*), without overt signs of PAC (IOP elevation or PAS) or glaucomatous optic nerve damage.

Although only a small percentage of PACS eyes develop angle-closure disease (acute PAC, PAC, or PACG), these eyes are at risk. The predictive value of gonioscopy is relatively poor even when the test is performed by experienced clinicians. When performing gonioscopy, the clinician should observe the effect that the examination light has on the angle recess. For example, pupillary constriction stimulated by the slit-lamp beam itself may open the angle, and the narrow recess may go unrecognized. AS-OCT imaging (Fig 9-2) can be

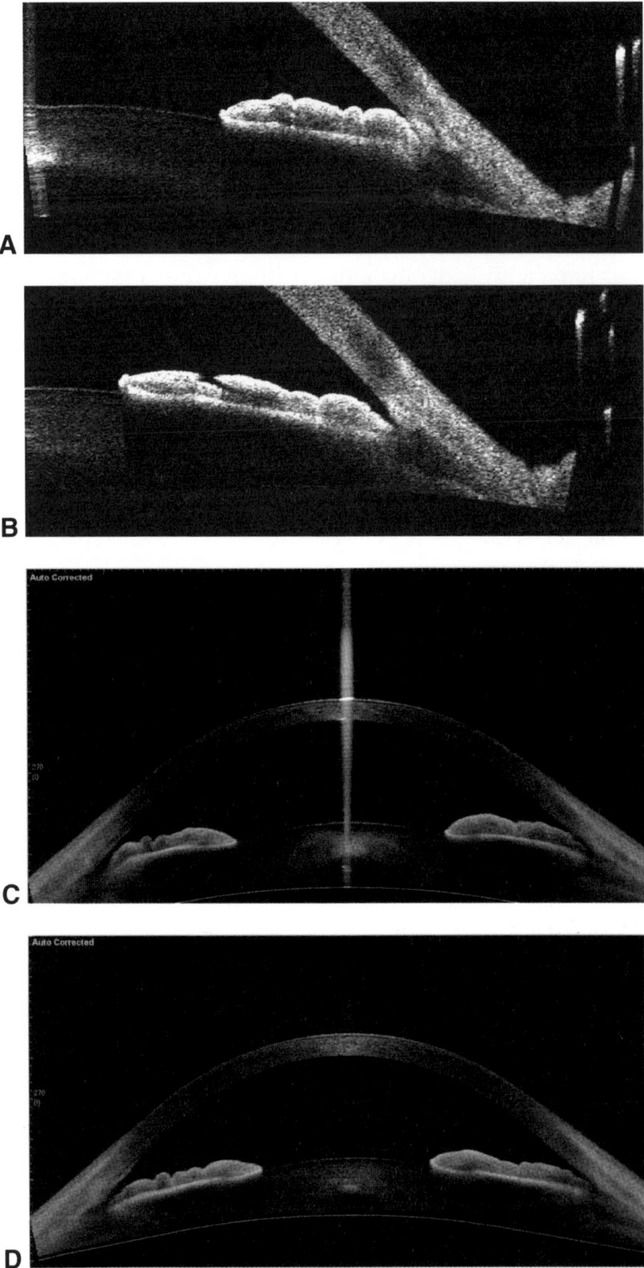

Figure 9-2 Anterior segment optical coherence tomography of a narrow angle. **A,** Angle closure is evident when the angle is imaged with lights off. **B,** The same angle is much more open when it is imaged with lights on. **C,** Narrow angles due to plateau iris (before laser peripheral iridotomy [LPI]). **D,** The same meridian with persistent narrow angles after LPI. *(Parts A and B courtesy of Yaniv Barkana, MD; parts C and D courtesy of David A. Lee, MD.)*

used to evaluate potential angle closure. The substantial change in angle configuration that may occur when the angle is imaged by AS-OCT in dark versus light conditions is demonstrated in Figures 9-2A and 9-2B, respectively. In Video 9-1, ultrasound biomicroscopy captures this dynamic change in the angle.

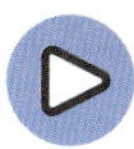

VIDEO 9-1 Angle apposition with light to dark adaptation.
Courtesy of Shan C. Lin, MD.
Available at: aao.org/bcscvideo_section10

Provocative tests such as pharmacologic pupillary dilation and the darkroom prone provocative test (DRPPT) can precipitate a limited form of angle closure and thus have been used in an attempt to predict which patients might develop angle closure and benefit from iridotomy. However, findings from the Zhongshan Angle-Closure Prevention (ZAP) study (see Treatment Controversies sidebar) suggested that provocative testing (15-minute darkroom prone position) is not predictive of an angle-closure attack or glaucoma development (although patients were excluded from the study if there was an elevation in IOP of >15 mm Hg on either mydriatic dilation or the DRPPT). Anterior segment imaging is under investigation to determine whether this modality can better predict PACD (see the section Anterior Segment Imaging in Chapter 4).

He M, Jiang Y, Huang S, et al. Laser peripheral iridotomy for the prevention of angle closure: a single-centre, randomized controlled trial. *Lancet.* 2019;393(10181):1609–1618.

TREATMENT CONTROVERSIES

Laser Peripheral Iridotomy

Whether to perform a laser peripheral iridotomy (LPI) in patients who meet the criteria for primary angle-closure suspect (PACS) remains controversial. The Zhongshan Angle-Closure Prevention (ZAP) trial randomly assigned 1 eye of participants with PACS to LPI, with the contralateral eye serving as a control. The study results showed that very few cases in either group progressed to primary angle-closure glaucoma (PACG) or an acute attack of angle closure. There was a significantly lower risk of conversion to primary angle closure (PAC) with treatment; however, most cases of conversion were attributed to formation of peripheral anterior synechiae (PAS) alone, without ocular hypertension. Overall, the study results suggest that prophylactic LPI is appropriate mainly for the high-risk PACS population. For the individual patient, the clinician needs to consider whether an LPI is appropriate based on the narrowness of the angle, the presence of symptoms such as eye discomfort consistent with elevated intraocular pressure (IOP), and other factors relevant to the individual, including the patient's preference given the available evidence.

An LPI should be considered for patients who have a narrow angle with PAS, increased segmental trabecular meshwork pigmentation, a history of previous acute angle closure, or other risk factors for angle closure (eg, strong family history such as a first-degree relative). The status of the

(Continued on next page)

(continued)

lens and the potential benefit of cataract surgery should also be taken into consideration.

For eyes in which most or all of the angle is closed with PAS, there is debate about whether an LPI should be performed. Such eyes have limited outflow facility and may have marked IOP elevation as a result of the dispersed pigment and iris debris. In some cases, the IOP elevation is refractory to medications and requires filtering surgery. Thus, caution should be exercised in such cases, and consideration of an alternative to LPI may be the better course of action.

Laser Iridoplasty

Another controversial area is whether to perform laser iridoplasty in patients with angle closure. There is evidence that laser iridoplasty is effective in further widening a narrow angle after iridotomy (Video 9-2). However, there is no strong evidence that laser iridoplasty is beneficial in preventing the development or progression of glaucoma.

VIDEO 9-2 Iridoplasty in the peripheral iris.
Courtesy of Robert Ritch, MD.
Available at: aao.org/bcscvideo_section10

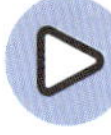

Bayliss JM, Ng WS, Waugh N, Azuara-Blanco A. Laser peripheral iridoplasty for chronic angle closure. *Cochrane Database Syst Rev.* 2021;(3): CD006746. doi:10.1002/14651858.CD006746.pub4

Lim DK, Chan HW, Zheng C, et al. Quantitative assessment of changes in anterior segment morphology after argon laser peripheral iridoplasty: findings from the EARL study group. *Clin Exp Ophthalmol.* 2019;47(1): 33–40.

Lens Extraction

Clear lens extraction (CLE) may be beneficial for certain patients with angle closure. The Effectiveness of Early Lens Extraction for the Treatment of Primary Angle-Closure Glaucoma (EAGLE) study was a prospective randomized controlled trial that evaluated the safety and efficacy of CLE in participants with no or non–visually significant cataracts, compared with standard treatment with LPI and medications. The participants enrolled were ≥50 years, without visually significant cataracts, and had either newly diagnosed PAC with IOP ≥30 mm Hg or PACG. Seventy percent of the participants were of non-Chinese ethnicity, and 30% were Chinese. The study found that CLE resulted in lower IOP, fewer medications used, and better quality of life than did standard treatment with LPI; visual field progression was similar in both groups.

Azuara-Blanco A, Burr J, Ramsay C, et al; EAGLE study group. Effectiveness of early lens extraction for the treatment of primary angle-closure glaucoma (EAGLE): a randomised controlled trial. *Lancet.* 2016;388 (10052):1389–1397.

Management

It is considered reasonable to perform a laser peripheral iridotomy (LPI) in an eye that meets the criteria for PACS (Videos 9-3, 9-4) (see Chapter 13 for LPI treatment parameters). However, iridotomy is not necessary for all PACS patients, and the decision of whether to treat an asymptomatic individual with narrow angles is based on an accurate assessment of the anterior chamber angle, the clinical judgment of the ophthalmologist, and the patient's preference. See the sidebar Treatment Controversies for further discussion. Any patient with narrow angles should be advised of the symptoms of acute angle closure (discussed in the subsection "Acute primary angle closure"), the need for immediate ophthalmologic attention if symptoms occur, and the value of long-term periodic follow-up.

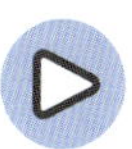

VIDEO 9-3 Angle apposition before laser peripheral iridotomy.
Courtesy of Shan C. Lin, MD.
Available at: aao.org/bcscvideo_section10

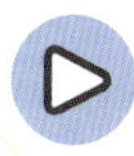

VIDEO 9-4 Angle status after laser peripheral iridotomy, with the angle opening.
Courtesy of Shan C. Lin, MD.
Available at: aao.org/bcscvideo_section10

Primary Angle Closure

Primary angle closure refers to an eye that has a narrow angle with ≥180° of iridotrabecular contact, along with PAS and/or statistically elevated IOP (>21 mm Hg). The angle can close gradually, with a slow increase in IOP as angle function progressively becomes compromised. Even in the absence of synechial angle closure, damage of the trabecular meshwork can occur from iridotrabecular contact, leading to elevated IOP. The chronic form of PAC, in which there is asymptomatic synechial angle closure, is the most common presentation of PACD.

Management

An LPI is usually necessary to relieve the pupillary block component and reduce the potential for further synechial angle closure. However, there is some debate about performing LPI in an eye with extensive synechiae, as IOP elevation may occur (see Treatment Controversies sidebar). Without an iridotomy, closure of the angle usually progresses, making the IOP more difficult to control. Even with a patent peripheral iridotomy, progressive angle closure can occur, and repeated periodic gonioscopy is imperative. An iridotomy with or without long-term use of ocular hypotensive medications controls the disease in most patients with PAC. However, the Effectiveness of Early Lens Extraction for the Treatment of Primary Angle-Closure Glaucoma (EAGLE) study suggests that in PAC cases with IOP of ≥30 mm Hg, clear lens extraction may be the preferred treatment (see Treatment Controversies sidebar).

Primary Angle-Closure Glaucoma

In *primary angle-closure glaucoma (PACG),* the conditions of PAC are met, and there is also optic nerve damage consistent with glaucoma. Because of the insidious nature of PACG, vision loss may be the presenting symptom. Accordingly, this disease, which is a major cause of blindness in Asia, tends to be diagnosed in its later stages. The clinical course of PACG usually resembles that of open-angle glaucoma in its lack of initial symptoms, modest elevation of IOP, progressive glaucomatous optic nerve damage, and characteristic patterns of visual field loss. Thus, the diagnosis of PACG is frequently overlooked, and this condition is commonly confused with primary open-angle glaucoma. Over time, however, IOP can rise precipitously and become more difficult to control. As previously noted, gonioscopic examination of all glaucoma patients is important to establish an accurate diagnosis.

Management

Laser peripheral iridotomy is considered standard treatment for PACG (see Chapter 13 for discussion of technique). However, as with PAC, there is some concern about performing LPI in PACG eyes with extensive synechiae, as a paradoxical rise in IOP may occur (see Treatment Controversies sidebar).

Medical treatment of PACG may include both aqueous suppressants and outflow drugs. Prostaglandin analogues are very effective for lowering IOP in angle-closure glaucoma, with efficacy similar to or exceeding that of β-blockers. The degree of IOP reduction does not seem to correlate with the amount of permanent angle closure. See Chapter 12 for further discussion of medical management of glaucoma.

Cataract surgery alone is beneficial in reducing IOP and medication use, and it compares favorably to cataract extraction combined with trabeculectomy. The EAGLE study showed that lens extraction can be an effective option in treating PACG (see also Treatment Controversies sidebar).

Tham CC, Kwong YY, Leung DY, et al. Phacoemulsification versus combined phacotrabeculectomy in medically uncontrolled chronic angle closure glaucoma with cataracts. *Ophthalmology.* 2009;116(4):725–731, 731.e1–3.

Symptomatic Primary Angle Closure

Intraocular pressure elevation with acute or subacute blockage of most of the angle can cause symptomatic angle closure.

Subacute primary angle closure

Subacute, or *intermittent, angle closure* is characterized by episodes of blurred vision, halos, and mild pain caused by elevated IOP. Vague symptoms of pain or headache not associated with visual symptoms have a low specificity for angle closure. The visual symptoms resolve spontaneously, especially during sleep-induced miosis, and the IOP is usually normal between episodes, which occur periodically over days, months, or years. These episodes are often confused with headaches or migraines, so obtaining a careful history is required. The correct diagnosis can be made only with a high index of suspicion and gonioscopy. The typical history and the gonioscopic appearance of a narrow angle with or without PAS help establish the diagnosis. The management of subacute PAC is similar to that of PAC.

Acute primary angle closure

In *acute primary angle closure* (*APAC;* sometimes called *acute angle-closure crisis*), IOP rises rapidly as a result of relatively sudden blockage of the trabecular meshwork by the iris.

APAC is typically manifested by ocular pain, headache, blurred vision, and halos around lights. Signs of APAC include the following:

- high IOP
- mid-dilated, sluggish, and irregularly shaped pupil
- corneal epithelial edema
- congested episcleral and conjunctival blood vessels
- shallow peripheral anterior chamber
- mild amount of aqueous flare and cells

The rise in IOP to relatively high levels causes the corneal epithelial edema, which is responsible for the visual symptoms. Acute systemic distress may result in nausea and vomiting.

Diagnosis Definitive diagnosis depends on gonioscopic verification of angle closure. Gonioscopy should be possible in almost all cases of APAC, although clearing of corneal edema with topical IOP-lowering therapy, topical glycerin, or paracentesis may be necessary to allow visualization of the angle. Dynamic gonioscopy, with indentation of the central cornea, may help the clinician determine whether the iris–trabecular meshwork blockage is reversible *(appositional closure)* or irreversible *(synechial closure),* and it may also be therapeutic in breaking the attack of acute angle closure. Gonioscopy of the fellow eye in a patient with APAC usually reveals a narrow, occludable angle. The presence of a deep angle in the fellow eye should prompt the clinician to search for secondary causes of elevated IOP, such as a posterior segment mass, zonular insufficiency, anterior segment neovascularization, or iridocorneal endothelial syndrome. When performing gonioscopy, the clinician should note the effect of the examination light on the angle recess; the slit-lamp beam can cause pupillary constriction, thus artificially opening the inherently narrow angle recess (see Fig 9-2). Because some aspects of gonioscopy and the interpretation of gonioscopic findings are subjective and variable based on technique, minimizing factors that can cause this variability is important for correct diagnosis.

During an acute attack, the IOP may be high enough to cause glaucomatous optic nerve damage, ischemic optic neuropathy, and/or retinal vascular occlusion. PAS can form rapidly, and IOP-induced ischemia may produce sectoral atrophy of the iris, releasing pigment. This causes pigmentary dusting of the iris surface and corneal endothelium. Iris ischemia, specifically of the iris sphincter, may cause the pupil to become permanently fixed and dilated. *Glaukomflecken,* characteristic small anterior subcapsular lens opacities, may also develop as a result of necrosis (see BCSC Section 11, *Lens and Cataract*). These findings are sometimes helpful in the detection of previous episodes of APAC.

Management The definitive treatment of APAC associated with pupillary block is usually LPI (discussed in Chapter 13). Once an iridotomy has been performed, the pupillary block is relieved and the pressure gradient between the posterior and anterior chambers is normalized, which in most cases allows the iris to fall away from the trabecular meshwork. As a result, the anterior chamber deepens and the angle opens. However, corneal edema at presentation may interfere with the creation of a patent LPI, and medications or procedures may be needed to break the attack and clear the cornea until iridotomy can be performed.

If the APAC is mild, it may be broken by cholinergic agents (pilocarpine 1%–2%), which induce miosis that pulls the peripheral iris away from the trabecular meshwork. However, these agents may worsen some types of angle closure without pupillary block and exacerbate pupillary block in some eyes. Stronger miotics are ideally avoided, as they may increase the vascular congestion of the iris or rotate the lens–iris interface more anteriorly, increasing the pupillary block. Moreover, when the IOP is markedly elevated (eg, >40–50 mm Hg), the pupillary sphincter may be ischemic and unresponsive to miotic agents alone. Consequently, in most cases, the patient is treated with other topical agents, including β-adrenergic antagonists, α_2-adrenergic agonists, and prostaglandin analogues, and with topical, oral, or intravenous carbonic anhydrase inhibitors. If necessary, hyperosmotic agents may be administered orally or intravenously. Nonselective adrenergic agonists or medications with significant α_1-adrenergic activity (eg, apraclonidine) should be avoided to prevent further pupillary dilation and iris ischemia.

Techniques for quickly lowering the IOP in order to clear the corneal edema include globe compression over the central cornea, dynamic gonioscopy, and careful paracentesis with a 30-gauge needle or sharp blade. Care must be taken with these maneuvers, as they can easily injure the lens or iris in an eye with a shallow anterior chamber.

Once the attack is broken and the cornea is of adequate clarity, typically an LPI is performed. Lens extraction is also a viable treatment option, although LPI may be more easily accomplished in acute episodes, especially if the eye is inflamed. Laser iridoplasty is another option. In rare cases, a surgical iridectomy is required. These procedures are discussed in Chapter 13. Following resolution of the acute attack, it is important to reevaluate the angle by gonioscopy to assess the degree of residual synechial angle closure and to confirm the reopening of at least part of the angle.

Improved IOP does not necessarily mean that the angle has opened. Because of ciliary body ischemia and reduced aqueous production, the IOP may remain low for weeks following acute angle closure. Thus, IOP may be a poor indicator of angle function or configuration. A second gonioscopy or serial gonioscopy is essential for follow-up.

In most cases of APAC, the fellow eye shares the anatomical predisposition for increased pupillary block and is at high risk of developing the same condition, especially if the inciting mechanism included a systemic sympathomimetic agent such as a nasal decongestant or an anticholinergic agent. If a similar angle configuration is present, it is recommended that an LPI be performed in the fellow eye.

Lam DS, Leung DY, Tham CC, et al. Randomized trial of early phacoemulsification versus peripheral iridotomy to prevent intraocular pressure rise after acute primary angle closure. *Ophthalmology.* 2008;115(7):1134–1140.

Plateau Iris as a Mechanism of Angle Closure

Plateau iris is an atypical configuration of the anterior chamber angle that may result in PACD (Case Study 9-1). It is a common finding in younger individuals with angle closure. Evidence suggests that the configuration results from anteriorly positioned ciliary processes, which appear as an absence of the ciliary sulcus on ultrasound biomicroscopy imaging, or anterior insertion of the iris on the ciliary body.

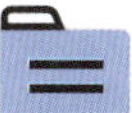

CASE STUDY 9-1 The patient with angle closure.
Courtesy of Shan C. Lin, MD.
Available at: aao.org/bcsccasestudy_section10

Plateau iris is suspected when the central anterior chamber appears to be of normal depth and the iris plane appears flat for an eye with angle closure. This suspicion can be confirmed by the presence of the *"double-hump" sign* on dynamic gonioscopy, in which the iris is held forward by the anteriorly situated ciliary processes, creating the appearance of a hump in the iris contour ("peripheral roll") (Fig 9-3). The condition will be missed if the examiner relies solely on slit-lamp examination or the Van Herick method of angle examination. The term *plateau iris configuration* refers to an eye that has a narrow angle due to an anteriorly positioned ciliary body, with a deep central anterior chamber.

The term *plateau iris syndrome* refers to an eye that has a narrow angle due to an anteriorly positioned ciliary body, a deep central anterior chamber, and persistent iridotrabecular contact despite a patent LPI (see Fig 9-2). In eyes with this syndrome, pharmacologic mydriasis may induce IOP elevation of 6 mm Hg or more. Formation of PAS has been reported

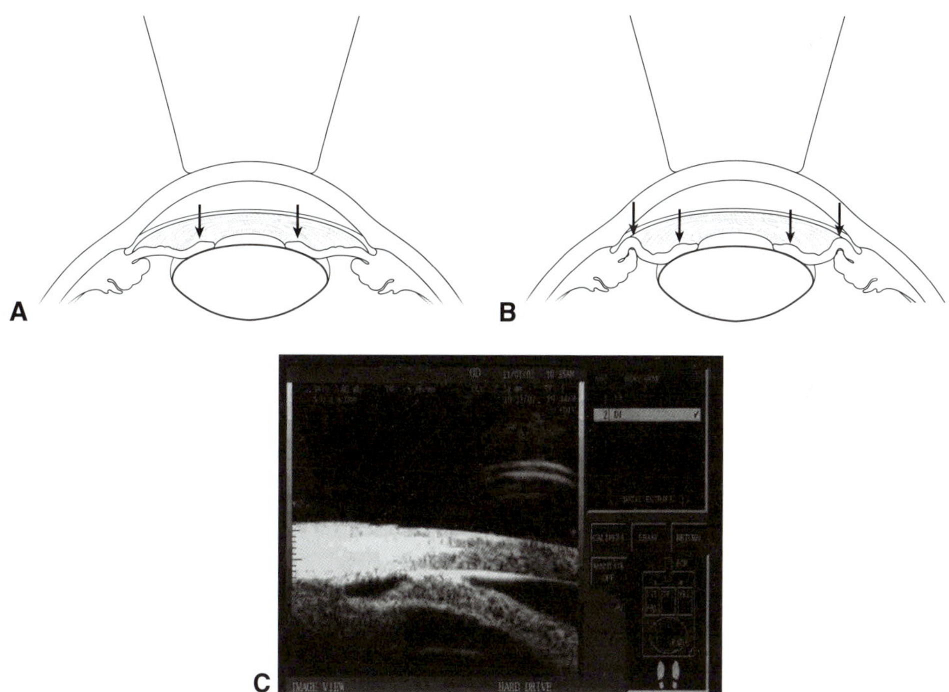

Figure 9-3 Plateau iris configuration and syndrome. **A,** Dynamic (compression) gonioscopy in an eye with pupillary block. A single hump, which is the iris circumferentially draping over the anterior lens capsule, is observed on both sides of the pupil in the diagram *(arrows)*. The angle is deep because of the increased pressure in the anterior chamber. **B,** Dynamic (compression) gonioscopy in an eye with plateau iris syndrome demonstrates the classic "double-hump" sign *(arrows to each hump)*. The hump at the angle is due to the peripheral iris roll, which is typically caused by the relative anterior position of the ciliary body. **C,** Ultrasound biomicroscopy shows peripheral iris contact with the Schwalbe line, anterior to the angle recess, in an eye with plateau iris configuration. *(Illustrations by Mark Miller; part C courtesy of Robert Ritch, MD.)*

to begin at the Schwalbe line (see Fig 9-3) and then to extend in a posterior direction over the trabecular meshwork, scleral spur, and angle recess. The reverse is seen in pupillary block–induced angle closure, in which synechiae form in a posterior-to-anterior direction.

In eyes with plateau iris, angle closure is most often caused by the anteriorly positioned ciliary processes pushing the peripheral iris forward, severely narrowing the anterior chamber angle recess. A component of pupillary block may also be present. The angle may be further compromised after pupillary dilation, as the peripheral iris crowds and obstructs the trabecular meshwork.

In patients with angle closure, the cause of the narrow or closed angle ranges from pure pupillary block to primarily plateau iris; however, the cause is often a combination of pupillary block and plateau iris.

Kumar RS, Tantisevi V, Wong MH, et al. Plateau iris in Asian subjects with primary angle closure glaucoma. *Arch Ophthalmol.* 2009;127(10):1269–1272.

Li Y, Wang YE, Huang G, et al. Prevalence and characteristics of plateau iris configuration among American Caucasian, American Chinese and mainland Chinese subjects. *Br J Ophthalmol.* 2014;98(4):474–478.

Ritch R, Chang BM, Liebmann JM. Angle closure in younger patients. *Ophthalmology.* 2003;110(10):1880–1889.

Management

The initial management of plateau iris includes either LPI to remove any component of pupillary block or lens extraction if cataract is present. Eyes with plateau iris configuration may be monitored without further intervention. Because of the peripheral iris anatomy, eyes with plateau iris syndrome remain predisposed to angle closure—and possible acute attack—despite a patent iridotomy. Plateau iris syndrome is the most common reason for a persistently narrow or occludable angle after LPI or cataract surgery. Thus, following LPI or lens extraction, careful assessment of the angle is necessary to determine whether additional treatment is required to further deepen the angle.

Patients with plateau iris syndrome may be treated with long-term miotic therapy; however, laser iridoplasty may be more useful in these individuals to flatten and thin the peripheral iris (see Chapter 13). Repeated gonioscopy at regular intervals is necessary because the risk of chronic angle closure remains despite measures to deepen the angle recess. The management of plateau iris syndrome is evolving, and further research is needed to determine the optimal management of this condition.

Pavlin CJ, Foster FS. Plateau iris syndrome: changes in angle opening associated with dark, light, and pilocarpine administration. *Am J Ophthalmol.* 1999;128(3):288–291.

CHAPTER 10

Secondary Angle Closure

Highlights

- Secondary angle closure can occur in a variety of settings, including anterior segment neovascularization, inflammation, and after surgery.
- Secondary angle closure can be divided into types with pupillary block and those without pupillary block.
- Detection of iris and angle neovascularization requires careful observation with the slit lamp and gonioscopy.
- Management of neovascular glaucoma has changed with the use of anti–vascular endothelial growth factor therapy, which when combined with panretinal photocoagulation, can sometimes delay the need for surgical intervention and reduce the risk of significant bleeding.
- It is important to ask patients presenting with acute bilateral angle closure about the use of drugs, including topiramate, that can induce secondary angle closure.

Introduction

Secondary angle closure can be divided mechanistically into types with pupillary block and those without pupillary block. Non–pupillary block secondary angle closure can be further categorized as angle closure caused by "pushing" or "pulling" mechanisms; that is, mechanisms that push the iris forward from behind or those that pull the iris forward into contact with the trabecular meshwork. Non–pupillary block angle closure can also be caused by a combination of pushing and pulling or other mechanisms. Table 10-1 presents conditions associated with the pushing and pulling mechanisms of secondary non–pupillary block angle closure.

Secondary Angle Closure With Pupillary Block

As discussed in Chapter 9, in eyes with *pupillary block,* the flow of aqueous humor from the posterior chamber through the pupil to the anterior chamber is impeded at the level of the lens–iris interface. Aqueous is trapped in the posterior chamber, which causes a relative increase in pressure compared with that in the anterior chamber. This results in the peripheral iris bowing forward against the trabecular meshwork (see Chapter 9, Fig 9-1A).

Table 10-1 Conditions Associated With the Pulling and Pushing Mechanisms of Non–Pupillary Block Angle Closure

Conditions that can pull the iris forward into contact with the trabecular meshwork
Contraction of inflammatory membrane or fibrovascular tissue
Migration of abnormal corneal endothelium (iridocorneal endothelial syndrome)
Fibrous ingrowth
Epithelial ingrowth
Iris incarceration in traumatic wound or surgical incision
Conditions that can push the iris forward from behind into contact with the trabecular meshwork
Malignant glaucoma (also referred to as *aqueous misdirection*)
Ciliary body swelling, inflammation, or cysts
Anteriorly oriented ciliary processes (plateau iris configuration/syndrome)
Serous or hemorrhagic uveal effusions
Posterior segment tumors or space-occupying substances (silicone oil, gas bubble)
Contraction of retrolental tissue (persistent fetal vasculature, retinopathy of prematurity)
Anteriorly displaced lens (eg, due to trauma, zonular laxity)
Encircling bands placed with scleral buckles

Lens-Induced Angle Closure

Phacomorphic glaucoma

The mechanism of phacomorphic glaucoma typically is multifactorial (pupillary block and posterior pushing), although by definition, a substantial component of the pathologic angle narrowing is related to the acquired mass effect of the cataractous lens itself. As in primary angle-closure disease (PACD), pupillary block often plays an important role in this condition. Narrowing of the angle generally occurs slowly with formation of the cataract. However, in some cases, the onset is acute and rapid, precipitated by marked lens swelling *(intumescence)* as a result of cataract formation and the development of pupillary block in an eye that is not otherwise anatomically predisposed to angle closure (Figs 10-1, 10-2).

Distinguishing between PACD and phacomorphic angle closure is not always straightforward, but differences in anterior chamber depth (ACD), gonioscopic appearance, and degree of cataract can help the clinician determine the etiology (see also BCSC Section 11, *Lens and Cataract*). Several anterior segment imaging techniques (anterior segment optical coherence tomography [AS-OCT], ultrasound biomicroscopy [UBM], and Scheimpflug imaging) provide ocular biometric parameters that are useful for diagnosis. For example, in 1 study, AS-OCT in eyes with phacomorphic angle closure showed that the ACD was approximately half that of control eyes (1.4 mm vs 2.8 mm) and that the lens vault was 3 times the value of controls (1.4 mm vs 0.4 mm). Of note, eyes that develop phacomorphic glaucoma are often predisposed to angle closure.

Laser peripheral iridotomy (LPI) may be performed before cataract extraction to relieve the pupillary block component. Laser iridoplasty can also be performed as a temporizing procedure to help expand the angle before cataract surgery. However, in many cases, the

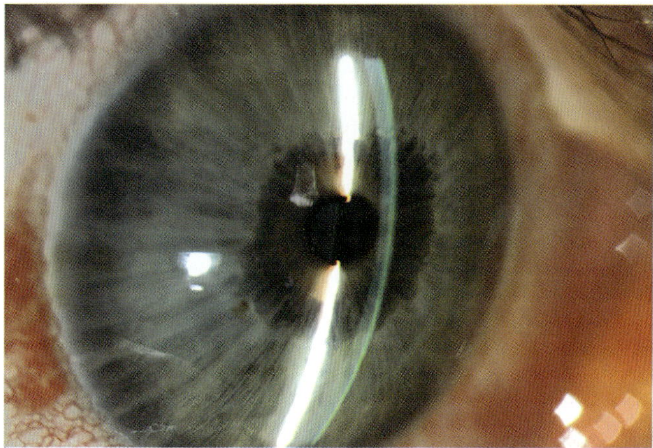

Figure 10-1 Phacomorphic glaucoma. An intumescent lens precipitates pupillary block and secondary angle closure in an eye that is not anatomically predisposed to angle closure. *(Courtesy of Wallace L. M. Alward, MD. From the* Iowa Glaucoma Curriculum. *© The University of Iowa.)*

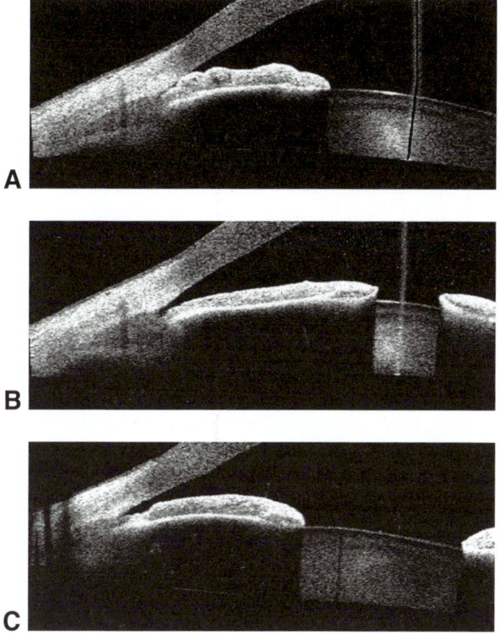

Figure 10-2 Phacomorphic glaucoma. **A,** The angle remains narrow despite a patent iridotomy. **B,** In bright light, the angle is transiently made deeper by pupillary constriction. **C,** Thinning the peripheral iris with laser iridoplasty (as shown) can also help to make the angle more open. However, lens extraction is the definitive treatment. *(Courtesy of Yaniv Barkana, MD.)*

iridotomy or iridoplasty is unnecessary, as cataract surgery is the definitive treatment in eyes that have the potential for improved or useful vision. Cholinergic agents have no role in the treatment of this condition because they may further narrow the angle (by increasing the pupillary block and causing forward movement of the lens–iris interface as a result of zonular laxity) and worsen vision in the presence of cataract. In addition, the miotic pupil makes subsequent cataract surgery more challenging.

Ectopia lentis

Ectopia lentis is defined as displacement of the crystalline lens from its normal anatomical position caused by broken or absent zonular fibers. With forward displacement, pupillary block may occur, resulting in an anteriorly bowed iris, narrowing of the anterior chamber angle, and secondary angle closure. Common causes of lens subluxation include the following:

- pseudoexfoliation syndrome
- trauma
- Marfan syndrome
- homocystinuria
- microspherophakia
- Weill-Marchesani syndrome
- Ehlers-Danlos syndrome
- sulfite oxidase deficiency

The most common cause of acquired zonular insufficiency and crystalline lens subluxation is *pseudoexfoliation syndrome* (Fig 10-3).

The treatment of choice is the creation of 2 laser iridotomies 180° apart so that both will not be occluded simultaneously by the lens. This relieves the pupillary block and is a temporizing measure until the definitive procedure, lens extraction, can be performed (if indicated to improve visual function). Lens extraction is usually indicated to restore vision and to reduce the risk of recurrent pupillary block and formation of peripheral anterior synechiae (PAS).

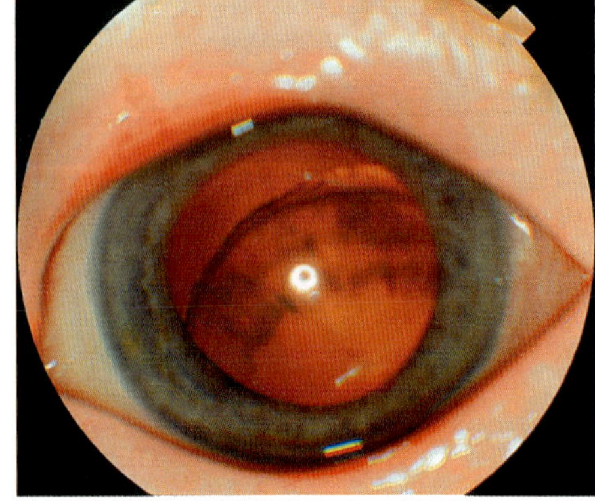

Figure 10-3 Pseudoexfoliation syndrome is a common cause of subluxation of the crystalline lens. The image shows the left eye of a patient with subluxation of the lens. *(Courtesy of Thomas W. Samuelson, MD.)*

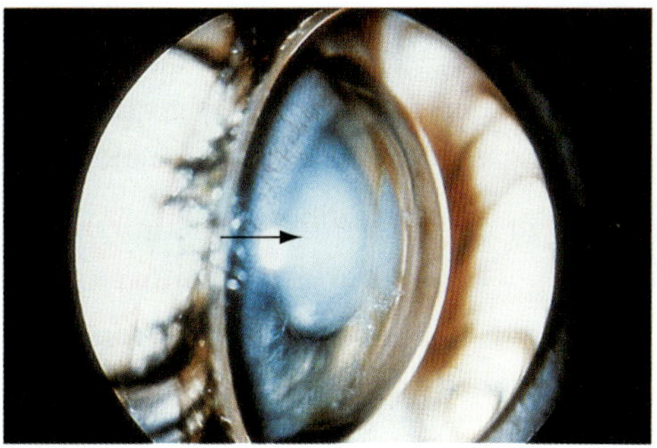

Figure 10-4 Ectopia lentis due to microspherophakia. The lens *(arrow)* is trapped anteriorly by the pupil, resulting in anterior iris bowing and a dramatic shallowing of the anterior chamber. *(Courtesy of G. L. Spaeth, MD.)*

Microspherophakia

Microspherophakia, a congenital disorder in which the lens has a spherical or globular shape, may cause ectopia lentis and subsequent pupillary block with resultant angle closure (Fig 10-4). Treatment with cycloplegia may tighten the zonular fibers, flatten the lens, and pull it posteriorly, breaking the pupillary block. Miotics may make the condition worse by increasing the pupillary block and by rotating the ciliary body forward, loosening the zonular fibers and allowing the lens to become more globular. Microspherophakia is often genetic and may occur as an isolated condition or as part of Weill-Marchesani or Marfan syndrome.

Aphakic or pseudophakic angle closure

Pupillary block may occur in aphakic and pseudophakic eyes. Vitreous can block the pupil and/or an iridotomy site in aphakic or pseudophakic eyes or in a phakic eye with a dislocated lens. Generally, the anterior chamber shallows, and the iris bows forward. Treatment with mydriatic and cycloplegic agents may restore aqueous flow through the pupil but may also make performing an LPI difficult initially. Topical β-adrenergic antagonists, α_2-adrenergic agonists, carbonic anhydrase inhibitors, and hyperosmotic agents can be effective in reducing intraocular pressure (IOP) before an iridotomy is performed. One or more LPIs may be required.

Pupillary block may also occur in eyes with anterior chamber intraocular lenses (ACIOLs). To prevent pupillary block, an iridectomy should be done when an ACIOL is implanted, or an early postoperative LPI should be performed. Pupillary block can develop as a result of apposition of the iris to the ACIOL optic or apposition of the vitreous face to the pupil–optic complex. If pupillary block occurs, the peripheral iris bows forward around the ACIOL and occludes the angle. In this situation, the central anterior chamber remains deep relative to the peripheral chamber because the ACIOL itself prevents the central portions of the iris and vitreous face from moving forward. LPIs, often multiple, are required in order to relieve the pupillary block. In rare cases, pupillary block occurs in the presence of an iridectomy if the lens haptic or vitreous obstructs the iridectomy site or the pupil.

In addition, pupillary block can occur following posterior capsulotomy when vitreous obstructs the pupil. A condition referred to as *capsular block* may also be seen, wherein retained viscoelastic or fluid in the capsular bag pushes a posterior chamber IOL anteriorly, which may narrow the angle.

Secondary Angle Closure Without Pupillary Block

A number of conditions can lead to angle closure without pupillary block. This form of secondary angle closure occurs primarily through 1 of 2 mechanisms (see Table 10-1):

- a *pulling* mechanism, caused by contraction of an inflammatory, hemorrhagic, cellular, or vascular membrane, band, or exudate in the angle, leading to PAS formation
- a *pushing* mechanism, caused by forward displacement of the lens–iris interface, often accompanied by swelling and anterior rotation of the ciliary body

Secondary angle closure without pupillary block can also occur as a result of a combination of pushing and pulling or other mechanisms.

Conditions Associated With a Pulling Mechanism

Anterior segment neovascularization

Anterior segment neovascularization is a common cause of a severe type of secondary angle-closure glaucoma known as *neovascular glaucoma.* The neovascularization is accompanied by the formation of a fibrovascular membrane on the iris surface, pupillary margin, and trabecular meshwork. Anterior segment neovascularization is caused by a variety of conditions that involve retinal or ocular ischemia or ocular inflammation (Table 10-2), most commonly diabetic retinopathy, central retinal vein occlusion (CRVO), branch retinal vein occlusion

Table 10-2 Conditions Predisposing to Neovascularization of the Iris and Angle

Systemic vascular conditions	**Other ocular diseases**
Carotid stenosis	Chronic uveitis
Carotid artery ligation	Chronic retinal detachment
Carotid-cavernous fistula	Endophthalmitis
Giant cell arteritis	Stickler syndrome (hereditary progressive arthro-ophthalmopathy)
Takayasu arteritis (pulseless disease)	Retinoschisis
Ocular vascular diseases	Pseudoexfoliation syndrome
Diabetic retinopathy[a]	**Intraocular tumors**
Central retinal vein occlusion[a]	Uveal melanoma
Central retinal artery occlusion	Metastatic carcinoma
Branch retinal vein occlusion	Retinoblastoma
Ocular ischemic syndrome[a] (eg, due to carotid occlusive disease)	Lymphoma
	Reticulum cell sarcoma
	Medulloepithelioma
Sickle cell retinopathy	**Ocular therapy**
Coats disease	Radiation therapy
Eales disease	**Trauma**
Retinopathy of prematurity	
Persistent fetal vasculature	
Syphilitic vasculitis	
Anterior segment ischemia	

[a]Most common causes.

(BRVO), and ocular ischemic syndrome. Anterior segment neovascularization can also occur with metastatic or other tumors of the eye, such as retinoblastomas, medulloepitheliomas, and choroidal melanomas, as well as following radiation treatment, resulting in neovascular glaucoma.

The pathophysiology of neovascular glaucoma most often involves secretion of angiogenic factors, especially vascular endothelial growth factor (VEGF), from ischemic retinal tissue. These angiogenic factors can diffuse into the anterior chamber and promote neovascularization of the iris (NVI) and neovascularization of the angle (NVA). In rare instances, anterior segment neovascularization occurs without demonstrable retinal ischemia, as in Fuchs uveitis syndrome and other types of uveitis, pseudoexfoliation syndrome, or isolated iris melanomas. When an ocular cause cannot be found, carotid artery occlusive disease should be considered.

Clinically, patients with neovascular glaucoma often present with acute IOP elevation, along with reduced vision, ocular pain, conjunctival hyperemia, and microcystic corneal edema. In establishing a diagnosis, the clinician should distinguish dilatated iris vessels associated with inflammation from neovascularization. In the classic pattern of development, neovascularization of the anterior segment usually begins with fine vascular tufts at the pupillary margin. Often, these vessels are difficult to observe in darkly pigmented eyes or in eyes with corneal edema due to high IOP. Conversely, in lightly pigmented eyes, NVI can be more readily detected, but it is important to distinguish normal vessels from NVI (Fig 10-5A). As neovascular vessels grow, they extend radially over the iris (Fig 10-5B). Unlike dilatated stromal vessels, neovascular vessels are delicate and lacy and do not adhere to the normal anterior segment vasculature. Further, when neovascularization involves the angle, the vessels cross the ciliary body face and scleral spur as fine single vessels that branch as they reach the trabecular meshwork (Fig 10-6). Often, the trabecular meshwork takes on a reddish color. With contraction of the fibrovascular membrane, PAS develop and coalesce, gradually closing the angle (Fig 10-7). Although the fibrovascular membrane can cause ectropion uveae, it typically does not grow over healthy corneal endothelium. Thus, the PAS end at the Schwalbe line, distinguishing this condition from iridocorneal endothelial syndrome, which also features ectropion uveae. When performing gonioscopy in patients with possible neovascularization, the clinician may find it helpful to use a bright slit-lamp beam and high magnification to better visualize the fine vessels.

Because the prognosis for neovascular glaucoma typically is poor, prevention and early diagnosis are essential. In CRVO, NVA develops without NVI in approximately 4% of patients. Thus, gonioscopy is important for early diagnosis.

Management Because the most common cause of NVI is retinal ischemia, the definitive treatment when the ocular media are clear is panretinal photocoagulation (PRP). Ablation of ischemic areas of the retina reduces the angiogenic stimulus. However, intravitreal anti-VEGF therapy can be used to more quickly reduce the neovascular stimulus. The regression of neovascularization after PRP, anti-VEGF therapy, or both may reduce or normalize the IOP, depending on the extent of PAS formation. Even in the presence of total synechial angle closure, PRP may improve the success rate of subsequent glaucoma surgery by eliminating the angiogenic stimulus and may decrease the risk of hemorrhage at the time of surgery. More recently, anti-VEGF agents have been successfully employed to promote regression

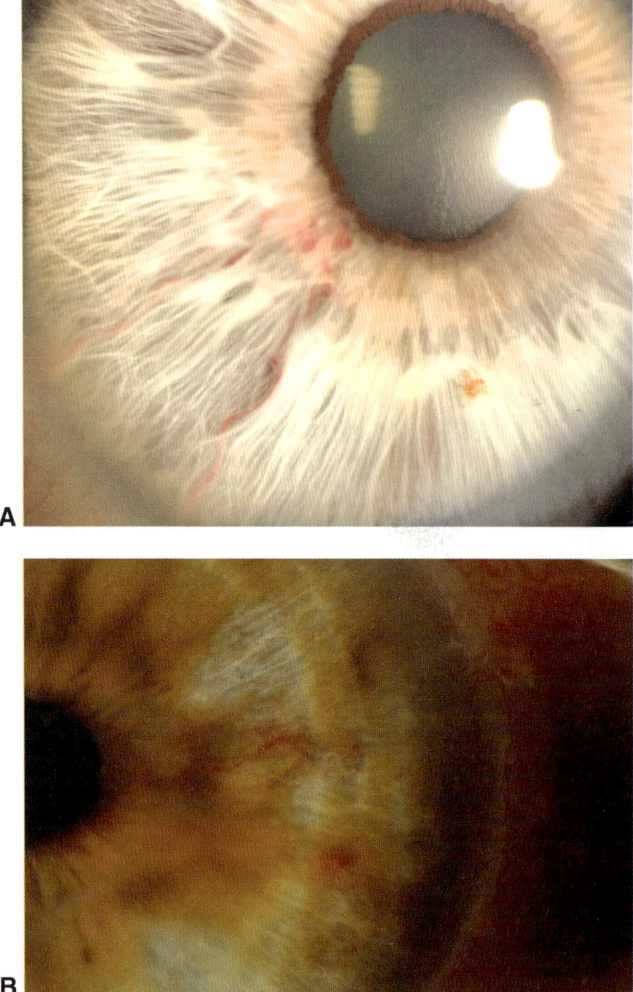

Figure 10-5 Distinguishing normal iris vessels from iris neovascularization. **A,** Prominent normal iris vessels in a lightly pigmented eye. Vessels are typically large and relatively straight. **B,** Iris neovascularization usually begins at the pupillary margin. In this eye, there is more extensive iris neovascularization with radial extension along the iris surface. Note the fine, lacy, branching pattern of the neovascular vessels. *(Part A courtesy of Shan C. Lin, MD; part B courtesy of Angelo P. Tanna, MD.)*

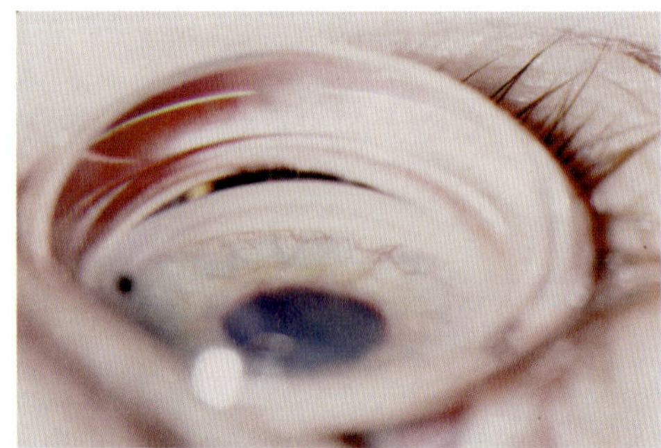

Figure 10-6 Iris neovascularization. With progressive angle involvement, peripheral anterior synechiae (PAS) develop with contraction of the fibrovascular membrane, resulting in secondary angle closure. *(Courtesy of H. Dunbar Hoskins, MD. From the Glaucoma Center of San Francisco archives.)*

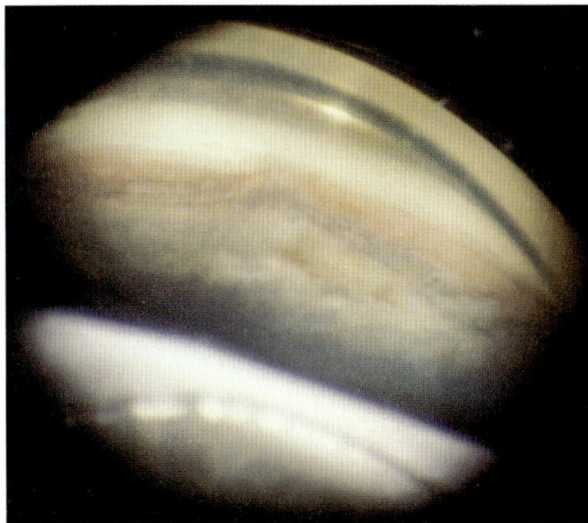

Figure 10-7 With end-stage neovascular glaucoma, total angle closure occurs, obscuring the iris neovascularization. The PAS end at the Schwalbe line because the fibrovascular membrane does not grow over healthy corneal endothelium. *(Courtesy of Wallace L. M. Alward, MD. From the* Iowa Glaucoma Curriculum. *© The University of Iowa.)*

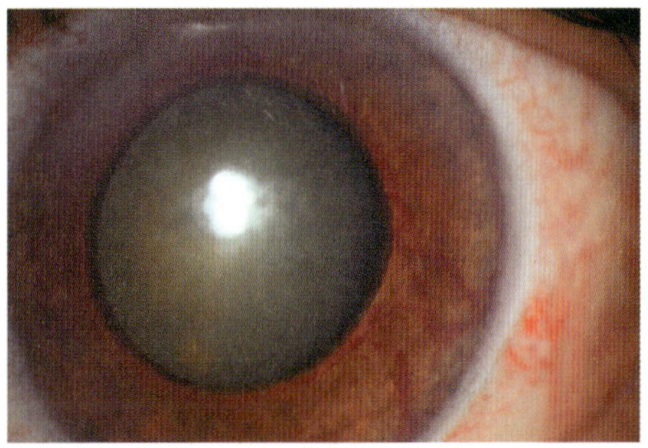

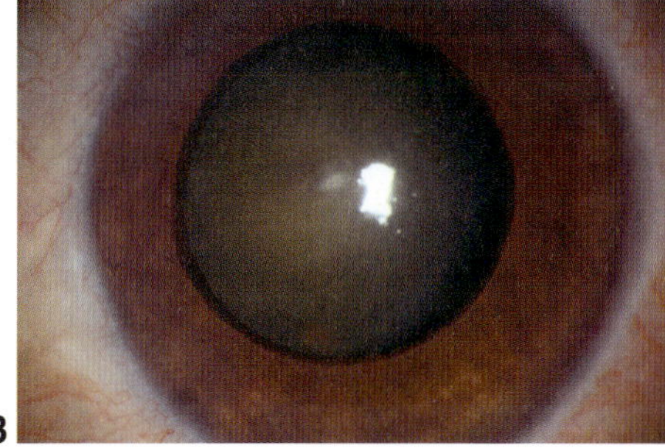

Figure 10-8 Effect of bevacizumab on iris neovascularization. **A,** Slit-lamp photograph of florid iris neovascularization taken before the injection of bevacizumab. **B,** Regression of iris neovascularization 4 days after treatment with bevacizumab. *(Courtesy of Nicholas P. Bell, MD.)*

of the neovascular tissue before filtering surgery (Fig 10-8) and to improve outcomes. Although anti-VEGF treatment can substantially delay the need for surgery, studies have shown that PRP is the most important factor in obviating the need for IOP-lowering surgery for neovascular glaucoma.

Medical management of neovascular glaucoma yields variable success and is sometimes only a temporizing measure until more definitive incisional or laser surgery is undertaken. Topical β-adrenergic antagonists, α_2-adrenergic agonists, carbonic anhydrase inhibitors, prostaglandin analogues, cycloplegics, and corticosteroids may be useful in reducing IOP and decreasing inflammation, either as a long-term therapy or prior to filtering surgery. Incisional glaucoma surgery is more likely to be successful if performed after the neovascularization has regressed following PRP or anti-VEGF therapy. In many cases, tube shunt surgery, usually with a valved device, is the surgical procedure of choice. If these therapies fail or if the eye has poor visual potential, either endoscopic or transscleral cyclophotocoagulation may be considered as an alternative. See Chapter 13 for discussion of these procedures.

Havens SJ, Gulati V. Neovascular glaucoma. *Dev Ophthalmol.* 2016;55:196–204.

Iridocorneal endothelial syndrome

Iridocorneal endothelial (ICE) syndrome is a disorder with variable presentation resulting from abnormal corneal endothelial cells that acquire characteristics of epithelial cells: they proliferate, migrate, and fail to exhibit contact inhibition. These abnormal endothelial cells cause various degrees of iris atrophy, secondary angle closure, and corneal edema. (See also BCSC Section 8, *External Disease and Cornea.*) Three clinical presentations have been described:

- Chandler syndrome
- essential (progressive) iris atrophy
- iris nevus syndrome (also known as *Cogan-Reese syndrome*)

Chandler syndrome is the most common type, accounting for approximately 50% of the cases of ICE syndrome.

ICE syndrome most commonly presents between 20 and 50 years of age, occurs more often in women, and is clinically unilateral. No consistent association has been found with other ocular or systemic diseases, and familial cases are very rare. A viral etiology has been postulated for ICE syndrome and is supported by studies demonstrating the presence of viral DNA in the corneas and aqueous humor of some eyes with this syndrome.

Patients typically present with elevated IOP, decreased vision due to corneal edema, secondary chronic angle-closure glaucoma, or an abnormal iris appearance. In each of the 3 clinical variants, the abnormal corneal endothelium takes on a "beaten bronze" appearance similar to cornea guttata, as seen in Fuchs endothelial corneal dystrophy. Microcystic corneal edema may be present without elevated IOP, especially in Chandler syndrome. The unaffected eye may have subclinical irregularities of the corneal endothelium, detectable with confocal or specular microscopy, without other manifestations of the disease.

High PAS are common in ICE syndrome (Fig 10-9), and they often extend anterior to the Schwalbe line. The extent of angle closure does not always correlate with the IOP because some angles may be functionally closed by the endothelial membrane without overt PAS formation.

Various degrees of iris atrophy and corneal changes distinguish the 3 clinical entities, but there is no evidence that each entity has a different pathophysiology. The *essential iris atrophy variant* is characterized by severe, progressive iris atrophy resulting in heterochromia, corectopia, ectropion uveae, iris stromal and pigment epithelial atrophy, and hole formation

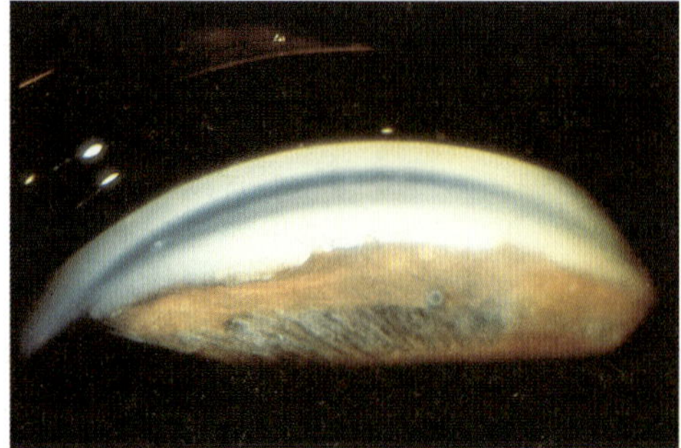

Figure 10-9 The classic high PAS of iridocorneal endothelial (ICE) syndrome. These PAS extend anterior to the Schwalbe line. *(Courtesy of Steven T. Simmons, MD.)*

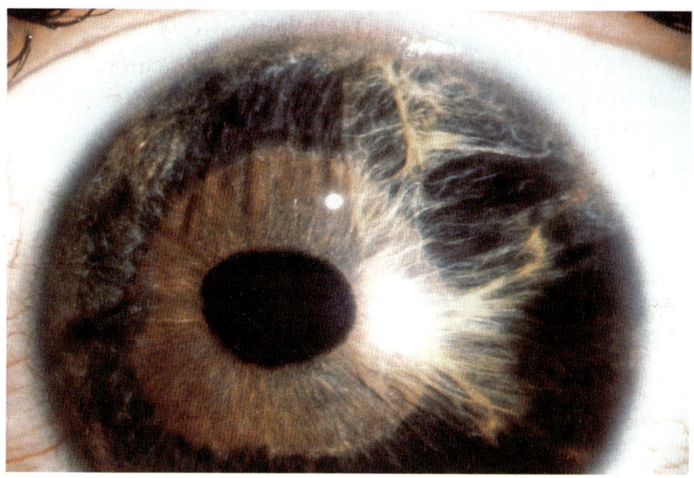

Figure 10-10 Clinical photograph showing corectopia and hole formation, typical findings in the essential iris atrophy variant of ICE syndrome. *(Courtesy of Steven T. Simmons, MD.)*

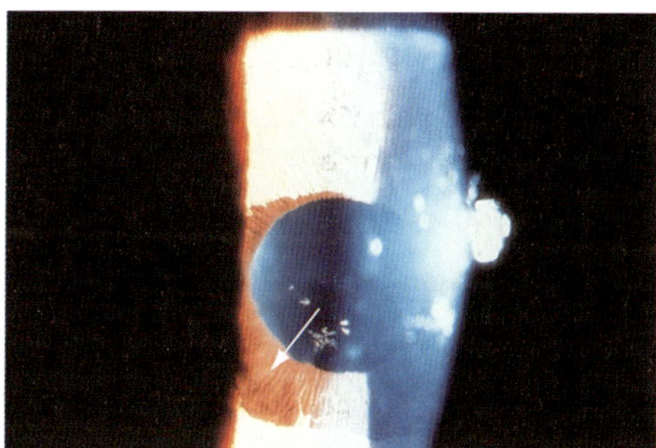

Figure 10-11 Clinical photograph showing ectropion uveae *(arrow)* in a patient with ICE syndrome. *(Courtesy of Steven T. Simmons, MD.)*

(Figs 10-10, 10-11). In *Chandler syndrome,* minimal iris atrophy and corectopia occur, and the corneal and angle findings predominate. Corneal endothelial proliferation can cause corneal edema, as well as possible glaucoma and iris changes. Iris atrophy also tends to be less severe in *iris nevus syndrome,* a condition distinguished by tan pedunculated nodules or diffuse pigmented lesions on the anterior iris surface.

Glaucoma develops in approximately 50% of patients with ICE syndrome and may be more severe in those with essential iris atrophy or iris nevus syndrome. In ICE, the corneal endothelium migrates posterior to the Schwalbe line, onto the trabecular meshwork and iris. Electron microscopy has shown the endothelium to vary in thickness, with areas of single and multiple endothelial cell layers and surrounding collagenous and fibrillar tissue. Unlike normal corneal endothelium, filopodial processes and cytoplasmic actin filaments are present, allowing cellular motility. PAS are formed when this migratory endothelium and its surrounding collagenous fibrillar tissue contract.

The diagnosis of ICE syndrome must always be considered in young to middle-aged patients who present with unilateral secondary angle closure. It is particularly important to maintain a high index of suspicion for this condition because it can mimic primary open-angle glaucoma when the iris and corneal features are subtle. The diagnosis can be confirmed by specular microscopy, which demonstrates an asymmetric loss of endothelial cells and atypical endothelial cell morphology in the involved eye.

Therapy is directed toward the corneal edema and IOP reduction. Hypertonic saline solution and medications to reduce the IOP, when elevated, can be effective in controlling the corneal edema. IOP can be lowered with aqueous suppressants and prostaglandin analogues. Miotics are often ineffective. When medical therapy fails, trabeculectomy or tube shunt surgery can be effective. Late failures due to endothelialization of the fistula have been reported with trabeculectomy. The fistula can be reopened with the Nd:YAG laser in some cases. Laser trabeculoplasty has no therapeutic role in ICE syndrome.

Epithelial and fibrous ingrowth

Epithelial ingrowth and fibrous ingrowth are rare complications of surgery or of penetrating trauma in which epithelium, fibroblasts, or both invade the anterior chamber through a surgical incision or traumatic wound. These proliferations can result in severe secondary glaucoma. Fortunately, improved surgical and wound closure techniques have greatly reduced the incidence of these entities. Both types are potential causes of corneal graft failure, with fibrous ingrowth being more common than epithelial ingrowth. Risk factors for developing ingrowth include prolonged inflammation, wound dehiscence, delayed wound closure, and Descemet membrane tear. Epithelial ingrowth has also been reported after Descemet-stripping automated endothelial keratoplasty.

Epithelial ingrowth presents as a grayish, sheetlike membrane on the trabecular meshwork, iris, ciliary body, and posterior surface of the cornea (Fig 10-12). Radical surgery is sometimes necessary to remove the intraocular epithelial membrane and affected tissues and to repair the fistula, but the prognosis remains poor. Unlike epithelial proliferation, *fibrous ingrowth* progresses slowly and is often self-limited. Fibrous ingrowth appears as a thick, gray-white, vascular retrocorneal membrane with an irregular border. The ingrowth often involves the angle, resulting in PAS formation with destruction of the trabecular meshwork and ectropion uveae. Surgery may also be required in some cases of fibrous ingrowth.

Trauma

Angle closure without pupillary block may develop after trauma, as a result of PAS formation associated with angle recession or from contusion, hyphema, and inflammation. See Chapter 8 for discussion of trauma.

Conditions Associated With a Pushing Mechanism

Tumors

Posterior segment tumors or anterior uveal cysts may cause unilateral secondary angle closure. Primary choroidal melanomas, ocular metastases, and retinoblastoma are the tumors most commonly responsible. The mechanism of the angle closure is determined by the size, location, and pathology of the tumor. For example, choroidal and retinal tumors tend to shift the lens–iris interface forward as the tumors enlarge, whereas breakdown of

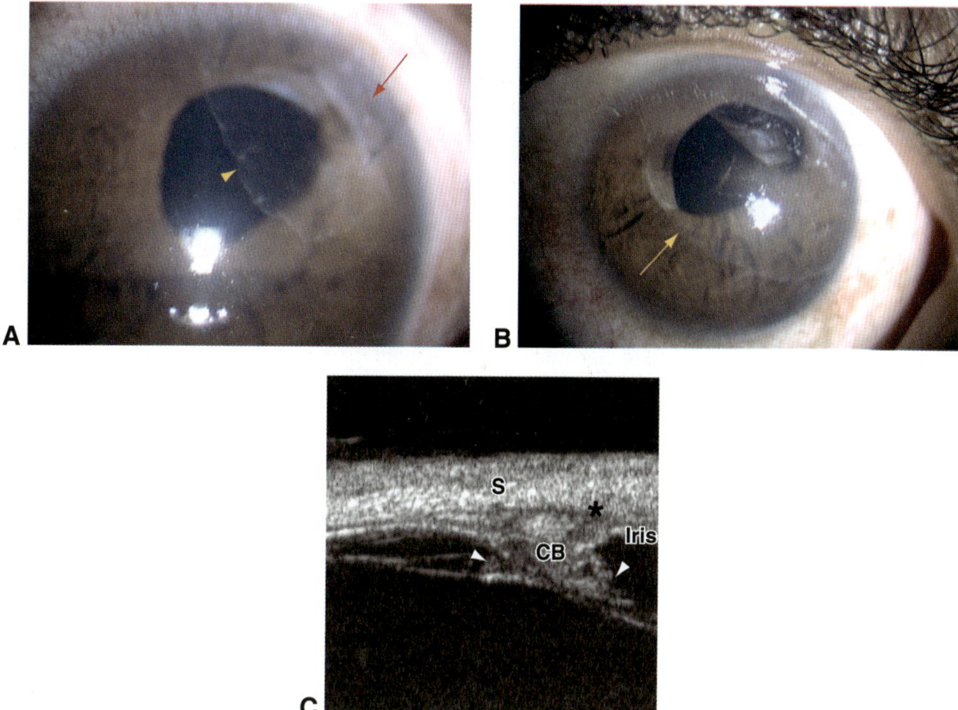

Figure 10-12 Epithelial ingrowth appears as a grayish, sheetlike membrane on the endothelial surface of the cornea, usually originating from a surgical incision or traumatic wound. **A,** The epithelial ingrowth shown here originated from a traumatic wound *(arrow),* causing PAS formation (deep to the incision) and corectopia. The *arrowhead* marks the edge of the epithelial ingrowth. **B,** The epithelial ingrowth spread across the central cornea *(arrow at leading edge).* **C,** Ultrasound biomicroscopy image of structures of the anterior chamber angle shows angle closure and growth of the epithelial membrane over the posterior iris, ciliary process *(arrowheads),* and pars plana region. The scleral spur *(asterisk)* is also depicted. CB = ciliary body; S = sclera. *(Courtesy of Herbert P. Fechter III, MD.)*

the blood–aqueous barrier and inflammation from tissue necrosis can result in posterior synechiae and PAS formation, further exacerbating other underlying mechanisms of angle closure.

Ocular tumors can also cause anterior segment neovascularization leading to angle closure (see the section "Anterior segment neovascularization").

Malignant glaucoma

Malignant glaucoma (also called *aqueous misdirection* or *ciliary block glaucoma*) is a rare but potentially devastating form of glaucoma that usually presents following ocular surgery in patients with a history of angle closure. In rare instances, it can occur spontaneously in eyes with an open angle or after cataract surgery or various laser procedures. The disease presents with uniform shallowing of both the central and peripheral anterior chamber (Fig 10-13).

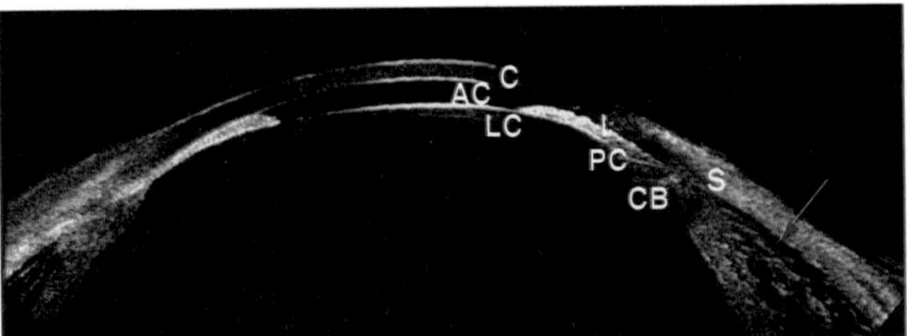

Figure 10-13 Ultrasound biomicroscopy of an eye with malignant glaucoma. The lens–iris diaphragm is pushed forward, causing a uniform shallowing of the anterior chamber (AC). The central portion of the anterior lens capsule (LC) is nearly in contact with the cornea (C). Note the ciliary body (CB) detachment due to choroidal effusion *(arrow)*, which is commonly seen in malignant glaucoma. I = iris; PC = posterior chamber; S = sclera. *(Courtesy of Robert Ritch, MD.)*

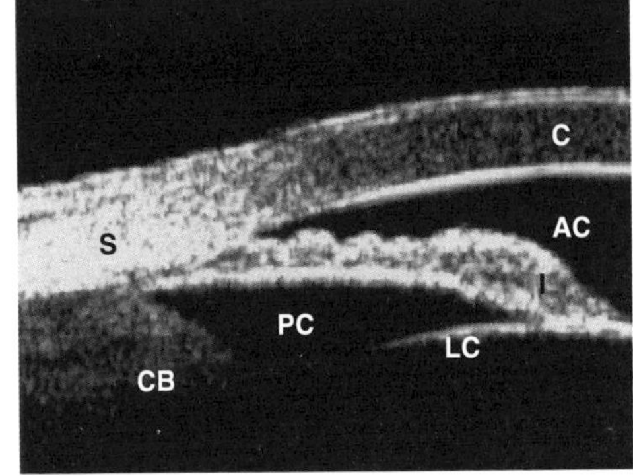

Figure 10-14 Ultrasound biomicroscopy of an eye with acute primary angle closure. Pupillary block leads to forward bowing of the peripheral iris. The peripheral anterior chamber is shallow, whereas the central anterior chamber is relatively deep by comparison. AC = anterior chamber; C = cornea; CB = ciliary body; I = iris; LC = lens capsule; PC = posterior chamber; S = sclera. *(From Lundy DC. Ciliary block glaucoma.* Focal Points: Clinical Modules for Ophthalmologists. *American Academy of Ophthalmology; 1999, module 3. Courtesy of Jeffrey M. Liebmann, MD.)*

This is in contrast to acute primary angle closure (PAC), which presents with an anteriorly bowed iris and a shallow peripheral anterior chamber (Fig 10-14). In malignant glaucoma, typically there is marked asymmetry between the affected anterior chamber and the anterior chamber of the fellow eye.

Classically, the condition has been thought to result from anterior rotation of the ciliary body and posterior misdirection of the aqueous, in association with blockage of forward aqueous movement at the level of the lens equator, vitreous face, and ciliary processes. However, this explanation is controversial. Some have argued that (a) it is not physically plausible given the proposed one-way valve permitting aqueous humor to flow only posteriorly; and (b) malignant glaucoma may result from the simultaneous presence of several factors, including a small, anatomically predisposed eye; an eye's propensity for choroidal expansion; and reduced vitreous fluid conductivity.

Clinically, the anterior chamber is shallow or flat, with anterior displacement of the lens, IOL, or vitreous face. Optically clear zones may be seen in the vitreous. Some experts argue that these clear zones represent aqueous humor trapped in the vitreous cavity; however, this is controversial. In the early postoperative setting, malignant glaucoma is often difficult to distinguish from choroidal effusion, pupillary block, or suprachoroidal hemorrhage. Often, the level of IOP, time frame after surgery, patency of an iridotomy, or presence of a choroidal effusion or suprachoroidal hemorrhage helps the clinician make the appropriate diagnosis. In some cases, the clinical picture is difficult to interpret, and surgical intervention may be required to establish the diagnosis.

Medical management includes the triad of intensive cycloplegic therapy; aggressive aqueous suppression with β-adrenergic antagonists, α_2-adrenergic agonists, and carbonic anhydrase inhibitors; and dehydration of the vitreous with hyperosmotic agents. Miotics can make malignant glaucoma worse and should not be used. In aphakic and pseudophakic eyes, the anterior vitreous can be disrupted with the Nd:YAG laser. Laser photocoagulation of the ciliary processes reportedly has been helpful in treating this condition; this procedure may alter the adjacent vitreous face. In some patients, malignant glaucoma can be controlled with medical management; however, many patients may require surgical intervention for control. The definitive surgical treatment is pars plana vitrectomy with anterior hyaloido-zonulectomy combined with iridectomy, ultimately creating a unicameral eye. BCSC Section 12, *Retina and Vitreous,* discusses vitrectomy in detail.

Foreman-Larkin J, Netland PA, Salim S. Clinical management of malignant glaucoma. *J Ophthalmol.* 2015;2015:283707. doi:10.1155/2015/283707

Uveal effusions and retinal pathologies

The terms *uveal effusion* and *uveal hemorrhage* refer to the abnormal accumulation of serous fluid or blood, respectively, in the potential space between the uvea (choroid and ciliary body) and the sclera. Causes include certain sulfonamide medications (see the section "Drug-induced secondary angle-closure glaucoma"), inflammation, infection, PRP, penetrating surgery, scleral buckle (see the section "Vitreoretinal surgery"), trauma, retinal vein occlusion, tumor, and uveal effusion syndrome. The mass effect of a suprachoroidal or supraciliary effusion may result in secondary angle closure related to forward displacement of the lens–iris interface.

In addition, exudative retinal detachments can act as space-occupying lesions, which may progressively compress the vitreous, moving it forward and resulting in angle closure. Potential causes of exudative retinal detachment include retinoblastoma, Coats disease, metastatic carcinoma, choroidal melanoma, suprachoroidal hemorrhage, choroidal effusion or detachment, infections (eg, HIV), and subretinal neovascularization in age-related macular degeneration with extensive effusion or hemorrhage.

Vitreoretinal surgery

Scleral buckles (especially the encircling bands) used for retinal detachment repair can produce angle narrowing and frank angle closure, often accompanied by choroidal effusion and anterior rotation of the ciliary body that result in flattening of the peripheral iris with a relatively deep central anterior chamber. Vortex vein compression may be responsible for the choroidal effusion. With medical therapy (cycloplegics, anti-inflammatory agents, β-adrenergic antagonists, carbonic anhydrase inhibitors, and hyperosmotic agents), the anterior chamber usually deepens with opening of the angle over days to weeks. If medical management is unsuccessful, laser iridoplasty, drainage of suprachoroidal fluid, or adjustment of the scleral buckle may be required. The scleral buckle can impede venous drainage by compressing a vortex vein, thus elevating episcleral venous pressure and IOP. Such cases may respond only to moving the scleral buckle or releasing tension on the encircling band. LPI is usually of no benefit in this condition as the mechanism is not pupillary block.

Injection of *air,* long-acting *gases* such as sulfur hexafluoride and perfluorocarbons (perfluoropropane and perfluoroethane), or *silicone oil* into the eye after pars plana vitrectomy may lead to angle closure by pushing the lens and/or iris forward. A surgical iridectomy can be done at the time of the vitrectomy. If a component of pupillary block is present, an LPI may be subsequently performed and beneficial. If performed, the iridotomy or iridectomy should be located inferiorly to prevent obstruction of the opening by the gas or oil, given that these substances are less dense than aqueous and rise to the top of the eye when the patient is upright.

Patients who have undergone complicated vitreoretinal surgery and have elevated IOP require individualized treatment plans. Therapeutic options include removal of the silicone oil; release of the encircling band; removal of expansile gases; and primary glaucoma surgery, such as trabeculectomy, tube shunt surgery, or a cyclodestructive procedure.

Following *PRP,* IOP may become elevated by an angle-closure mechanism. The ciliary body is thickened and rotated anteriorly, and often, an anterior annular choroidal effusion occurs. Generally, this secondary angle closure is self-limited, and therapy consists of temporary medical management with cycloplegic agents, topical corticosteroids, and aqueous suppressants.

Nanophthalmos

A nanophthalmic eye is normal in shape but unusually small, with a shortened axial length (<20 mm), shallow anterior chamber, small corneal diameter, and relatively large lens for the volume of the eye. These eyes are markedly hyperopic and highly susceptible to angle closure, which occurs at an earlier age than in typical PAC. Intraocular surgery is frequently complicated by choroidal effusion and nonrhegmatogenous retinal detachment. Choroidal effusion may occur spontaneously and may induce angle closure.

LPI, laser iridoplasty, and medical therapy are initial options to manage IOP elevation in these patients. Surgery should be avoided, if possible, because of the high rate of complications. When intraocular surgery is performed, prophylactic posterior sclerotomies may reduce the severity of intraoperative choroidal effusion. If the angles remain compromised despite a patent iridotomy, lens extraction is an additional treatment option. In such cases, a limited core vitrectomy is sometimes necessary to provide adequate anterior chamber depth for safe lens removal. Many clinicians consider early lens extraction in patients with nanophthalmos to avoid the development of angle closure. In these cases, the surgeon should consider prophylactic measures to reduce the risk of clinically significant choroidal effusion, including sclerotomies, decompression of the eye with a Honan balloon, and systemic hyperosmotic agents such as mannitol.

Persistent fetal vasculature and retinopathy of prematurity

The contraction of retrolental fibrovascular tissue seen in *persistent fetal vasculature* (*PFV;* formerly known as *persistent hyperplastic primary vitreous*) and in *retinopathy of prematurity (ROP)* can cause progressive narrowing of the anterior chamber angle with subsequent angle closure. In PFV, the onset of this complication is usually at 3–6 months of age, during the cicatricial phase of the disease, although angle closure may occur later in childhood.

Cataract may be associated with PFV, and cataractous swelling of the lens can also cause angle closure. PFV is usually unilateral and often associated with microphthalmos and elongated ciliary processes.

Eyes with ROP have a steeper cornea and a higher lens thickness to axial length ratio compared with healthy eyes. These features contribute to angle closure in ROP, leading to elevated IOP. NVI is also occasionally associated with ROP and may contribute to the development of angle closure. LPI may be performed as the first-line treatment of the angle closure. However, if the IOP cannot be controlled medically, lens extraction, trabeculectomy, or tube shunt surgery may be necessary.

For further discussion of PFV and ROP, see BCSC Section 6, *Pediatric Ophthalmology and Strabismus;* Section 11, *Lens and Cataract;* and Section 12, *Retina and Vitreous.*

Drug-induced secondary angle-closure glaucoma

A variety of drugs, both ocular and systemic, can lead to angle-closure glaucoma. They include and can be categorized as follows:

- ophthalmic (eg, dilating agents, pilocarpine)
- psychiatric (eg, selective serotonin reuptake inhibitors, benzodiazepines)
- neurologic (eg, topiramate)
- respiratory (eg, adrenergics, antihistamines, oseltamivir [Tamiflu])
- antibiotics (eg, sulfamethoxazole)
- diuretics (eg, acetazolamide, hydrochlorothiazide)
- anticoagulants (eg, heparin)
- neuromuscular blocking agents (eg, botulinum toxin)

Topiramate, a sulfamate-substituted monosaccharide, is an oral medication prescribed in the treatment of epilepsy, depression, headaches, and idiopathic intracranial hypertension. In some patients, this medication causes a syndrome characterized by acute myopic shift and acute bilateral angle closure. Patients with this syndrome experience sudden bilateral vision loss with acute myopia, bilateral ocular pain, and headache, usually within 1 month of starting topiramate. In addition to myopia, ocular findings in this syndrome include a uniformly shallow anterior chamber with anterior displacement of the iris and lens, microcystic corneal edema, elevated IOP (40–70 mm Hg), a closed anterior chamber angle, and choroidal effusion (Fig 10-15).

Other medications associated with uveal effusion and secondary angle closure include *acetazolamide, methazolamide, bupropion,* and *trimethoprim-sulfamethoxazole.* Some recreational drugs, including *MDMA* (3,4-methylenedioxymethamphetamine, or "ecstasy"), can also cause bilateral secondary angle closure.

When clinicians encounter a bilateral presentation of this type of angle closure, they should consider the possibility of an idiosyncratic response to topiramate or other drugs and should ask their patients about the use of drugs that can induce secondary angle closure.

Treatment of this syndrome involves immediate discontinuation of the inciting medication and initiation of medical therapy, generally in the form of aqueous suppressants, to decrease the IOP. In addition, systemic corticosteroids may hasten recovery. Aggressive cycloplegia may help deepen the anterior chamber and relieve the attack. The angle closure usually resolves within 24–48 hours with medical treatment, and the myopia resolves within

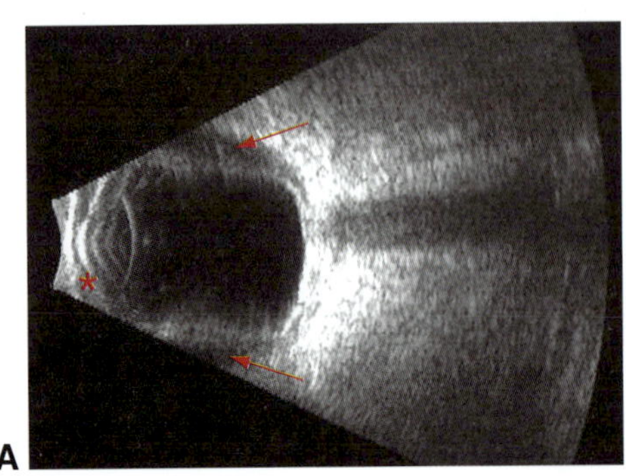

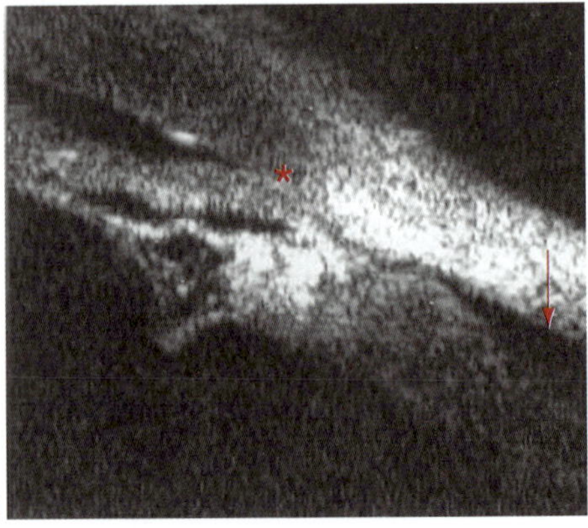

Figure 10-15 Topiramate-induced angle closure. **A,** B-scan ultrasonogram of an eye with a very shallow anterior chamber *(asterisk)* and topiramate-induced angle closure. The choroidal effusion is clearly evident *(arrows)*. **B,** Ultrasonographic view of an extremely shallow anterior chamber and closed angle *(asterisk)*. The posterior choroidal effusion is clearly visible *(arrow)*. *(Courtesy of Jonathan Eisengart, MD.)*

1–2 weeks of discontinuing topiramate. Because pupillary block is not an underlying mechanism of this syndrome, LPI is not indicated.

Murphy RM, Bakir B, O'Brien C, Wiggs JL, Pasquale LR. Drug-induced bilateral secondary angle-closure glaucoma: a literature synthesis. *J Glaucoma.* 2016;25(2):e99–e105. doi:10.1097/IJG.0000000000000270

Conditions Associated With Combined Pushing and Pulling or Other Mechanisms

Ocular inflammation

Secondary angle closure can occur as a result of ocular inflammation. Due to the breakdown of the blood–aqueous barrier, fibrin is released, and serum protein enters the aqueous, increasing the aqueous humor protein concentration, which may predispose to formation of posterior synechiae (Fig 10-16) and PAS. If left untreated, these posterior synechiae can lead to a secluded pupil and secondary angle closure (Fig 10-17). Complete (360°) posterior synechiae leading to pupillary block is properly referred to as *iris bombé*. Since the mechanism in iris bombé is pupillary block, LPI (possibly more than one) may be necessary to relieve the angle closure.

Peripheral iris edema, organization of inflammatory debris in the angle, and bridging of the angle by large keratic precipitates (seen in sarcoidosis) may accompany the ocular inflammation and lead to formation of PAS. These PAS form most often in the inferior angle, unlike the PAS in PAC, which typically occur in the superior angle. The PAS are usually not uniform in shape or height, further distinguishing inflammatory disease from PAC (Fig 10-18). In rare instances, ischemia secondary to inflammation may cause rubeosis iridis and neovascular glaucoma.

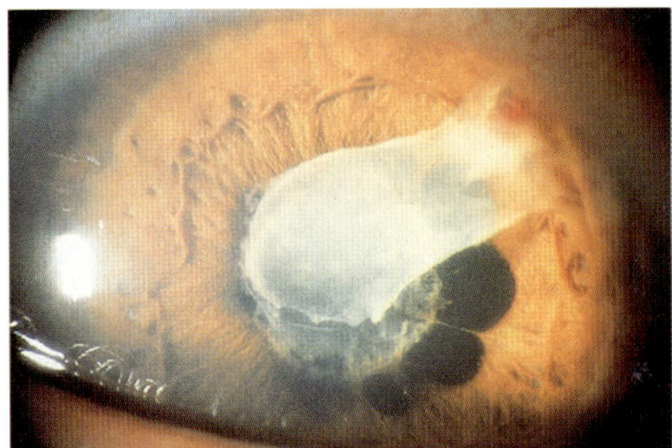

Figure 10-16 Inflammatory glaucoma in a patient with ankylosing spondylitis. A fibrinous anterior chamber reaction and posterior synechiae formation are evident. *(Courtesy of Steven T. Simmons, MD.)*

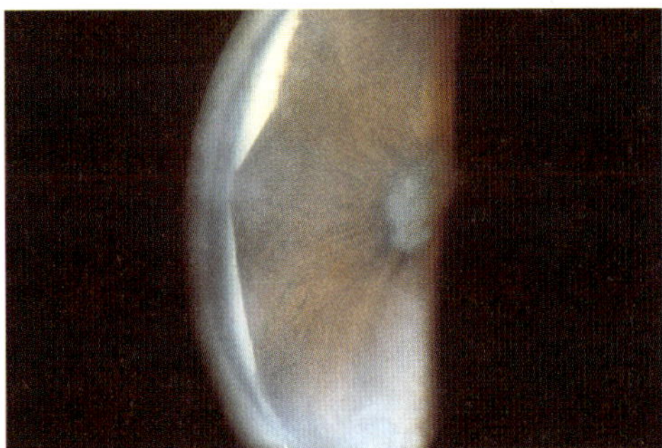

Figure 10-17 Clinical photograph showing inflammatory glaucoma. A secluded pupil is seen in a patient with long-standing uveitis with classic iris bombé and secondary angle closure. *(Courtesy of Steven T. Simmons, MD.)*

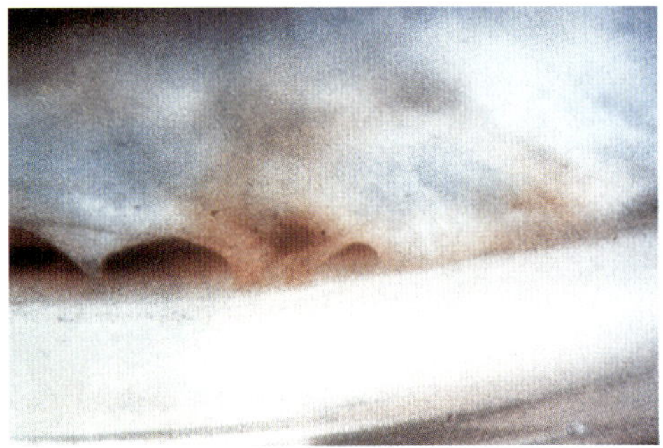

Figure 10-18 Inflammatory glaucoma. PAS in uveitis typically occur in the inferior anterior chamber angle and are not uniform in height or shape, as shown in this photograph. *(Courtesy of Joseph Krug, MD.)*

Ocular inflammation can lead to anterior chamber shallowing and to angle closure by other mechanisms as well, such as uveal effusion and subsequent anterior rotation of the ciliary body. Significant posterior uveitis can cause massive exudative retinal detachment or choroidal effusions that push the lens–iris interface forward, resulting in secondary angle closure. Treatment is primarily directed at the underlying cause of the uveitis. Aqueous suppressants and corticosteroids are the primary agents for reducing IOP and preventing synechial angle closure in this situation. Although prostaglandin analogues can cause increased inflammation in some eyes, they may be considered for control of IOP, if needed.

Interstitial keratitis may be associated with open-angle glaucoma or angle closure. The angle-closure component may be caused by chronic inflammation and PAS formation or by multiple cysts of the iris pigment epithelium.

Sng CC, Barton K. Mechanism and management of angle closure in uveitis. *Curr Opin Ophthalmol.* 2015;26(2):121–127.

Flat anterior chamber after surgery

A flat anterior chamber from any cause can result in the formation of PAS. Hypotony in an eye with a flat chamber after cataract surgery or filtering surgery indicates an aqueous leak or overfiltration unless proven otherwise. A Seidel test should be performed to locate a leak. Simple pressure patching or bandage contact lens application will sometimes seal the leak and allow the anterior chamber to re-form. If the chamber does not re-form, the leak should be repaired surgically to prevent synechial angle closure or other complications of hypotony.

Debate continues concerning how long a postoperative flat chamber should be managed conservatively before surgical intervention is undertaken. Some ophthalmologists repair the wound leak and re-form a flat chamber following cataract surgery within 24 hours. Others prefer observation in conjunction with corticosteroid therapy for several days to prevent formation of synechiae. Although iridocorneal contact is well tolerated, contact between the cornea and the hyaloid face or an IOL requires re-formation of the chamber without delay to minimize corneal endothelial damage. Early intervention should also be considered in the presence of corneal edema, excessive inflammation, or posterior synechiae formation.

Secondary angle closure after corneal endothelial transplant

Secondary angle closure, including an acute angle-closure attack, may occur after corneal endothelial transplant. At the end of such procedures, an air bubble is injected into the anterior chamber to help maintain adherence of the graft to the recipient corneal stroma. If the air moves into the posterior chamber, the iris can be pushed forward, resulting in angle closure. Another mechanism of angle closure after corneal endothelial transplant is pupillary block, which can occur when air in the anterior chamber obstructs the flow of aqueous humor at the pupil. Treatment modalities include LPI, medical therapies to lower the IOP, cycloplegia, and air removal.

CHAPTER 11

Glaucoma in Children and Adolescents

This chapter includes related videos. Go to aao.org/bcscvideo_section10 or scan the QR codes in the text to access this content.

Highlights

- Pediatric glaucomas can cause damage to the optic nerve, visual field, and up to approximately age 4 years, the cornea and other structures.
- Examination of a child can be challenging, so best results may be obtained with a systematic approach that includes the use of general anesthesia.
- For most cases of primary congenital glaucoma, surgery is the preferred, definitive treatment. The angle is frequently the first site of surgical intervention in children.

Classification

The glaucomas of childhood and adolescence (herein called *pediatric glaucomas*) are a heterogeneous group of disorders associated with elevated intraocular pressure (IOP). These rare disorders, which have various presentations and etiologies, can cause damage to the optic nerve, visual field, and up to approximately age 4 years, the cornea and other structures. The Childhood Glaucoma Research Network and the World Glaucoma Association have defined both glaucoma and glaucoma suspect for pediatric populations (Table 11-1). Although pediatric glaucomas share many characteristics with adult-onset glaucomas, there are numerous management issues that are unique to the pediatric and adolescent populations.

Typically, pediatric glaucoma is classified as primary or secondary (Table 11-2). Isolated abnormalities of the anterior chamber angle are seen in the primary pediatric glaucomas. In *primary congenital glaucoma (PCG),* angle dysgenesis leads to outflow resistance and elevated IOP, which in turn leads to the classic features of PCG: enlarged and/or cloudy corneas, Haab striae, and an enlarged globe (buphthalmos). In *juvenile open-angle glaucoma (JOAG),* another high-pressure primary glaucoma, the angle appearance may be normal. This type of glaucoma develops later in childhood (generally after 4 years of age) or in early adulthood.

Table 11-1 Definitions of Pediatric Glaucoma and Glaucoma Suspect

Finding	Pediatric Glaucoma: IOP-Related Damage to the Eye; at Least 2 of the Following Criteria Required for Diagnosis	Pediatric Glaucoma Suspect: No IOP-Related Damage; at Least 1 of the Following Criteria Required for Diagnosis
IOP	IOP >21 mm Hg	IOP >21 mm Hg on 2 separate occasions
Optic disc (also called *optic nerve head*)	Optic disc cupping: progressive increase in cup–disc ratio	Optic disc appearance suggestive of glaucoma (ie, increased cup–disc ratio for size of optic disc)
	Cup–disc ratio asymmetry of ≥0.2 between the 2 eyes when the optic discs are similar in size	
	Focal rim thinning	
Cornea	Haab striae	Increased corneal diameter or axial length in eyes with normal IOP
	Diameter ≥11 mm in newborn infants, >12 mm in children <1 year, or >13 mm at any age	
Visual field	Reproducible visual field defect consistent with glaucomatous optic neuropathy with no other observable reason for defect	Visual field suggestive of glaucoma
Myopia	Progressive myopia, myopic shift, or an increase in ocular dimensions inconsistent with normal growth	–

IOP = intraocular pressure.

Information adapted from Beck AD, Chang TCP, Freedman SF. Definition, classification, differential diagnosis. In: Weinreb RN, Grajewski AL, Papadopoulos M, Grigg J, Freedman S, eds. *Childhood Glaucoma.* Kugler Publications; 2013:3–10. *World Glaucoma Association Consensus Series—9.*

Secondary pediatric glaucomas are associated with other ocular or systemic conditions. These glaucomas are further classified according to whether the associated condition is acquired after birth or is present at birth (nonacquired) (Tables 11-3, 11-4; see also Table 11-2). Nonacquired pediatric glaucoma is categorized according to whether the signs of the associated condition are mainly ocular or systemic. Glaucoma following extraction of a congenital cataract is its own category. See BCSC Section 6, *Pediatric Ophthalmology and Strabismus,* for additional discussion of many of the topics covered in this chapter.

Thau A, Lloyd M, Freedman S, Beck A, Grajewski A, Levin AV. New classification system for pediatric glaucoma: implications for clinical care and research registry. *Curr Opin Ophthalmol.* 2018;29(5):385–394.

Genetics

Some pediatric glaucomas are inherited and associated with known pathogenic genetic variants (mutations). Genetic testing and counseling should be considered for parents of pediatric glaucoma patients and for adults with onset of glaucoma in childhood or early

Table 11-2 Classification of Pediatric Glaucoma

Primary Pediatric Glaucoma

Primary congenital glaucoma

Neonatal onset (age 0–1 month)

Infantile onset (age 1–24 months)

Late onset or late recognized (age ≥24 months)

Comments: Isolated angle anomalies, with or without mild congenital iris anomalies

Meets glaucoma definition; usually with ocular enlargement

Spontaneously arrested cases have normal IOP but typical signs of primary congenital glaucoma

Juvenile open-angle glaucoma (age 4–40 years)

Comments: Open angle, usually normal angle appearance

Meets glaucoma definition; no corneal enlargement

No congenital ocular anomalies or syndromes

Usually very elevated IOP

Secondary Pediatric Glaucoma

Glaucoma associated with nonacquired ocular anomalies

Comments: Includes predominantly ocular anomalies present at birth that may be associated with nonocular findings

Meets glaucoma definition

Glaucoma associated with nonacquired systemic disease or syndrome

Comments: Includes predominantly systemic diseases present at birth that may be associated with ocular findings

Meets glaucoma definition

Glaucoma associated with acquired conditions[a]

Comments: Meets glaucoma definition after acquired condition is recognized

Glaucoma diagnosed based on gonioscopy results:

- open-angle glaucoma: angle ≥50% open (<180° ITC)
- angle-closure glaucoma: angle <50% open (≥180° ITC) or acute angle closure

Glaucoma following cataract surgery

Comments: Meets glaucoma definition only after cataract surgery is performed and is categorized on the basis of the type of cataract removed:

- congenital idiopathic cataract
- congenital cataract associated with ocular anomalies/systemic disease; no previous glaucoma
- acquired cataract; no previous glaucoma

Glaucoma diagnosed based on gonioscopy results:

- open-angle glaucoma: angle ≥50% open (<180° ITC)
- angle-closure glaucoma: angle <50% open (≥180° ITC) or acute angle closure

ITC = iridotrabecular contact.

[a] An acquired condition is one that is not inherited or present at birth.

Information adapted from Beck AD, Chang TCP, Freedman SF. Definition, classification, differential diagnosis. In: Weinreb RN, Grajewski AL, Papadopoulos M, Grigg J, Freedman S, eds. *Childhood Glaucoma.* Kugler Publications; 2013:3–10. *World Glaucoma Association Consensus Series—9.* Also adapted from Beck AD, Chang TCP. Glaucoma: definitions and classification. *Disease Reviews.* Pediatric Ophthalmology Education Center. American Academy of Ophthalmology; 2015. Accessed January 29, 2024. aao.org/disease-review/glaucoma-definitions-classification

Table 11-3 Secondary Glaucomas Associated With Nonacquired Conditions

Predominantly ocular anomalies present at birth that may be associated with systemic findings

Anterior segment abnormalities
- Aniridia
- Axenfeld-Rieger anomaly (Axenfeld-Rieger syndrome if systemic abnormalities present)
- Congenital corneal opacification
- Congenital ectropion uveae
- Congenital iris hypoplasia
- Ectopia lentis: simple ectopia lentis (no systemic associations; possible type 1 fibrillin *[FBN1]* pathogenic variant), ectopia lentis et papillae
- Microcornea
- Microphthalmos
- Microspherophakia
- Oculodermal melanocytosis (nevus of Ota)
- Peters anomaly (syndrome if systemic associations)
- Posterior polymorphous corneal dystrophy
- Primary congenital aphakia
- Tumors of the iris

Posterior segment abnormalities
- Familial exudative vitreoretinopathy
- Persistent fetal vasculature (if glaucoma present before cataract surgery)
- Retinopathy of prematurity
- Tumors of the ciliary body or retina

Known syndromes, systemic anomalies, or systemic diseases present at birth that may be associated with ocular findings

Chromosomal disorders such as trisomy 21 (Down syndrome)

Congenital rubella

Connective tissue disorders: Marfan syndrome, osteogenesis imperfecta, Stickler syndrome, Weill-Marchesani syndrome

Klippel-Trénaunay-Weber syndrome

Metabolic disorders: homocystinuria, Lowe (oculocerebrorenal) syndrome, mucopolysaccharidoses

Nail-patella syndrome

Phakomatoses: neurofibromatosis 1, Sturge-Weber syndrome

Rubinstein-Taybi syndrome

Information adapted from Beck AD, Chang TCP, Freedman SF. Definition, classification, differential diagnosis. In: Weinreb RN, Grajewski AL, Papadopoulos M, Grigg J, Freedman S, eds. *Childhood Glaucoma.* Kugler Publications; 2013:3–10. *World Glaucoma Association Consensus Series—9.*

adulthood. See Chapter 1, Table 1-2, which lists important mendelian genes associated with the more common pediatric glaucomas and glaucoma syndromes.

Primary Congenital Glaucoma

Although most cases of PCG occur sporadically, up to 40% of cases are inherited in an autosomal recessive pattern with incomplete or variable penetrance. Increased rates of familial

Table 11-4 Secondary Glaucomas Associated With Acquired Conditions

Childhood Glaucoma Research Network classification of glaucoma criteria met; glaucoma not present at birth and can be either open-angle or angle-closure type
Uveitic
Traumatic (hyphema, angle recession, ectopia lentis)
Steroid/medication induced
Glaucoma secondary to tumor (benign/malignant, ocular/orbital)
Glaucoma secondary to retinopathy of prematurity, familial exudative vitreoretinopathy, persistent fetal vasculature
Prior ocular surgery, *excluding* cataract surgery

Information adapted from Beck AD, Chang TCP, Freedman SF. Definition, classification, differential diagnosis. In: Weinreb RN, Grajewski AL, Papadopoulos M, Grigg J, Freedman S, eds. *Childhood Glaucoma.* Kugler Publications; 2013:3–10. *World Glaucoma Association Consensus Series—9.*

inheritance are seen in children from the Middle East and central Europe among families with a history of consanguinity. PCG can be caused by an alteration of transcription factors or signaling pathways that are essential for anterior segment development. This includes alterations in retinoic acid, transforming growth factor β, and angiopoietin signaling, as well as transcriptional networks involving *PAX6, FOXC1,* and *PITX2.*

PCG is most commonly caused by autosomal recessive pathogenic variants in *CYP1B1* within the *GLC3A* locus. *CYP1B1* encodes cytochrome P450 oxygenase, an enzyme that converts retinol (vitamin A) to retinal and then to retinoic acid. This enzyme is thought to be important in development of the anterior segment and regulation of aqueous humor secretion. Less commonly, PCG is associated with pathogenic variants in *LTBP2* (within the *GLC3C/GLC3D* loci), also inherited in an autosomal recessive pattern. *LTBP2* encodes an extracellular matrix protein associated with cell adhesion and microfibril assembly. *LTBP2* variants have been associated with other ocular conditions, including megalocornea, microspherophakia, and ectopia lentis, as well as Weill-Marchesani syndrome. Pathogenic variants in *ANGPT1* and *TEK* (also known as *TIE2*) within *GLC3E* are inherited in an autosomal dominant pattern. The angiopoietin-tie (ANG-TIE) signaling pathway is an essential regulator of blood and lymphatic development. Pathogenic variants in *ANGPT1* or *TEK* result in loss of protein function that affects development of the Schlemm canal and can lead to PCG.

Lewis CJ, Hedberg-Buenz A, DeLuca AP, Stone EM, Alward WLM, Fingert JH. Primary congenital and developmental glaucomas. *Hum Mol Genet.* 2017;26(R1):R28–36.

Zhao Y, Sorenson CM, Sheibani N. Cytochrome P450 1B1 and primary congenital glaucoma. *J Ophthalmic Vis Res.* 2015;10(1):60–67.

Pediatric Glaucoma Without Anterior Segment Dysgenesis

Families with autosomal dominant inheritance of early-onset glaucoma without anterior segment dysgenesis (eg, JOAG) may have pathogenic variants in *MYOC (GLC1A),* the gene coding for myocilin. Aggregation of abnormal myocilin (formerly called TIGR), a protein found in the trabecular meshwork and ciliary body, is thought to result in trabecular meshwork dysfunction. Approximately 20% of these families will have *MYOC* pathogenic variants. The confirmed presence of an *MYOC* variant in a patient can prompt earlier screening and monitoring of their family members for glaucoma.

Pediatric Glaucoma With Anterior Segment Dysgenesis

For patients with conditions involving anterior segment dysgenesis, the proband should be tested for pathogenic variants in *FOXC1, PITX2, PAX6,* and *LMX1B.* These genes are important in the development of the eye and other structures. The order of the genetic testing is prioritized according to the patient's clinical features. Once a pathogenic variant has been identified, the entire family (both affected and unaffected members) can be screened. Unaffected family members may be identified as carriers of the pathogenic variant and informed of the potential risk to any future offspring. Together, *PITX2* and *FOXC1* pathogenic variants account for 50% of the glaucoma cases associated with anterior segment dysgenesis.

Balikov DA, Jacobson A, Prasov L. Glaucoma syndromes: insights into glaucoma genetics and pathogenesis from monogenic syndromic disorders. *Genes (Basel).* 2021;12(9):1403. doi:10.3390/genes12091403

Chen HY, Lehmann OJ, Swaroop A. Genetics and therapy for pediatric eye diseases. *EBioMedicine.* 2021 May;67:103360. doi:10.1016/j.ebiom.2021.103360

Primary Congenital Glaucoma

Incidence

Primary congenital glaucoma (PCG) accounts for most primary pediatric glaucoma cases, and newborn PCG accounts for approximately 25% of PCG cases. PCG is bilateral in 70% of patients and is diagnosed within the first year of life in over 75% of cases. It occurs more frequently in males (65%) than females. The incidence varies with race and ethnicity, and consanguinity greatly increases the risk. Without a family history of PCG, an affected patient has a 2% chance of having a child with PCG.

Ko F, Papadopoulos M, Khaw PT. Primary congenital glaucoma. *Prog Brain Res.* 2015; 221:177–189.

Pathophysiology

The pathogenesis of PCG is undetermined. Clinically, the angle appears immature, which is thought to result from developmental arrest of tissues derived from cranial neural crest cells. This is believed to subsequently cause increased resistance to aqueous outflow through the trabecular meshwork. Barkan hypothesized that this resistance was caused by a membrane covering the anterior chamber angle. Although this membrane has never been identified, developmental anomalies of the angle are found in eyes with PCG, with dysgenesis and compression of the trabecular meshwork and an anterior insertion of the iris root (Fig 11-1). In cases with pathogenic variants in *ANGPT1* or *TEK,* the etiology is thought to be maldevelopment of the Schlemm canal.

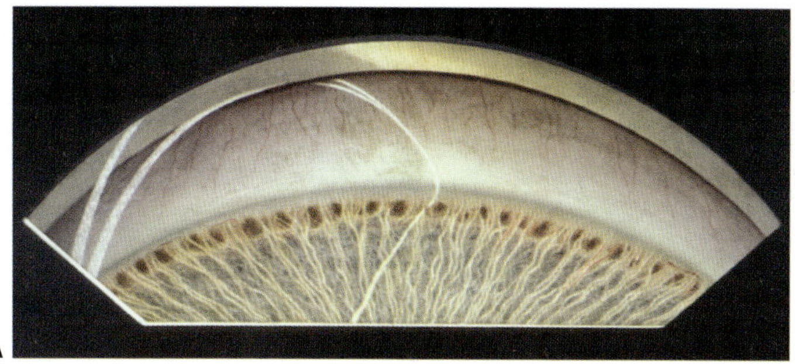

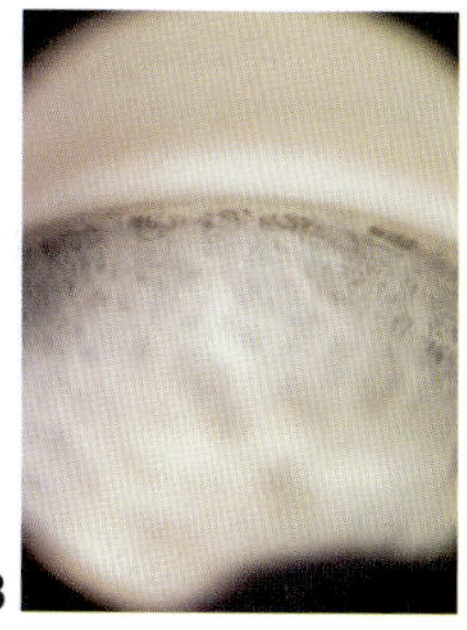

Figure 11-1 Anterior chamber angle in primary congenital glaucoma (PCG). **A,** Illustration of a gonioscopic view of the anterior chamber angle in PCG reveals a deep angle with no angle recess due to compression of the trabecular meshwork and an anterior insertion of the iris root. The iris root appears as a scalloped line with reduced density of the iris fibers (rarefaction). **B,** Goniophotograph of the angle shows a similar view with scalloped edges. *(Part A courtesy of Lee Allen and Wallace L. M. Alward, MD; part B courtesy of Faruk Orge, MD.)*

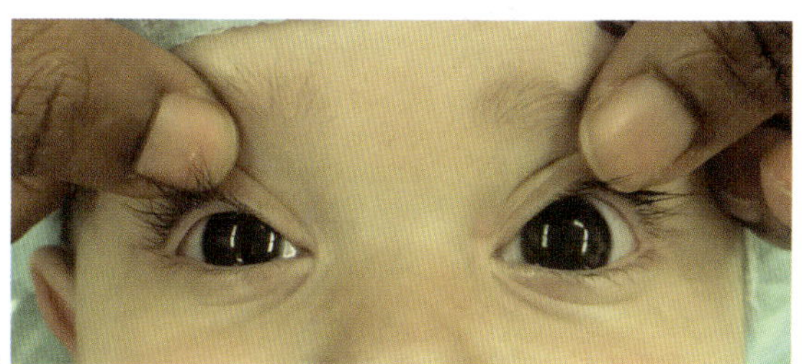

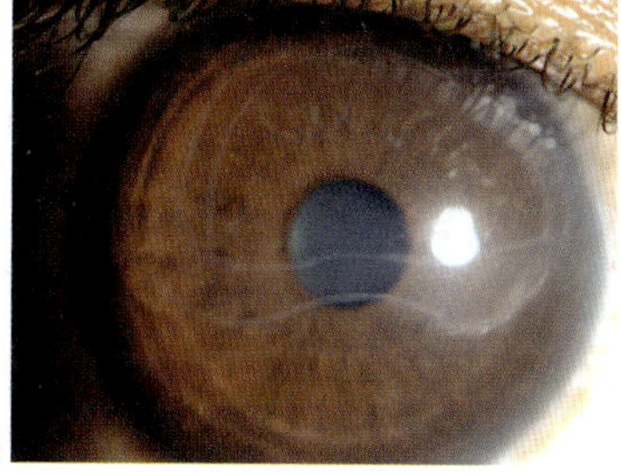

Figure 11-2 Primary congenital glaucoma. **A,** Child with unilateral buphthalmos resulting from uncontrolled elevated intraocular pressure (IOP) in the left eye prior to surgery. **B,** Haab striae, or breaks in Descemet membrane, which are visible after corneal edema clears. The striae are both horizontal and circumferential. *(Part A courtesy of JoAnn A. Giaconi, MD; part B courtesy of Deepak Edward, MD.)*

Clinical Features

In infants, PCG presents with the classic triad of epiphora, photophobia, and blepharospasm. Elevated IOP causes the cornea to stretch, leading to increased corneal diameter and enlargement of the globe (buphthalmos; Fig 11-2A), along with stretching of the scleral canal, through which the optic nerve passes. The corneal stretching produces breaks in Descemet membrane, known as *Haab striae,* and may lead to corneal edema and corneal opacification (Fig 11-2B; see also BCSC Section 6, *Pediatric Ophthalmology and Strabismus*). As the cornea swells, the child may become irritable and photophobic. After age 3–4 years, the cornea ceases to enlarge further; however, scleral stretching can continue up to 10 years of age. Sustained IOP elevation may result in continued optic nerve damage.

Differential Diagnosis

The extensive differential diagnosis for PCG is presented in Table 11-5. Figure 11-3 presents an algorithm for the classification of childhood glaucoma. PCG should be considered in the

Table 11-5 Differential Diagnosis for Symptoms and Signs of Primary Congenital Glaucoma

Conditions associated with epiphora
Nasolacrimal duct obstruction
Corneal epithelial defect or abrasion
Conjunctivitis
Keratitis
Ocular inflammation (due to uveitis, trauma)
Epiblepharon with eyelash–corneal touch
Conditions associated with corneal enlargement or apparent enlargement
X-linked megalocornea
Exophthalmos
Shallow orbits (eg, craniofacial dysostoses)
Axial myopia
Conditions associated with corneal clouding
Birth trauma with breaks in Descemet membrane
Keratitis (secondary to maternal rubella, herpes, phlyctenules)
Corneal dystrophies: congenital hereditary endothelial dystrophy, posterior polymorphous corneal dystrophy
Corneal malformations: dermoids, sclerocornea, choristomas, Peters anomaly
Congenital corneal opacification
Keratomalacia
Lysosomal storage diseases with associated corneal abnormalities: mucopolysaccharidosis, sphingolipidosis, cystinosis
Skin disorders affecting the cornea: congenital ichthyosis, congenital dyskeratosis
Nonglaucomatous optic nerve abnormalities
Pit
Coloboma
Hypoplasia
Malformation
Atrophy
Physiologic cupping, particularly in a large optic nerve
Periventricular leukomalacia

differential diagnosis of epiphora in children. PCG is a relatively rare disease and may go undetected or be misdiagnosed by primary care doctors and general ophthalmologists. Mild cases may be misdiagnosed as nasolacrimal duct obstruction, resulting in a delayed PCG diagnosis and irreversible damage. Physicians must be vigilant in their examination and refer infants presenting with the classic triad of epiphora, photophobia, and blepharospasm to a specialist without delay. Left untreated, PCG will progress to blindness in nearly all cases.

Treatment and Prognosis

Treatment of PCG typically requires surgical intervention following a thorough examination with the patient under anesthesia (see the section Surgical Management later in this

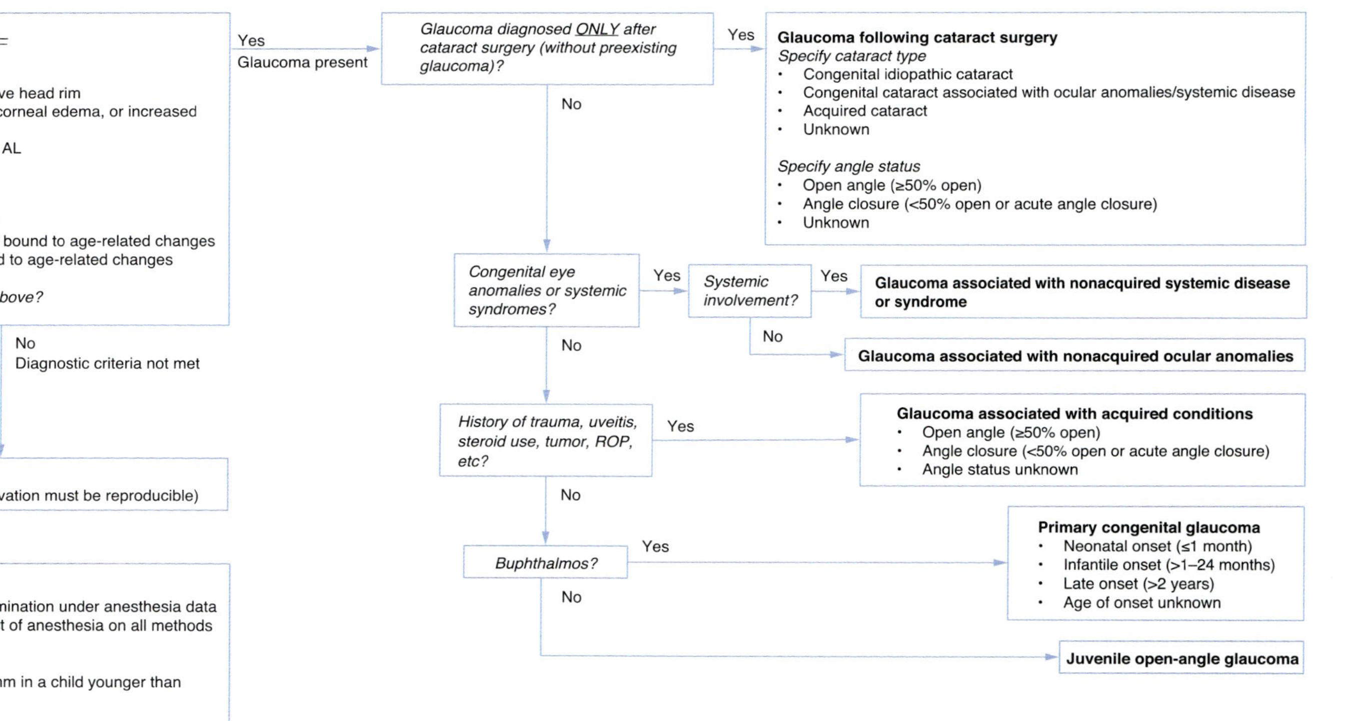

Figure 11-3 Modified Childhood Glaucoma Research Network/World Glaucoma Association algorithm for the classification of childhood glaucoma. *(Courtesy of Ta Chen Peter Chang, MD, on behalf of the Childhood Glaucoma Research Network (CGRN) and the Samuel & Ethel Balkan International Pediatric Glaucoma Center, Bascom Palmer Eye Institute, University of Miami.)*

chapter). Medical therapy has limited long-term value but may be used to temporize or reduce corneal edema for improved visualization during surgery.

PCG generally has a better visual prognosis than most secondary pediatric glaucomas. In retrospective reviews in the United States, approximately two-thirds of patients with PCG have a visual acuity of 20/70 or better at final follow-up.

A poorer prognosis is associated with the following:

- newborn PCG (50% of patients progress to legal blindness)
- PCG diagnosed after 1 year of age
- corneal diameter >14 mm (severe dysgenesis may make IOP control difficult, or late-stage optic nerve damage may be present at time of diagnosis)

The prognosis is best for patients diagnosed between 3 and 12 months of age, as most of these cases respond well to angle surgery (goniotomy, trabeculotomy).

Juvenile Open-Angle Glaucoma

Juvenile open-angle glaucoma (JOAG) is a form of primary open-angle glaucoma that presents between the ages of 4 and 40 years, usually with very elevated IOP and normal-appearing angles. Because most cases of JOAG are inherited as an autosomal dominant trait, many families may be aware of their risk of developing this condition, leading to earlier screening and detection. Although the IOP is elevated, it does not cause corneal enlargement or Haab striae because of the later age at onset; however, progressive myopia may result and continue until 10 years of age.

The first-line treatment of JOAG is medical therapy, but many cases are refractory to maximal medical treatment and may require incisional glaucoma surgery. Angle procedures may be helpful in select cases. However, the response to angle surgery may be reduced in eyes with JOAG compared with PCG, because of the presence of other angle abnormalities in JOAG. Although trabeculectomy has been effective in JOAG, tube shunt surgery may be preferable in these eyes because of the risks associated with antimetabolites, which are typically used with trabeculectomy surgery, and the greater tendency for fibrosis in younger patients. Also, high myopia is associated with an increased likelihood of hypotony after trabeculectomy.

Secondary Glaucomas Associated With Nonacquired Conditions

Pediatric glaucomas may be associated with various ocular and systemic abnormalities that are present at birth (see Table 11-3). The following sections discuss some of the more common conditions that are associated with glaucoma. For further discussion of these entities, see BCSC Section 6, *Pediatric Ophthalmology and Strabismus,* and Section 8, *External Disease and Cornea.*

Axenfeld-Rieger Syndrome

Axenfeld-Rieger syndrome (ARS) is a spectrum of disorders characterized by anomalous development of the neural crest–derived anterior segment structures, including the angle,

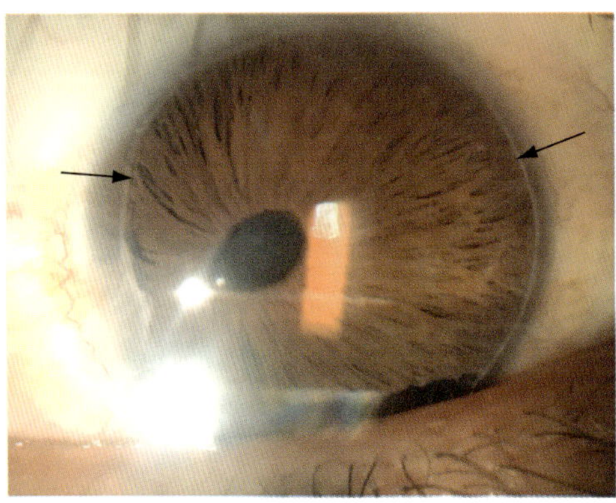

Figure 11-4 An eye with Axenfeld-Rieger syndrome with prominent posterior embryotoxon *(arrows)* and corectopia. The term *posterior embryotoxon* refers to the displacement of the Schwalbe line anterior to the corneal limbus. *(Courtesy of Jonathan Young, MD, PhD.)*

iris, and trabecular meshwork. ARS is bilateral, and there is no sex predilection. Most cases of ARS are inherited in an autosomal dominant manner, but sporadic cases can occur.

Classic clinical manifestations include the following:

- *posterior embryotoxon* of the cornea, seen as a prominent and anteriorly displaced Schwalbe line (Fig 11-4)
- *iris adhesions* to the Schwalbe line that may be focal or broad (see Fig 11-4)
- *iris changes,* including hypoplasia, corectopia, holes, and ectropion uveae

The term *Axenfeld anomaly* previously referred to a condition characterized by the first 2 clinical manifestations, while *Rieger anomaly* was used for an entity characterized by all 3 findings. The term *Rieger syndrome* was used to describe Rieger anomaly occurring with developmental defects of the teeth or facial bones, including maxillary hypoplasia; redundant periumbilical skin; pituitary abnormalities; or hypospadias. Axenfeld anomaly, Rieger anomaly, and Rieger syndrome are now recognized as variations of the same clinical entity, ARS. See BCSC Section 4, *Ophthalmic Pathology and Intraocular Tumors,* and Section 8, *External Disease and Cornea,* for additional discussion. Table 11-6 outlines the differential diagnosis of ARS to help distinguish it from other conditions involving abnormalities of the iris, cornea, and anterior chamber.

Approximately 50% of cases of ARS are associated with glaucoma, which typically occurs in middle or late childhood. Glaucoma is thought to develop because of the abnormal formation of the trabecular meshwork or Schlemm canal. The development of glaucoma correlates with the height of the iris insertion in the angle, not to the number of iris processes or the degree of iris abnormality. Treatment is generally the same as for an OAG; however, angle surgery may not be possible if there are many iris processes. Possible treatments for glaucoma associated with ARS include medications, goniotomy, trabeculotomy, trabeculectomy, tube shunt surgery, and cyclodestructive procedures.

Peters Anomaly

Peters anomaly is a rare developmental condition presenting with an annular corneal opacity (leukoma) in the central visual axis (Fig 11-5), often accompanied by iris strands that originate at the iris collarette and adhere to the corneal opacity. The leukoma corresponds to a defect in the corneal endothelium and underlying Descemet membrane and posterior

Table 11-6 Differential Diagnosis for Axenfeld-Rieger Syndrome

Condition	Differentiating Features
Iridocorneal endothelial syndrome	Unilateral Middle-age onset Corneal endothelial abnormalities Progressive changes
Isolated posterior embryotoxon	Lack of glaucoma-associated or iris changes
Aniridia	Iris hypoplasia Associated corneal and macular changes
Iridoschisis	Splitting of iris layers with atrophy of anterior layer
Peters anomaly	Corneal leukoma
Ectopia lentis et pupillae	Lens subluxation Pupillary displacement Axial myopia Retinal detachment Enlarged corneal diameter Cataract Prominent iris processes in the anterior chamber angle
Oculodentodigital dysplasia	Microphthalmos Microcornea Iris abnormalities Cataracts

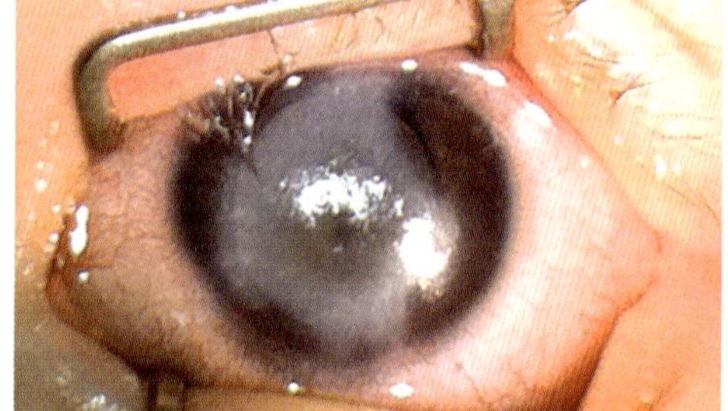

Figure 11-5 An eye with Peters anomaly exhibiting a central leukoma, which can be confused with corneal edema. *(Courtesy of JoAnn A. Giaconi, MD.)*

stroma. The lens may be in its normal position, with or without a cataract, or the lens may be adherent to the posterior layers of the cornea. Patients with corneolenticular adhesions have an increased likelihood of other ocular abnormalities, such as microcornea and angle anomalies, and of systemic abnormalities, including those of the heart, genitourinary tract, musculoskeletal system, ear, palate, and spine.

Peters anomaly is usually sporadic, although autosomal dominant and autosomal recessive forms have been reported. Most cases are bilateral, and angle abnormalities leading to glaucoma occur in approximately 50% of affected patients. Development of glaucoma is more common in patients with cataracts or corneolenticular adhesions. Glaucoma is thought to result from a malformed trabecular meshwork or Schlemm canal and/or formation of peripheral anterior synechiae. Secondary glaucoma may also occur after penetrating keratoplasty or with long-term steroid use. Elevated IOP typically presents in infancy but can also arise later in life.

Treatment of glaucoma associated with Peters anomaly can be difficult because of the iridocorneal dysgenesis. If possible, angle surgery is performed. Alternative treatments include medications, trabeculectomy, tube shunt surgery, and cyclodestructive procedures.

Aniridia

Aniridia is a panocular, bilateral congenital disorder characterized by iris hypoplasia (Fig 11-6). Most patients with aniridia have only a rudimentary stump of iris; however, the iris appearance may vary greatly, with some patients having nearly complete but thin irides. Aniridia is associated with other ocular anomalies, including microcornea, anterior polar cataracts that may present at birth or develop later in life, and optic nerve and foveal hypoplasia resulting in pendular nystagmus and reduced vision.

It had been thought that glaucoma develops in patients with aniridia after the rudimentary iris stump rotates anteriorly to progressively cover the trabecular meshwork, resulting in synechial angle closure. However, one study showed that aniridia patients without previous intraocular surgery did not have angle closure even when they had glaucoma. This suggests that intraocular surgery, especially angle surgery, may trigger closure of the angle. IOP elevation in aniridia may not occur until the second decade of life or later. Occasionally, however, aniridia is associated with congenital glaucoma; primary maldevelopment of the drainage angle may result in elevated IOP at a younger age.

Patients with aniridia may have limbal stem cell abnormalities that eventually result in a corneal pannus, which begins in the peripheral cornea and slowly extends centrally. If corneal opacification threatens vision, keratolimbal stem cell transplantation can be performed.

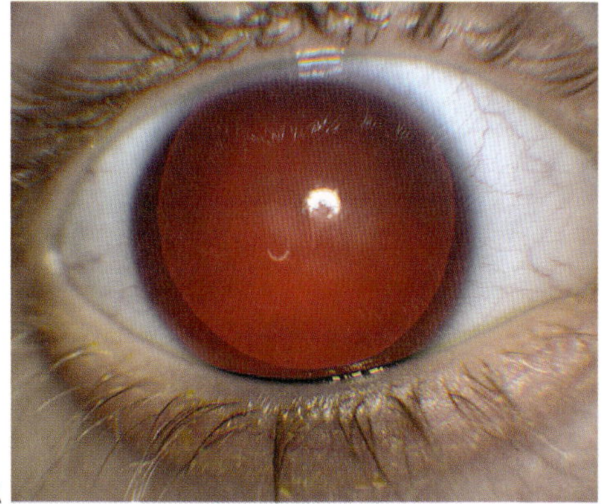

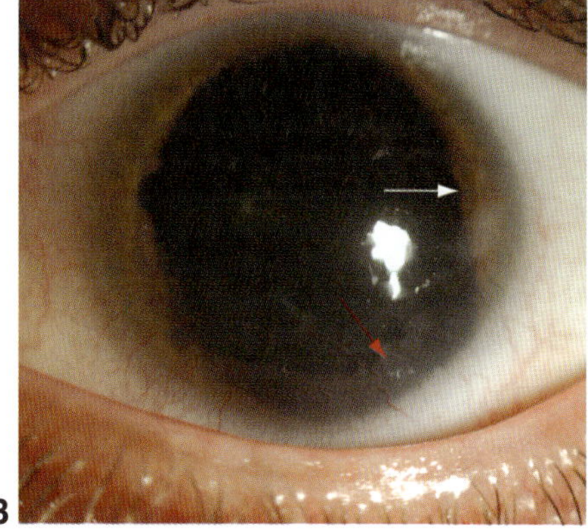

Figure 11-6 Iris morphology in aniridia in 2 patients with documented *PAX6* pathogenic variants. **A,** An eye with aniridia with no iris visible on slit-lamp biomicroscopy, exposing zonular fibers and lens edge. **B,** An eye with aniridia in which remnants of rudimentary, hypoplastic iris tissue are present *(white arrow)*. Peripheral aniridic keratopathy, a classic finding in aniridia involving thickening and vascularization of the peripheral cornea, is also present *(red arrow)*. *(Courtesy of Peter A. Netland, MD, PhD.)*

Implantation of an artificial iris can be performed for cosmesis; however, this implant is not recommended for children younger than 16 years.

Most cases of aniridia are inherited and transmitted in an autosomal dominant pattern (66% of cases); however, approximately one-third of cases result from isolated sporadic pathogenic variants in *PAX6* on band 11p13. Approximately 20%–30% of the sporadic cases are associated with a large chromosomal deletion that includes *PAX6* and the adjacent Wilms tumor 1 gene *(WT1),* a tumor suppressor gene. These patients have a 50% chance of developing a Wilms tumor and require abdominal ultrasonography to screen for tumor development. Relatively few cases of Wilms tumor are seen in the inherited form.

In addition to isolated aniridia without systemic involvement, there are 2 less common phenotypes of aniridia that are associated with systemic abnormalities. *WAGR* (Wilms tumor, aniridia, genitourinary anomalies, and cognitive disability) *syndrome* is an autosomal dominant disorder that occurs in 13% of patients with aniridia. *Gillespie syndrome* is an autosomal recessive form of aniridia associated with cerebellar ataxia and intellectual disability that occurs in 2% of persons with aniridia.

Sturge-Weber Syndrome

Sturge-Weber syndrome (SWS; *encephalofacial angiomatosis*) is a phakomatosis characterized by a facial cutaneous hemangioma (port-wine birthmark), with ipsilateral choroidal cavernous hemangioma, and ipsilateral leptomeningeal angioma associated with cerebral calcifications, seizures, focal neurologic deficits, and a variable degree of cognitive impairment. The syndrome is sporadic, usually unilateral (rarely bilateral), and has no race or sex predilection.

Glaucoma is the most common ocular complication, occurring in 30%–70% of patients with SWS. It has a bimodal presentation, with 60% of cases presenting from age 0 to 3 years and 40% presenting later in life. Glaucoma is more common when the cutaneous hemangioma involves the upper eyelid skin (Fig 11-7) but is also often associated with the presence of choroidal hemangioma, iris heterochromia, and/or episcleral hemangioma. When glaucoma occurs in infants with SWS, congenital angle dysgenesis (similar to that seen in cases of PCG) is thought to be responsible. In these cases, treatment typically consists of angle surgery. However, the success rate of this surgery is generally lower in SWS than in PCG. Combined trabeculotomy-trabeculectomy surgery has also been utilized as initial surgery for early-onset glaucoma to address possible distal resistance to aqueous outflow.

Glaucoma that develops after the first decade of life may be caused by elevated episcleral venous pressure. Trabeculectomy, or preferably tube shunt surgery, should be performed with caution because of the increased pressure gradient across the choroidal vasculature and the increased risk of choroidal effusion and suprachoroidal hemorrhage in patients with SWS. To reduce the risk of suprachoroidal hemorrhage, suggested prophylactic measures may include the following: maximum preoperative IOP control, intraoperative maintenance of the anterior chamber, surgical modifications such as posterior sclerotomy, and radiotherapy or laser photocoagulation of the choroidal hemangioma.

Hassanpour K, Nourinia R, Gerami E, Mahmoudi G, Esfandiari H. Ocular manifestations of the Sturge-Weber syndrome. *J Ophthalmic Vis Res.* 2021;16(3):415–431.

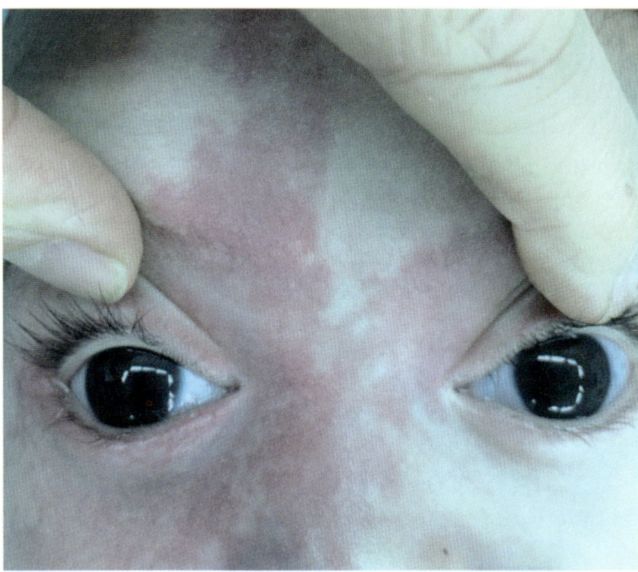

Figure 11-7 Patient with Sturge-Weber syndrome and glaucoma. The facial hemangioma involves both upper eyelids. *(Courtesy of JoAnn A. Giaconi, MD.)*

Other Nonacquired Conditions Associated With Secondary Glaucoma

Other notable causes of pediatric glaucoma include neurofibromatosis, nail-patella syndrome, Stickler syndrome (hereditary progressive arthro-ophthalmopathy), and osteogenesis imperfecta.

Neurofibromatosis is the most common phakomatosis and has 2 recognizable forms: neurofibromatosis 1 (NF1; also called *peripheral neurofibromatosis*), which is the most frequent type, and neurofibromatosis 2 (NF2; also called *central neurofibromatosis*). NF1 is an autosomal dominant disorder (approximately 50% of cases) caused by a pathogenic variant in the neurofibromin 1 gene *(NF1)*; the other 50% of cases are sporadic. In individuals with NF1, the neurofibromin gene, which is a tumor suppressor gene, is abnormal; loss of tumor suppressor function leads to proliferation of neural tumors.

Ocular findings associated with NF1 include Lisch nodules, ectropion uveae, choroidal lesions, optic nerve gliomas, eyelid neurofibromas, and glaucoma. Systemic melanocytic lesions seen with NF1 include cutaneous café-au-lait spots, cutaneous neurofibromas, and axillary or inguinal freckling. Although the incidence of glaucoma in individuals with NF1 is low overall, the presence of an eyelid neurofibroma is strongly associated with glaucoma on the ipsilateral side. When glaucoma is present at birth, it is thought to result from abnormal formation of angle structures. When glaucoma develops later in life, the mechanism is thought to be either infiltration of the angle with neurofibromatous tissue or angle closure caused by thickening of the ciliary body and choroid. Surgical treatment is often necessary, but its success rate is lower in NF1-associated glaucoma than in PCG. NF2 is characterized by the presence of bilateral acoustic neuromas and is not associated with glaucoma.

Nail-patella syndrome is a rare autosomal dominant disease characterized by nail dysplasia, aplastic or hypoplastic patellae, elbow dysplasia, and the presence of iliac horns. The syndrome is caused by pathogenic variants in *LMX1B,* which lead to loss of function of proteins essential for normal development of the anterior segment. In addition to the association with glaucoma, ocular findings include microcornea, sclerocornea, and congenital cataract.

Both Stickler syndrome and osteogenesis imperfecta are systemic connective tissue disorders affecting collagen production and typically are inherited in an autosomal dominant pattern. *Stickler syndrome* produces pathologic maxillofacial, ocular, auditory, and joint manifestations. Ocular findings include vitreous syneresis, retinal lattice degeneration, axial myopia, and glaucoma due to anterior segment dysgenesis. *Osteogenesis imperfecta* is characterized by bone fragility, skeletal deformities, ligament hyperlaxity, cardiovascular disease, and hearing loss. Typical ocular findings include blue sclera (due to scleral thinning), low ocular rigidity, short axial length, retinal detachment, and glaucoma.

Pallozzi Lavorante N, Iester M, Bonzano C, Bagnis A, Traverso CE, Cutolo CA. Nail-patella syndrome and glaucoma: a case report and review of the literature. *Case Rep Ophthalmol.* 2022;13(3):984–990. doi:10.1159/000527234

Secondary Glaucomas Associated With Acquired Conditions

Many of the causes of secondary glaucoma in infants and children are similar to the causes in adults, including uveitis, lens-associated disorders, trauma, steroid use, tumors, and posterior segment disorders, as well as topiramate-induced angle closure (see Table 11-4). The signs and symptoms at presentation will depend on the age of the child (whether the child is younger than or older than 3–4 years), the extent of the IOP elevation, and the severity of vision loss.

Juvenile idiopathic arthritis–associated uveitis is the most common pediatric uveitis. Uveitic glaucomas may be a result of open-angle mechanisms (trabecular meshwork obstruction/damage/dysfunction, altered vascular permeability and/or corticosteroid response) or angle-closure mechanisms (central posterior synechiae, peripheral anterior synechiae, forward rotation of the ciliary body). Due to the multifactorial nature of the mechanisms, IOP control may be difficult and require surgical management with trabeculectomy or tube shunt surgery. Patients who have undergone these procedures are at higher risk of postoperative hypotony.

The most common lens-associated disorders that cause angle-closure glaucoma may occur in patients with Marfan syndrome, homocystinuria, Weill-Marchesani syndrome, and microspherophakia. Blunt or penetrating ocular trauma can lead to glaucoma, which has 2 peak incidences: less than 1 year and more than 10 years from the time of the traumatic incident. Posterior segment abnormalities such as persistent fetal vasculature, retinopathy of prematurity ([ROP]; largely angle closure due to cicatricial ROP), familial exudative vitreoretinopathy, and tumors of the retina or ciliary body can also result in glaucoma. The intraocular tumors known to lead to secondary glaucoma in infants and children include retinoblastoma, juvenile xanthogranuloma, and medulloepithelioma.

Glaucoma Following Cataract Surgery

Glaucoma or signs suggestive of glaucoma frequently develop in children who have undergone surgery for congenital cataract. The glaucoma is predominantly an open-angle type. In some cases, angle closure occurs as a late consequence of an enlarging Sommering ring that pushes the iris forward. The term "aphakic glaucoma" is commonly used to refer to this group of glaucomas, although it may be considered outdated because many of these young patients receive intraocular lens implants.

Risk factors for the development of glaucoma include cataract surgery in the first year of life (risk is greatest in individuals who have undergone surgery in the first 6 weeks of life), postoperative complications, and small corneal diameter. The risk of developing glaucoma is the same whether patients are left aphakic or receive an intraocular lens implant at the time of cataract extraction. The risk of glaucoma-related adverse events continues to increase with longer follow-up after congenital cataract surgery; therefore, these patients require lifelong follow-up for glaucoma. The underlying mechanism is unclear, but likely etiologies for open-angle cases include congenital anomalies of the outflow pathway, surgically induced inflammation, and altered intraocular anatomy postoperatively. Removing all residual cortex during cataract surgery may reduce the risk of IOP elevation.

For treatment of glaucoma, tube shunt surgery may be preferred because trabeculectomy has a higher risk of failure in aphakia, and there is a high risk of bleb-related infection in patients who require contact lenses.

Freedman SF, Beck AD, Nizam A, et al; Infant Aphakia Treatment Study Group. Glaucoma-related adverse events at 10 years in the Infant Aphakia Treatment Study. *JAMA Ophthalmol.* 2021;139(2):165–173.

Evaluating the Pediatric Glaucoma Patient

Evaluation of a pediatric glaucoma patient differs from examination of an adult glaucoma patient. Ophthalmologists should proceed with an orderly system of examination and have the appropriate equipment for evaluating infants and young children in both the office and the operating room (Table 11-7). For examinations under anesthesia (EUAs), efficiency in measuring ocular biometric parameters and recording data in the operating room is optimized by having all necessary equipment ready and gathered in a single place (Video 11-1). Given concerns about the effect of general anesthetics on pediatric brain development, cumulative time under anesthesia should be minimized.

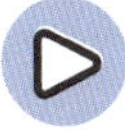

VIDEO 11-1 Examination under anesthesia of a pediatric glaucoma patient.
Courtesy of Shalini Sood, MD.
Available at: aao.org/bcscvideo_section10

Ing C, Warner DO, Sun L, et al. Anesthesia and developing brains: unanswered questions and proposed paths forward. *Anesthesiology*. 2022;136(3):500–512.

International Anesthesia Research Society. SmartTots. Accessed January 29, 2024. smarttots.org

Table 11-7 Supplies for Examining Children Under Anesthesia

Examination form/checklist
Topical medications
Proparacaine or tetracaine
Mydriatics (Do not use if proceeding with angle surgery.)
Viscous eyedrops or gel for gonioscopy
Glycerol
Pilocarpine and apraclonidine if proceeding with angle surgery
Tonometer: Tono-Pen, Perkins, iCare, or Pneumatonometer
(Measure IOP as soon as possible after induction because induction and anesthetics can lower IOP.)
Calipers to measure corneal diameter
Koeppe or other gonioscopy lens
Portable slit lamp
Pachymeter
Ultrasonographic system to image the posterior segment
Direct ophthalmoscope
Retinoscope and lenses for refraction
Indirect ophthalmoscope and lens
Portable fundus camera

History

For the evaluation of infants or school-aged children, it is important to ask the caregiver about the following:

- gestational history (maternal infection, delivery)
- developmental milestones
- family history (glaucoma, ocular and systemic conditions, parental consanguinity)
- prior ocular, medical, and surgical history
- medication use, particularly steroids of any form, and allergies
- general well-being, irritability, poor feeding, weight loss, crying when outside in the sunshine
- intermittent or persistent corneal clouding
- school-aged children: routine vision screenings, changes in academic performance, difficulty seeing in the classroom
- names of previous physicians consulted

Visual Acuity

Testing of visual acuity in infants and young children is discussed in BCSC Section 6, *Pediatric Ophthalmology and Strabismus.* Refraction should be performed to identify any myopia from axial enlargement and/or astigmatism from corneal irregularity. Decreased vision may be due to significant glaucomatous optic nerve damage, amblyopia, corneal scarring, or other associated ocular conditions (eg, retinal detachment, macular edema, cataract, lens dislocation).

External Examination

It is important that the ophthalmologist observe the child before looking through a slit lamp. Buphthalmos (see Fig 11-2A) and other signs and symptoms of PCG, including epiphora and blepharospasm, can be seen by observing a child from a distance. Systemic features that may be associated with primary and secondary glaucomas other than PCG should also be looked for, including features associated with chromosomal abnormalities, phakomatoses, connective tissue disorders, and ARS.

Anterior Segment Examination

As discussed previously, corneal enlargement and opacification are important signs associated with glaucoma in patients younger than 4 years. Corneal diameter can be measured with calipers or a ruler (see Video 11-1). Normal horizontal corneal diameter is 9.5–10.5 mm in full-term newborns, increasing to 11–12 mm by 2 years of age. Table 11-8 compares normal pediatric measurements with adult measurements. A corneal diameter of 11 mm or more in a newborn, greater than 12 mm in a child younger than 1 year, or greater than 13 mm at any age is suggestive of glaucoma. A difference in corneal diameter of 0.5 mm or greater between both eyes of the same patient may also be suggestive of glaucoma. Corneal edema may be due to elevated IOP or Haab striae and may range from a mild haze to dense opacification of the corneal stroma (Fig 11-8). Retroillumination after pupillary dilation may help

Table 11-8 Measurements in Healthy Pediatric and Adult Eyes

	Axial Length, mm	Horizontal Corneal Diameter, mm
Newborn	17.5–19.5	9.5–10.5
2-year-old	19.5–20.5	11.0–12.0
Adult	23.0–24.0	11.0–12.0

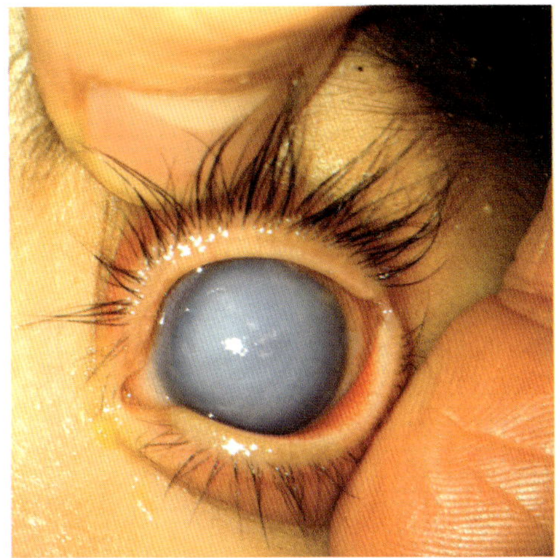

Figure 11-8 Severe corneal edema due to elevated IOP in a newborn with glaucoma. *(Courtesy of JoAnn A. Giaconi, MD.)*

make Haab striae visible. Evaluation for other anterior segment anomalies, such as aniridia, iridocorneal adhesions, and corectopia, may provide insight into the underlying diagnosis.

Tonometry

Accurate tonometry is important in the assessment of pediatric glaucoma but not always possible, especially in infants and very young children. A normal IOP measurement in newborns ranges from 10 mm Hg to the low teens; by middle childhood, IOP increases to adult levels of 10–21 mm Hg. Glaucoma should be suspected when IOPs are elevated or asymmetric in a cooperative or anesthetized child; in an uncooperative or struggling child, IOP measurements may be falsely elevated.

The clinician may be able to successfully measure the IOP of an infant younger than 6 months by performing the measurement while the infant is feeding or immediately thereafter. In this group of patients, IOP can be measured with the following devices if the palpebral fissure is sufficiently wide: the iCare rebound tonometer (iCare; iCare Finland OY), the Tono-Pen (Reichert Technologies), a pneumotonometer, or a Perkins handheld applanation tonometer.

For children who are relatively cooperative in the clinic but too young for Goldmann tonometry, the rebound tonometer is very useful because it does not require topical anesthesia and newer versions can measure IOP with the patient seated or supine. This device has been shown to reduce the number of EUAs performed to obtain pressure measurements. However, despite these advantages, initial reports indicate that measurements in patients with congenital glaucoma were higher when taken with the rebound tonometer than when taken with the Perkins tonometer, especially at higher levels of IOP.

General anesthesia is usually required for accurate IOP assessment in older infants (≥6 months) and young children, but the steps involved in and agents used for producing general anesthesia can affect IOP. Intubation and extubation generally increase IOP, possibly because of laryngeal spasm and sympathetic stimulation. In general, a laryngeal mask airway affects IOP less than does endotracheal intubation. Most anesthetic agents affect IOP measurements. Halothane, propofol, sevoflurane, isoflurane, and enflurane decrease IOP, whereas ketamine and suxamethonium (succinylcholine) generally increase IOP. Midazolam and chloral hydrate do not appear to affect IOP. It is best to coordinate with the anesthesiologist before the child is brought to the operating room and arrange to measure IOP immediately after induction of general anesthesia (preferably before intubation), which ideally minimizes the effects of anesthesia on IOP. Also, it is preferable for a patient to receive the same general anesthetic in serial examinations.

Fayed MA, Chen TC. Pediatric intraocular pressure measurements: tonometers, central corneal thickness, and anesthesia. *Surv Ophthalmol.* 2019;64(6):810–825.

Martinez-de-la-Casa JM, Garcia-Feijoo J, Saenz-Frances F, et al. Comparison of rebound tonometer and Goldmann handheld applanation tonometer in congenital glaucoma. *J Glaucoma.* 2009;18(1):49–52.

Pachymetry

The role of pachymetry in the diagnosis and management of pediatric glaucoma is unclear, as the range for central corneal thickness (CCT) values for eyes without glaucoma varies depending on the device used. In children without glaucoma, the average CCT obtained with ultrasound pachymetry is approximately 540–560 µm. In patients with certain ocular conditions associated with glaucoma, CCT is thicker than normal, which may lead to artifactually high IOP readings. These conditions include aphakia, aniridia, Sturge-Weber syndrome, and microcornea. In patients with these conditions, the effect of CCT on the accuracy of IOP measurements is unclear, and nomograms cannot accurately correct IOP measurements for differences in CCT measurements.

Bradfield YS, Melia BM, Repka MX, et al; Pediatric Eye Disease Investigator Group. Central corneal thickness in children. *Arch Ophthalmol.* 2011;129(9):1132–1138.

Gonioscopy

Gonioscopy can provide important information about the mechanism of a patient's glaucoma, as well as evidence of any prior angle surgeries. This information assists the surgeon in making surgical plans. For gonioscopic examination of young children, an EUA is usually required. A Koeppe lens or other direct gonioscopy lens allows visualization of the angle structures. Alternatively, indirect gonioscopy performed with the operating room microscope or certain ophthalmic cameras can be used to visualize and photograph the anterior chamber angle. In older children, indirect gonioscopy can be performed with a 4-mirror goniolens at the slit lamp.

The normal anterior chamber angle of an infant differs from the normal angle of an adult in several ways. The trabecular meshwork is less pigmented; the Schwalbe line is less prominent; and the junction between the scleral spur and the ciliary body band is less distinct (Fig 11-9A) compared with an adult angle. In PCG, the anterior chamber is deep, with a high anterior iris insertion. Also, the angle recess is absent, and the iris root appears as a scalloped line of glistening tissue (Fig 11-9B). Although this tissue is not a true membrane, it has been referred to as the *Barkan membrane* and likely represents thickened and compacted trabecular meshwork (see Fig 11-1).

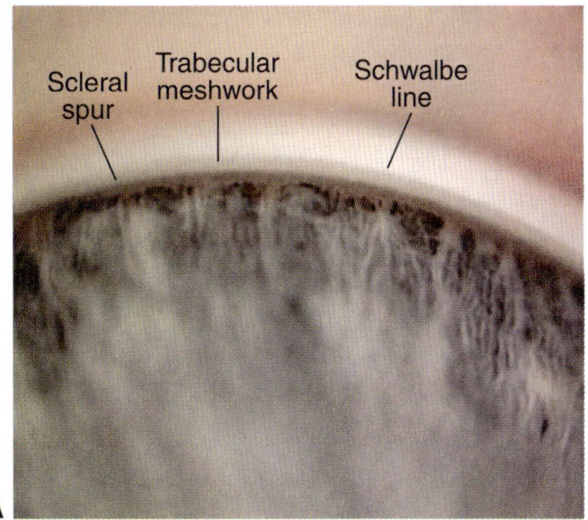

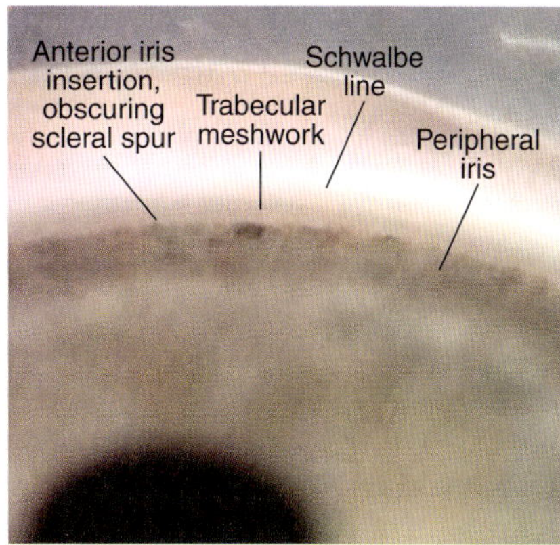

Figure 11-9 Gonioscopy of the anterior chamber angle. **A,** Angle of a nonglaucomatous infant eye, as seen by direct gonioscopy with a Koeppe lens. **B,** Typical appearance of the angle of an infant with PCG. Note the scalloped appearance of the peripheral iris root. The anterior iris insertion obscures the scleral spur. *(Courtesy of Ken K. Nischal, MD.)*

In eyes with JOAG, the angle usually appears normal. In patients with aniridia, gonioscopy reveals a rudimentary iris root.

Optic Nerve and Fundus Evaluation

Visualization and documentation of the optic nerve are crucial in the evaluation and management of pediatric glaucomas. A highly magnified view of the nerve is ideal. Often, this can be achieved with direct ophthalmoscopy, which may be done in the office or operating room. In patients with small pupils, viewing through a direct ophthalmoscope can be enhanced with a Koeppe lens (see Video 11-1). Alternatively, a stereoscopic view can be achieved by viewing the optic nerve head through the central lens of a 4-mirror gonioprism, used in conjunction with an operating microscope. Indirect ophthalmoscopy can be used, but this method may lead to underestimation of the cup–disc ratio (CDR). Slit-lamp biomicroscopy can be performed in older children with a dilated pupil. Photographs provide the best documentation and facilitate evaluation of changes over time.

Optic nerve imaging is possible in older, cooperative children, and the information obtained can be useful for longitudinal evaluation. Although normative databases for children do not yet exist in commercially available imaging platforms, it has been found that the retinal nerve fiber layer (RNFL) thickness in children older than 5 years is similar to adult values; therefore, adult normative values can be used for comparison. Of note, in children and adults, ocular parameters such as RNFL thickness captured with optical coherence tomography (OCT) vary with age, axial length, and race. OCT has demonstrated that RNFL and macular thickness in pediatric patients with glaucoma is reduced compared with that in pediatric patients without glaucoma. Nonetheless, OCT should be used with other conventional diagnostic tools and not as a standalone screening test for pediatric glaucoma.

A typical newborn without glaucoma has a small physiologic cup (CDR <0.3) with a pink rim. In individuals with PCG, the optic canal is stretched under high IOP, and the lamina cribrosa is bowed backward, causing generalized enlargement of the cup. Enlarged or increasing CDR or CDR asymmetry of 0.2 or greater between the 2 eyes is suggestive of glaucoma. Cupping may be reversible if the IOP is lowered before the child is 3 years of age; however, lowering IOP does not reverse any existing atrophy of the optic nerve axons. Studies in which OCT is performed in children with PCG show diffuse RNFL loss rather than loss localized to the superior and inferior poles of the optic nerve head.

In children without glaucoma, CDR increases slightly from birth until approximately 10 years of age. The CDR of older children without glaucoma is similar to that seen in adults. Racial differences in CDR are present even at birth. Children of African, Middle Eastern, Hispanic, and East Asian descent have larger average CDRs than do children of European descent. Cupping in older children is similar to that seen in adult patients with glaucoma; more focal defects are present, and there is greater loss in the superior and inferior neural rims because their scleral canals do not stretch.

Allingham MJ, Cabrera MT, O'Connell RV, et al. Racial variation in optic nerve head parameters quantified in healthy newborns by handheld spectral domain optical coherence tomography. *J AAPOS.* 2013;17(5):501–506.

Samarawickrama C, Pai A, Tariq Y, Healey PR, Wong TY, Mitchell P. Characteristics and appearance of the normal optic nerve head in 6-year-old children. *Br J Ophthalmol.* 2012;96(1):68–72.

Visual Field Testing

Assessment of the visual field in children is useful, but the testing process can be challenging. Automated testing can be performed, starting at age 5 years; the results become more reliable as the child approaches 7–8 years of age. For adults, abnormalities should be confirmed with repeated testing. Although there is no normative database for children, the age correction for mean deviation is small (0.7 dB/decade). Other indices—the pattern standard deviation, the glaucoma hemifield test, and glaucoma change probability—are largely unaffected by age.

Patel DE, Cumberland PM, Walters BC, Russell-Eggitt I, Cortina-Borja M, Rahi JS; OPTIC Study Group. Study of optimal perimetric testing in children (OPTIC): normative visual field values in children. *Ophthalmology.* 2015;122(8):1711–1717.

A-Scan Ultrasonography

Serial measurements of axial length using A-scan ultrasonography can document progressive globe enlargement in patients younger than 4 years (Fig 11-10; see also Video 11-1).

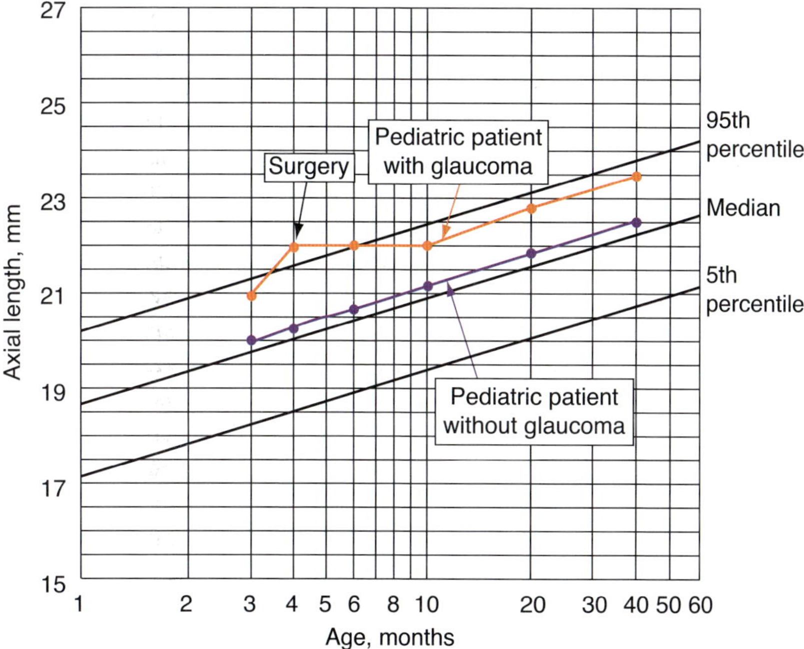

Figure 11-10 Graph of axial length showing normal pediatric growth with 95% confidence intervals. Charting axial length on a graph helps identify abnormally long eyes or eyes that are growing at abnormal rates. *(Courtesy of JoAnn A. Giaconi, MD.)*

Axial length may stabilize or decrease with control of IOP and thus serves as a critical marker for successful control of IOP.

Law SK, Bui D, Caprioli J. Serial axial length measurement in congenital glaucoma. *Am J Ophthalmol.* 2001;132(6):926–928.

Other Testing

If media opacities, particularly corneal edema, preclude fundus evaluation, B-scan ultrasonography can be performed.

Treatment Overview

Surgical Management

Surgery is the preferred, definitive treatment of most cases of PCG; medications have limited long-term value. Although medication can better control IOP in other forms of pediatric glaucoma, a high percentage of these cases also eventually require surgery. Angle surgery (goniotomy or trabeculotomy) is the procedure of choice for the treatment of PCG. Either procedure is appropriate if the cornea is clear. If the cornea is cloudy, poor visualization of the target structures makes goniotomy difficult to perform; ab externo trabeculotomy is preferred in these eyes because it is more easily performed. Angle surgery has a high success rate in children with PCG, with the highest rates observed in children diagnosed between 3 and 12 months of age.

Angle surgery may also be used to treat other forms of pediatric glaucoma, including glaucoma following congenital cataract surgery and glaucoma associated with aniridia, ARS, or Sturge-Weber syndrome; however, the success rates are lower. Trabeculectomy and tube shunt surgery should be reserved for congenital glaucoma cases in which goniotomy or trabeculotomy has failed or for cases in which angle surgery is not appropriate. Cyclodestruction is necessary in some intractable cases.

Glaucoma surgery in children poses unique difficulties. For example, in PCG, the anatomical landmarks are distorted in the buphthalmic eye, and the thin sclera presents additional challenges in trabeculotomy and trabeculectomy, such as false passage of the catheter, scleral perforation, and hypotony. The surgeon performing glaucoma surgery in pediatric patients should be experienced in handling these challenges and able to provide the necessary environment for evaluating these patients postoperatively. Because additional surgery is often required, the surgeon should develop a long-term plan in order to keep surgical options available for the future.

The decision to proceed with angle surgery is often made during an EUA. Ideally, if glaucoma is diagnosed, angle surgery is performed during the same anesthesia session to minimize the number of exposures to general anesthesia. If glaucoma is uncontrolled in both eyes, performing bilateral surgery in the same session is appropriate. When angle surgery is anticipated, it is best not to dilate the eye during the EUA in order to protect the lens during the surgical procedure.

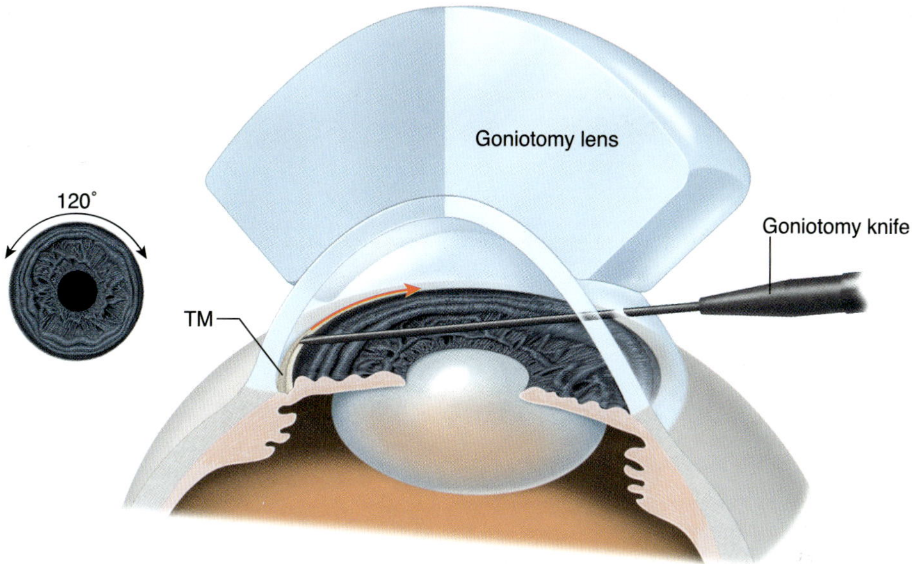

Figure 11-11 The illustration depicts a goniotomy incision as seen through a surgical contact lens. TM = trabecular meshwork. *(Illustration by Mark Miller.)*

Angle surgery

Both goniotomy and trabeculotomy open the abnormal trabecular meshwork to increase outflow. In a *goniotomy,* the angle is visualized with a gonioscopic contact lens. A needle or appropriate blade is then passed across the anterior chamber, and a superficial incision is made in the trabecular meshwork (Fig 11-11, Video 11-2). As previously mentioned, a clear cornea is required for visualization of the angle.

VIDEO 11-2 Goniotomy.
Courtesy of Ken K. Nischal, MD.
Available at: aao.org/bcscvideo_section10

In an *ab externo trabeculotomy,* the Schlemm canal is cannulated from an external approach, and the trabecular meshwork is opened by breaking through Schlemm canal into the anterior chamber. The procedure begins with creation of a conjunctival flap, beneath which a partial-thickness scleral flap is created, similar to flap creation in a trabeculectomy. Beneath that partial-thickness scleral flap, the surgeon identifies the Schlemm canal, either by creating a radial incision into the scleral–corneal junction or by dissecting a second, deep scleral flap and noting the canal at the edges of this flap. The surgeon can also identify the canal edges after unroofing the Schlemm canal by creating a single deep scleral flap. The surgeon inserts a rigid instrument (trabeculotome) into the Schlemm canal; passes it along the canal; and then rotates the instrument, which tears the trabecular meshwork, with the probe entering the anterior chamber (Fig 11-12, Video 11-3). Alternatively, a 6-0 polypropylene suture or a fiber-optic microcatheter can be placed in one end of the canal and fed through it for 360°,

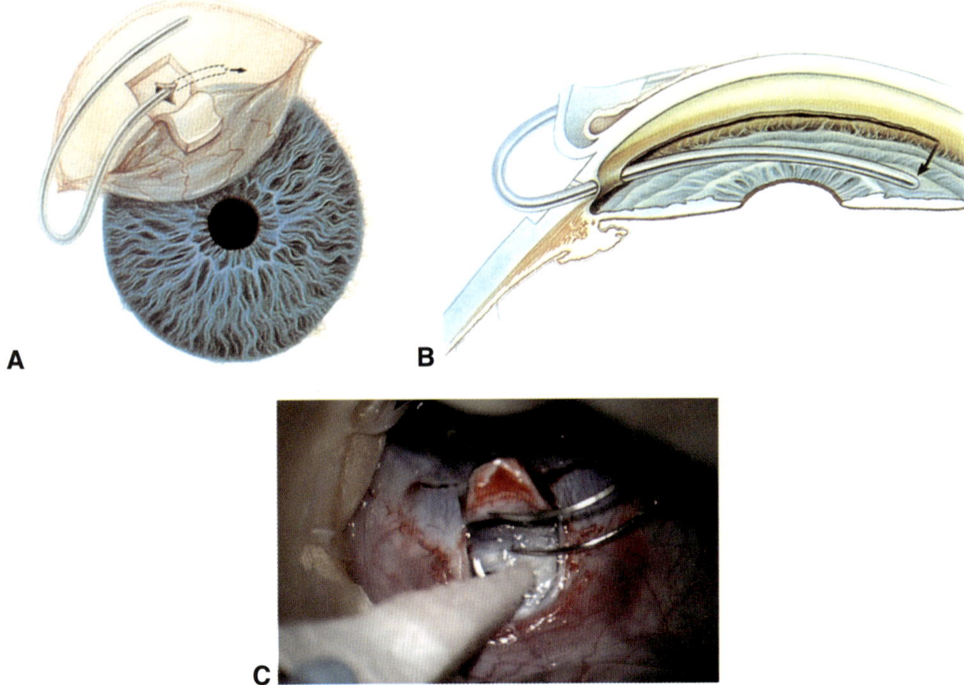

Figure 11-12 Trabeculotomy. **A,** Illustration of the probe as it is gently passed along Schlemm canal, with little resistance for 6–10 mm. **B,** By rotating the probe internally *(arrow),* the surgeon ruptures the trabecular meshwork and the probe appears in the anterior chamber with minimal bleeding. **C,** The trabeculotome used in ab externo trabeculotomy allows the surgeon to open the angle over 1 quadrant. *(Parts A and B reproduced and modified with permission from Kolker AE, Hetherington J, eds.* Becker-Shaffer's Diagnosis and Therapy of the Glaucomas. *5th ed. Mosby; 1983. Part C courtesy of JoAnn A. Giaconi, MD.)*

appearing at the other end of the canal. The surgeon then pulls the two ends of the suture or microcatheter to tear through the inner wall of the canal and the trabecular meshwork. If the cornea is clear, another approach is to insert the suture or fiber-optic microcatheter through a clear corneal incision, into a nasal goniotomy cleft, and cannulate Schlemm canal 360°, as may be done for treatment of adult glaucoma (Video 11-4).

VIDEO 11-3 Trabeculotomy with trabeculotome over 1 quadrant.
Courtesy of Young Kwon, MD, PhD.
Available at: aao.org/bcscvideo_section10

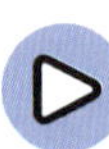

VIDEO 11-4 Trabeculotomy over 360° with a microcatheter.
Courtesy of JoAnn A. Giaconi, MD.
Available at: aao.org/bcscvideo_section10

An *ab interno trabeculotomy* can be performed by using other commercially available devices. When performing a trabeculotomy ab externo or ab interno, the surgeon must take care to avoid creating a false passage and entering the subretinal or suprachoroidal space.

Table 11-9 Comparison of Goniotomy and Trabeculotomy

Goniotomy	Trabeculotomy
Results in no postoperative conjunctival scarring	Ab externo approach may be more familiar to glaucoma surgeons who typically operate on adults
Is a faster procedure	Can be performed in opacified corneas
Causes less trauma to anterior segment tissues	Can be converted to a trabeculectomy if Schlemm canal cannot be cannulated

It is reasonable to inject viscoelastic into the anterior chamber at the start of goniotomy and trabeculotomy to prevent collapse of the chamber and to tamponade bleeding intraoperatively. To prevent a postoperative spike in IOP, thorough removal of the viscoelastic at the end of the procedure is necessary.

The success rates of goniotomy and trabeculotomy are similar, but each procedure has its advantages (Table 11-9). Complications associated with these procedures include hyphema, infection, iris damage, lens damage, and uveitis. The Descemet membrane may be detached during a trabeculotomy.

Angle surgery has a success rate of 70%–80% in infants diagnosed with PCG between 3 and 12 months of age; this rate includes repeated angle procedures, which are common for this disease. After the entire angle has been treated or when adjunctive medical therapy is inadequate, trabeculectomy or tube shunt surgery should be considered.

Barkan O. Goniotomy for the relief of congenital glaucoma. *Br J Ophthalmol.* 1948;32(9): 701–728.

Trabeculectomy, combined trabeculotomy-trabeculectomy, and tube shunt surgery

If angle surgery is not successful, the surgeon must take several factors into account when deciding between trabeculectomy and tube shunt surgery as the next procedure. The success rate of *trabeculectomy* is low in children younger than 2 years and in aphakic eyes. Failure rates are high without the use of antifibrotics, but serious risks of bleb leaks and bleb infections are associated with the use of these agents. Due to the risk of blebitis and endophthalmitis, mitomycin C (MMC)–augmented trabeculectomy should be performed with caution in pediatric patients who are too young to understand good hygiene, which is necessary to minimize the risk of infection.

An alternative to trabeculectomy alone is to combine it with a trabeculotomy. The principal argument for a *combined trabeculotomy-trabeculectomy* procedure is that in a single operation, resistance of the trabecular meshwork is reduced and a filtration procedure is performed, thereby increasing the likelihood of success. Indeed, combined trabeculotomy-trabeculectomy has a higher success rate than does primary trabeculectomy alone, although it also has a higher risk of complications. This combined procedure may be useful for advanced cases that have been poorly responsive to preoperative topical medications.

Compared with trabeculectomy, *tube shunt surgery* has higher success rates in children and is associated with a lower risk of bleb-related infections. However, success rates vary with different tube shunts, diagnoses, and patient ages. Also, IOPs are usually higher after implantation of these devices than after successful trabeculectomy, and most children need to continue using topical ocular hypotensive medications, as is the case for adults. Complications associated with tube shunt surgery include anterior migration of the tube with resultant corneal damage, tube occlusion, relative posterior tube migration with extrusion from the anterior chamber, tube erosion, infection, cataract, motility disturbances, bleb encapsulation with elevated IOP, and pupil distortion.

In small eyes, the surgeon must ensure that the posterior aspect of the drainage device plate does not compress the optic nerve. The Freedman-Margeta GDD (glaucoma drainage device) online calculator (available at people.duke.edu/~freed003/GDDCalculator) calculates the distance of the posterior edge of the plate from the optic nerve depending on the axial length of the eye and the quadrant of implantation and determines whether trimming of the plate is indicated for safe placement of the implant. In addition to this adjunct tool, smaller sizes of the tube shunt implants are available for pediatric eyes.

Margeta MA, Kuo AN, Proia AD, Freedman SF. Staying away from the optic nerve: a formula for modifying glaucoma drainage device surgery in pediatric and other small eyes. *J AAPOS.* 2017;21(1):39–43.e1. doi:10.1016/j.jaapos.2016.09.027

Cyclophotocoagulation

In children, cyclophotocoagulation (discussed in Chapter 13) is reserved for cases refractory to other surgical and medical treatments. When these procedures are performed in pediatric patients, general anesthesia is required. The complication rate is lower with cyclodestructive laser procedures than with cyclocryotherapy. Disadvantages of cyclophotocoagulation include difficulty in titrating the results and the risk of serious complications, such as hypotony, uveitis, retinal detachment, phthisis bulbi, and blindness. The most common cyclodestructive modalities currently used are transscleral cyclophotocoagulation and endoscopic cyclophotocoagulation (ECP). ECP is particularly useful in eyes with distorted anterior segment anatomy and in eyes with prior unsuccessful transscleral cyclophotocoagulation. Either procedure can be very useful for providing additional IOP lowering after tube shunt surgery.

Medical Management

Although surgery is the mainstay of treatment for most pediatric glaucomas, medications are also frequently required. Medications may be used to lower IOP before surgery in order to reduce corneal edema and improve visualization during surgery. They may also be used for additional IOP lowering after surgical procedures. Primary medical therapy is used to treat most patients with JOAG, inflammatory glaucoma, glaucoma following cataract surgery, and other secondary glaucomas. Of note, the safety and efficacy of most glaucoma medications approved by the US Food and Drug Administration (FDA) have not been studied specifically in children in controlled clinical trials. Topical β-blockers, topical carbonic anhydrase inhibitors (CAIs), and prostaglandin analogues are reasonable first-line agents in children. When the patient is a preadolescent or adolescent girl, clinicians must inquire about pregnancy before initiating any treatment that might affect a fetus. For a full discussion of glaucoma medications and their mechanisms of action, see Chapter 12. For a list of systemic and ocular adverse effects of glaucoma medications in children, see BCSC Section 6, *Pediatric Ophthalmology and Strabismus,* Table 21-4.

Chang L, Ong EL, Bunce C, Brookes J, Papadopoulos M, Khaw PT. A review of the medical treatment of pediatric glaucomas at Moorfields Eye Hospital. *J Glaucoma.* 2013;22(8): 601–607.

Coppens G, Stalmans I, Zeyen T, Casteels I. The safety and efficacy of glaucoma medications in the pediatric population. *J Pediatr Ophthalmol Strabismus.* 2009;46(1):12–18.

Maeda-Chubachi T, Chi-Burris K, Simons BD, et al; A6111137 Study Group. Comparison of latanoprost and timolol in pediatric glaucoma: a phase 3, 12-week, randomized, double-masked multicenter study. *Ophthalmology.* 2011;118(10):2014–2021.

β-Adrenergic antagonists

While topical β-adrenergic antagonists, or β-blockers, are reasonable choices as first-line agents in children, they should be used with caution. The systemic absorption of topical β-blockers is considerable and can cause bronchospasm, bradycardia, and systemic hypotension in susceptible children. Thus, β-Blockers should be avoided in children with asthma or significant cardiac disease. To reduce the risk of bronchospasm, the clinician may consider administering the cardioselective β-blocker betaxolol. Systemic absorption can also be diminished with nasolacrimal occlusion for 2 to 5 minutes after administration and use of the lowest effective dose (eg, timolol 0.25% or levobunolol 0.25% instead of 0.5%), particularly for young children. The clinician should teach the child's caregiver how to occlude the nasolacrimal drainage system for administration at home.

α_2-Adrenergic agonists

The α_2-adrenergic agonist brimonidine, which crosses the blood–brain barrier, is associated with a risk of central nervous system depression, apnea, hypotension, bradycardia, hypotonia, hypothermia, and somnolence. Infants and young children are particularly susceptible to this adverse effect; thus α_2-adrenergic agonists are contraindicated in children younger than 2 years. Although brimonidine is FDA approved for use in children older than 2 years, there is some debate about the age at which children can safely use this drug. In general, it should be used with caution in children younger than 6 years or with weight less than 20 kg. The lowest dose that reduces the IOP to an acceptable range should be used, and nasolacrimal occlusion should be employed to minimize systemic absorption.

The α_2-adrenergic agonist apraclonidine is better tolerated systemically in children, but the risk of follicular conjunctivitis increases with long-term use. In addition to acting as an ocular hypotensive agent, apraclonidine acts as a vasoconstrictor and can be used to minimize bleeding during surgery.

Carbonic anhydrase inhibitors

Topical use of dorzolamide or brinzolamide has a minimal risk of systemic adverse effects and is an excellent first-line therapy for pediatric glaucoma. Systemic CAIs (acetazolamide and methazolamide) provide slightly more IOP lowering than the topical preparations, but they are associated with numerous systemic adverse effects, including anorexia, diarrhea, weight loss, paresthesia, hypokalemia, risk of sickle cell crisis in patients with sickle cell anemia, and metabolic acidosis (which can affect bone growth). Children using other diuretics are particularly at risk for these adverse effects. Because of the risk of not only these adverse effects but also of rare but life-threatening reactions such as Stevens-Johnson syndrome and aplastic anemia, systemic CAIs are reserved for patients at great risk of vision loss due to highly elevated IOP.

Prostaglandin analogues

Prostaglandin analogues have minimal systemic adverse effects and are dosed once daily. They have been shown to effectively lower IOP in JOAG. Older children respond better to prostaglandin analogues than do younger children and infants. These drugs are well tolerated and effective in patients with uveitic glaucoma; however, in some cases, they may cause or exacerbate uveitis.

Parasympathomimetic agents

Parasympathomimetic agents, or *miotics,* are traditionally divided into direct-acting cholinergic agonists and indirect-acting anticholinesterase agents. *Cholinergic agonists* are seldom used for long-term glaucoma therapy, particularly in phakic eyes, because of induced myopia. Cholinergic agents can be used intraoperatively to induce miosis, which facilitates angle surgery. They are sometimes used for a limited period after angle surgery in order to prevent formation of peripheral anterior synechiae.

The indirect-acting agent *echothiophate iodide* is highly effective in many patients with aphakic glaucoma and can be dosed once daily. Its use in children has been associated with the development of iris pigment epithelial cysts, which resolve with cessation of the medication. Also, use of echothiophate can result in disruption of the blood–aqueous barrier; therefore, it must be discontinued well in advance of any surgical procedure in order to prevent postsurgical inflammation.

Rho kinase inhibitors

There are case reports on the use of Rho kinase inhibitors in pediatric patients, but to date, results of systemic studies on their use in this patient group have not been reported.

Prognosis and Follow-Up

The development of effective surgical techniques has greatly improved the long-term prognosis for patients with pediatric glaucoma, particularly PCG patients asymptomatic at birth who are diagnosed between 3 and 12 months of age. These patients typically have a good prognosis; many achieve visual acuity of at least 20/70 with 5-year follow-up, although multiple surgeries may be required, and vision may still decline with longer-term follow-up. When symptoms are present at birth or when the disease is diagnosed after 12 months of age, the prognosis is poor, and the risk of blindness is high. Children with secondary pediatric glaucomas tend to have the worst prognosis, with up to 50% losing light perception despite treatment. Early referral to vision rehabilitation may be helpful for patients and their family.

In pediatric patients with IOP controlled by surgery, morbidities related to previous IOP elevation may include amblyopia, corneal scarring, strabismus, anisometropia, cataract, lens subluxation, susceptibility to trauma due to scleral fragility, and recurrent IOP elevation in the affected or unaffected eye. These morbidities can cause serious long-term visual compromise and thus should be addressed promptly.

Amblyopia is a common cause of decreased vision, particularly in patients with unilateral glaucoma, corneal opacification, and/or anisometropia. It is important to treat amblyopia aggressively, addressing conditions contributing to its development, such as refractive error, strabismus, cataract, and corneal pathology. Haab striae and corneal scarring may cause astigmatism. Elevated IOP can lead to buphthalmos in patients with PCG, and progressive myopia and anisometropia in patients with JOAG. Refractive errors should be corrected with eyeglasses or contact lenses, and the use of protective eyewear should be encouraged, especially in monocular patients.

Strabismus may develop as a result of tube shunt surgery or amblyopia. When performing surgery to correct strabismus, the surgeon should be cognizant of the sites of prior trabeculectomies and tube shunt implants and should use techniques that will minimize conjunctival scarring (in anticipation of future glaucoma surgeries).

All cases of pediatric glaucoma require lifelong follow-up to monitor IOP, potential complications from prior surgeries, and secondary vision-threatening complications. Because IOP elevation may recur even years later, glaucoma specialists and pediatric ophthalmologists should coordinate care. A team approach to care will involve low vision rehabilitation specialists, pediatricians, genetic counselors, educators, and parents or caregivers. Educating parents or caregivers about the need for lifelong care of a child with glaucoma and involving these children in their own care as they become older will enhance the long-term management of this challenging disease. For discussion of low vision rehabilitation in pediatric patients, see BCSC Section 6, *Pediatric Ophthalmology and Strabismus.*

de Silva DJ, Khaw PT, Brookes JL. Long-term outcome of primary congenital glaucoma. *J AAPOS.* 2011;15(2):148–152.

Khitri MR, Mills MD, Ying GS, Davidson SL, Quinn GE. Visual acuity outcomes in pediatric glaucomas. *J AAPOS.* 2012;16(4):376–381.

CHAPTER 12

Medical Management of Glaucoma and Ocular Hypertension

Highlights

- Target pressure is an estimate of the intraocular pressure (IOP) level below which the rate of disease progression is expected to be reduced sufficiently to minimize the patient's risk of further vision loss. The target pressure is determined based on an assessment of various clinical factors that influence the future risk of progression.
- There are several classes of topical ocular hypotensive medications that are prescribed for long-term use. They are frequently used in combination. Clinicians should tailor their selection among these agents for each patient based on their efficacy, contraindications, adverse effect profile, and cost.
- Prostaglandin analogues, the most commonly used IOP-lowering agents, lower IOP primarily by increasing uveoscleral outflow.

Introduction

The goal of currently available glaucoma therapy is to preserve visual function by lowering intraocular pressure (IOP). The treatment regimen chosen should achieve this goal with the lowest risk, the fewest adverse effects, and the least disruption to the patient's life, taking into account the cost of treatment. Although the long-term effectiveness of treatment is judged by the stability of measures of optic nerve structure and function, it is ensured through regular assessments demonstrating adequate IOP reduction.

Target pressure is an IOP below which the clinician estimates the rate of disease progression will be reduced sufficiently to minimize the patient's risk of experiencing further loss of visual function in their lifetime. For a patient with glaucoma or ocular hypertension, establishing a target pressure after an initial evaluation period is beneficial in 2 ways: (1) it encourages thoughtful appraisal of the various clinical factors that influence the future risk of progression; and (2) it allows efficient assessment of the patient's IOP level at each subsequent visit. Even if the target pressure is achieved, the clinician must continue to evaluate the stability of the structural and functional measures that are important in glaucoma.

Target pressure should be individualized for each eye, based on the IOP level at which damage is believed to have occurred and the severity of that damage. It can be adjusted on the basis of several factors, including the previously observed rate of progression (if known); life expectancy of the patient; and risk factors such as a history of optic disc hemorrhages, a thinner cornea, or a family history of severe vision loss in the setting of glaucoma (see Chapter 7 for further discussion of risk factors for primary open-angle glaucoma.

Evidence suggests that the severity of optic nerve injury may increase the likelihood of continued disease progression. Therefore, the more advanced the disease is on initial presentation, the lower the target pressure will need to be in order to minimize the risk of further vision loss. Moreover, if severe vision loss is already present, further damage (loss of retinal ganglion cells) is likely to have a disproportionately greater impact on visual function and quality of life. Establishing a target IOP is part of the art of glaucoma management, as many different approaches can be used. Clinical trials to evaluate these approaches and the value of establishing a target pressure are impractical to conduct. Differences among groups would likely be small and would take a long time to detect because disease progression usually occurs slowly. In addition, simply establishing a target pressure does not guarantee it will be achieved, and it often takes time and many treatment adjustments to reach the target pressure.

Disease progression occurs in some patients despite reduction of IOP below the initial target pressure. If progression does occur at an unacceptable rate, lowering the target pressure may be required. Conversely, once a target pressure is established, it does not become a mandate. The risks of each sequential medical or surgical intervention believed to be required to achieve a given target pressure must be weighed against the potential benefit of further IOP reduction. Table 12-1 offers a general framework for estimating an appropriate target pressure; however, there is no universally agreed-upon system.

After determining the target pressure, the clinician must decide whether to achieve this goal medically or surgically. For either approach, the anticipated benefits of any therapeutic intervention should justify the risks; regimens associated with substantial adverse effects should be reserved for patients with a high probability of progressive vision loss. In some cases, it may be necessary to accept an IOP level above the established target pressure because the adverse effects or risks of additional therapy are unacceptable. Both the risks and adverse events associated with specific treatment options and the risks of disease progression on the patient's overall quality of life must be considered.

Initial treatment of ocular hypertension and most glaucomas typically involves the use of medications or laser trabeculoplasty. When starting a patient on a medication, some clinicians favor using a unilateral treatment trial to assess the medication's efficacy; however, evidence suggests that this may be of limited value because of asymmetric IOP fluctuation between the eyes.

Ocular hypotensive agents are divided into several classes based on chemical structure and pharmacologic action. The classes in common clinical use include the following:

- prostaglandin analogues, including 1 agent with a nitric oxide–donating moiety
- adrenergic drugs
  - β-adrenergic antagonists (nonselective and β_1-selective)
  - adrenergic agonists (nonselective and α_2-selective)

Table 12-1 Estimating Target Pressure

Initial target pressure
Ocular hypertension (normal visual field, optic nerve head, and retinal nerve fiber layer)
<25 mm Hg and 20% below baseline (if there is a decision to treat)
Mild glaucomatous damage (optic nerve head damage with normal visual field)
<21 mm Hg and 25% below baseline
Moderate glaucomatous damage (visual field damage in 1 hemifield outside the central 10°)
<18 mm Hg and 30% below baseline
Severe glaucomatous damage (visual field damage in both hemifields and/or affecting the central 10°)
<15 mm Hg and 30% below baseline
Risk factors that may necessitate lowering the target pressure
New optic disc hemorrhage
Thinner central cornea
History of rapid progression or severe vision loss in the fellow eye
Family history of blindness due to glaucoma
Early age at onset of glaucomatous damage
Factors that may allow raising the target pressure
Decreased life expectancy or other comorbidities
History of acute optic nerve injury at very high IOP
History of stable or slowly progressive damage
High central corneal thickness

IOP = intraocular pressure.

- carbonic anhydrase inhibitors (topical and systemic)
- parasympathomimetic (miotic) agents
  - direct-acting cholinergic agonists
  - indirect-acting anticholinesterase agents
- Rho kinase inhibitors
- hyperosmotic agents

Table 12-2 lists the actions and adverse effects of the various glaucoma medications. See also BCSC Section 2, *Fundamentals and Principles of Ophthalmology,* for additional discussion of the mechanisms of action of these medications.

European Glaucoma Society Terminology and Guidelines for Glaucoma, 5th Edition. *Br J Ophthalmol.* 2021;105(Suppl 1):1–169. doi:10.1136/bjophthalmol-2021-egsguidelines

Netland PA, Tanna AP, eds. *Glaucoma Medical Therapy: Principles and Management.* 3rd ed. Kugler; 2020.

Prostaglandin Analogues

Mechanism of Action

Ocular hypotensive prostaglandin (PG) analogues are prodrugs that penetrate the cornea and become biologically active after being hydrolyzed by corneal esterase. They lower IOP

Table 12-2 Glaucoma Medications

Class/Compound	Concentration	Typical Dosing	Mechanism of Action	IOP Reduction From Untreated Baseline	Adverse Effects: Ocular	Adverse Effects: Systemic	Comments, Including Time to Peak Effect and Washout
Prostaglandin analogues							
Bimatoprost	0.03%, 0.01%	Once daily	Increases uveoscleral outflow primarily; also increases conventional (trabecular meshwork) outflow	≈30%	Increased pigmentation of iris, lashes, and periocular skin; hypertrichosis; trichiasis; distichiasis; blurred vision; keratitis; anterior uveitis; conjunctival hyperemia; exacerbation of herpes keratitis; CME; prostaglandin-associated periorbitopathy	Flulike symptoms, joint/muscle pain, headache	±IOP-lowering effect with miotic Peak: 10–14 hours Washout: 4–6 weeks Maximum IOP-lowering effect may take up to 6 weeks to occur
Latanoprost	0.005%	Once daily	Same as above	Same as above	Same as above	Same as above	Same as above
Travoprost	0.004%	Once daily	Same as above	Same as above	Same as above	Same as above	Same as above
Tafluprost	0.0015%	Once daily	Same as above	Same as above	Same as above	Same as above	Same as above
Latanoprostene bunod	0.024%	Once daily	Increases uveoscleral outflow; nitric oxide may also increase conventional outflow	Same as above	Same as above	Same as above	Same as above
Bimatoprost sustained-release	10-µg sustained-release implant	FDA-approved for one-time use	Same as for bimatoprost	Same as above	Conjunctival hyperemia, pain, irritation, corneal endothelial cell loss, photophobia, intraocular inflammation, implant migration, macular edema, endophthalmitis	None	Intracameral implant containing bimatoprost in a poly(D,L-lactide-co-glycolide) polymer matrix
β-Adrenergic antagonists (β-blockers), nonselective							
Timolol maleate	0.25%, 0.5% solution 0.1%, 0.25%, 0.5% gel	Solutions: 1–2 times daily Gels: once daily	Decreases aqueous humor production	20%–30%	Blurred vision, irritation, corneal anesthesia, punctate keratitis, allergy; aggravation of myasthenia gravis	Bradycardia, heart block, bronchospasm, lowered blood pressure, decreased libido, CNS depression, mood swings, reduced exercise tolerance, masked symptoms of hypoglycemia, exacerbation of myasthenia gravis	May be less effective if patient is taking systemic β-blockers; short-term escape, long-term drift; diabetic patients may experience reduced glucose tolerance and masking of hypoglycemic signs/symptoms Peak: 2–3 hours Washout: 1 month

Class/Compound	Concentration	Typical Dosing	Mechanism of Action	IOP Reduction From Untreated Baseline	Adverse Effects: Ocular	Adverse Effects: Systemic	Comments, Including Time to Peak Effect and Washout
Levobunolol hydrochloride	0.25%, 0.5%	1–2 times daily	Same as above	Same as above	Same as above	Same as above	Same as above
Metipranolol hydrochloride	0.3%	2 times daily	Same as above	Same as above	Same as above	Same as above	Same as above
Carteolol hydrochloride	1%	1–2 times daily	Same as above	Same as above	Same as above	Intrinsic sympathomimetic	May have less effect on nocturnal pulse, blood pressure Peak: 4 hours Washout: 1 month
β-Adrenergic antagonists (β-blockers), selective							
Betaxolol hydrochloride	0.25%	2 times daily	Decreases aqueous humor production	15%–20%	Blurred vision, irritation, corneal anesthesia, punctate keratitis, allergy; aggravation of myasthenia gravis	Lower risk of pulmonary complications than with nonselective β-blockers	Peak: 2–3 hours Washout: 1 month
α_2-Adrenergic agonists							
Brimonidine tartrate preserved with benzalkonium chloride	0.15%, 0.2%	2–3 times daily	Decreases aqueous humor production; increases uveoscleral outflow	20%–30%	Blurred vision, foreign-body sensation, eyelid edema, dryness, less ocular sensitivity/allergy than with apraclonidine, miosis	Headache, lethargy, hypotension, insomnia, depression, syncope, dizziness, anxiety, dry mouth	Highly selective for α_2-receptor Brimonidine should not be used in infants and young children Peak: 2 hours Washout: 7–14 days
Brimonidine tartrate preserved with sodium chlorite (Purite)	0.1%, 0.15%	2–3 times daily	Same as above	Same as above	Same as above, except less allergy than with brimonidine 0.2%	Same as above, except less lethargy and depression than with brimonidine 0.2%	Same as above
Apraclonidine hydrochloride	0.5%, 1%	2–3 times daily	Decreases aqueous humor production	Same as above	Irritation, ischemia, allergy, eyelid retraction, conjunctival blanching, follicular conjunctivitis, pruritus, dermatitis, ocular ache, photopsia, mydriasis	Hypotension, vasovagal attack, dry mouth and nose, lethargy	Useful in pre- or post-laser or cataract surgery Tachyphylaxis may limit long-term use Peak: <1–2 hours Washout: 7–14 days

(Continued)

Table 12-2 *(continued)*

Class/Compound	Concentration	Typical Dosing	Mechanism of Action	IOP Reduction From Untreated Baseline	Adverse Effects: Ocular	Adverse Effects: Systemic	Comments, Including Time to Peak Effect and Washout
Carbonic anhydrase inhibitors, topical							
Dorzolamide	2%	2–3 times daily	Decreases aqueous humor production	15%–20%	Induced myopia, blurred vision, stinging, keratitis, punctate keratopathy, conjunctivitis, dermatitis	Less likely to induce systemic effects of CAI, but may occur; taste disturbance	Peak: 2–3 hours Washout: 48 hours
Brinzolamide	1%	2–3 times daily	Same as above	Same as above	Same as above	Same as above	Same as above
Carbonic anhydrase inhibitors, systemic							
Acetazolamide	125 mg 250 mg 500 mg (sustained release)	Seldom used for IOP-lowering therapy in adults 2–4 times daily 2 times daily	Decreases aqueous humor production	15%–35%	None	Lethargy, paresthesia, dehydration, renal stones, taste disturbance (especially with carbonated beverages), anorexia, weight loss, hypokalemia, enuresis, rare but serious blood dyscrasias (including aplastic anemia)	Use with caution in patients susceptible to ketoacidosis Contraindicated in patients with hepatic cirrhosis Reduce dose for renal insufficiency Caution for using an oral CAI with other drugs that cause potassium loss Peak: 3–6 hours (sustained release); 2–4 hours (oral) Indicated for long-term therapy only in rare cases
Acetazolamide (intravenous)	500 mg 5–10 mg/kg	3–4 times daily	Same as above	Same as above	Same as above	Same as above	Same as above
Methazolamide	25 mg, 50 mg	2–3 times daily	Same as above	Same as above	Same as above	Same as above	Same as above
Parasympathomimetic agents (miotics)							
Cholinergic agonist (direct acting)							
Pilocarpine hydrochloride	0.5%, 1%, 2%, 3%, 4%, 6%	2–4 times daily	Increases conventional outflow	15%–25%	Posterior synechiae, keratitis, miosis, brow ache, cataract growth, angle-closure potential, myopia, retinal tear/detachment, dermatitis, change in retinal sensitivity, color vision changes, epiphora	Increased salivation, increased secretion (gastric), abdominal cramps	Exacerbation of cataract effect; more effective in lighter irides Peak: 1½–2 hours Washout: 48 hours

Class/Compound	Concentration	Typical Dosing	Mechanism of Action	IOP Reduction From Untreated Baseline	Adverse Effects: Ocular	Adverse Effects: Systemic	Comments, Including Time to Peak Effect and Washout
Anticholinesterase agent (indirect acting)							
Echothiophate iodide	0.125%	1–2 times daily	Increases conventional outflow	15%–25%	Intense miosis, iris pigment epithelial cyst, myopia, cataract, retinal detachment, angle closure, punctal stenosis, pseudopemphigoid, epiphora	Same as pilocarpine; more gastrointestinal difficulties	Increased inflammation with ocular surgery; may be helpful in aphakia, anesthesia risks (prolonged recovery); useful in eyelid-lash lice, cataract surgery postoperatively
Rho kinase inhibitor							
Netarsudil	0.02%	Once daily	Increases conventional outflow; also decreases episcleral venous pressure	≈20%–25%	Conjunctival hyperemia, subconjunctival hemorrhage, cornea verticillata, reticular corneal edema, pain, blurred vision, increased lacrimation	None	—
Fixed-combination medications							
Dorzolamide hydrochloride/timolol maleate	2%/0.5%	2 times daily	Decreases aqueous humor production	25%–30%	Same as those of topical CAI, nonselective β-blocker	Same as those of topical CAI, nonselective β-blocker	Peak: 2–3 hours Washout: 1 month
Brimonidine tartrate/timolol maleate	0.2%/0.5%	2 times daily	Same as α-agonist and nonselective β-blocker	Same as above	Same as those of α-agonist and nonselective β-blocker	Same as those of α-agonist and nonselective β-blocker	—
Brinzolamide/brimonidine tartrate	1%/0.2%	2–3 times daily	Decreases aqueous humor production; may increase uveoscleral outflow	26%–36%	Same as those of the individual components	Same as those of the individual components	—
Netarsudil/latanoprost	0.02%/0.005%	Once daily (nighttime)	Same as those of the individual components	31%–37%	Same as those of the individual components	Same as those of the individual components	—
Brinzolamide/timolol maleate	1%/0.5%	2 times daily	Decreases aqueous humor production	25%–30%	Same as those of topical CAI, nonselective β-adrenergic antagonist	Same as those of topical CAI, nonselective β-adrenergic antagonist	Not currently available in the United States

(Continued)

Table 12-2 *(continued)*

Class/Compound	Concentration	Typical Dosing	Mechanism of Action	IOP Reduction From Untreated Baseline	Adverse Effects		Comments, Including Time to Peak Effect and Washout
					Ocular	Systemic	
Bimatoprost/ timolol maleate	0.03%/0.5%	Once daily (nighttime)	Same as bimatoprost and nonselective β-blocker	25%–30%	Same as those of bimatoprost and nonselective β-blocker	Same as those of bimatoprost and nonselective β-blocker	Not currently available in the United States
Latanoprost/ timolol maleate	0.005%/0.5%	Once daily (nighttime)	Same as latanoprost and nonselective β-blocker	Greater than monotherapy with each individually	Same as those of latanoprost and nonselective β-blocker	Same as those of latanoprost and nonselective β-blocker	Not currently available in the United States
Travoprost/timolol maleate	0.004%/0.5%	Once daily (nighttime)	Same as travoprost and nonselective β-blocker	25%–30%	Same as those of travoprost and nonselective β-blocker	Same as those of travoprost and nonselective β-blocker	Not currently available in the United States
Hyperosmotic agents							
Mannitol (parenteral)	20%	0.5–2.0 g/kg body weight	Creates osmotic gradient; dehydrates vitreous	—	IOP rebound, increased aqueous flare	Urinary retention, headache, acute congestive heart failure, diabetic complications, nausea, vomiting, diarrhea, electrolyte disturbance, confusion, backache, myocardial infarction	Contraindicated in patients in renal failure or on dialysis; caution in heart failure; useful in acute increased IOP
Glycerol (oral)	50%	1–1.5 g/kg body weight	Same as above	—	Similar to above	Similar to above; can cause problems in diabetic patients	Similar to above; may precipitate diabetic ketoacidosis

CAI = carbonic anhydrase inhibitor; CME = cystoid macular edema; CNS = central nervous system; FDA = Food and Drug Administration; IOP = intraocular pressure.

by increasing aqueous humor outflow primarily via the uveoscleral pathway and decreasing outflow resistance. The precise mechanism by which these changes occur has not been fully determined. It is thought that the ocular hypotensive PG analogues bind to various PG or prostamide receptors, triggering a cascade of events that lead to activation of matrix metalloproteinases. This in turn leads to remodeling of the ciliary body, trabecular meshwork, and possibly scleral extracellular matrix, so the flow rate of aqueous humor through these tissues is increased. Topical PG analogue therapy results in increased space between the muscle fascicles within the ciliary body, believed to be the primary location of uveoscleral outflow.

Available Agents

Currently, 5 PG analogues are in widespread clinical use: latanoprost, travoprost, bimatoprost, tafluprost, and latanoprostene bunod. These agents reduce IOP by approximately 30%. Latanoprostene bunod lowers mean diurnal IOP by 32% and is unique among these PG analogues in that it includes a *nitric oxide–donating* element in addition to latanoprost. Nitric oxide is thought to increase conventional (trabecular meshwork) outflow facility, with a resultant 1 mm Hg IOP-lowering advantage over latanoprost in 1 clinical trial. See also BCSC Section 2, *Fundamentals and Principles of Ophthalmology.*

PG analogues are used once daily and are less effective when used twice daily. Because some patients may respond better to 1 agent in this class than to another, switching drugs after a trial of 4–6 weeks may sometimes prove helpful.

Adverse Effects

An adverse effect unique to this class of drugs is the darkening of the iris and periocular skin as a result of an increased number of melanosomes within the melanocytes, without melanocyte proliferation. Increased iris pigmentation is permanent, and the frequency of this effect depends on the baseline iris color. Most published data relate to latanoprost and suggest a risk of up to 33% after 5 years of use. In particular, up to 79% of persons with green-brown irides and up to 85% of persons with hazel (yellow-brown) irides are affected, compared with 8% of persons with blue irides. There is no evidence to suggest that increased iris or periocular skin pigmentation is associated with any risk to the patient such as an increased risk of melanoma.

Other ocular adverse effects reported in association with the use of a topical PG analogue include conjunctival hyperemia (a result of vasodilation, more common with bimatoprost and travoprost), hypertrichosis of the eyelashes (Figs 12-1, 12-2), trichiasis, and distichiasis. These effects are reversible upon drug discontinuation.

Use of PG analogue eyedrops has also been associated with the development of *PG-associated periorbitopathy* (see Fig 12-2), a complex of abnormalities that includes deepening of the upper eyelid sulcus, upper eyelid ptosis, enophthalmos, inferior scleral show, and possibly a tight orbit. These abnormalities appear to be the result of periorbital fat atrophy. It is not clear whether this condition is reversible.

A link between PG analogues and intraocular inflammation, including cystoid macular edema, has been proposed but is not clear from available data. Reactivation of herpetic keratitis has been reported. Nongranulomatous anterior uveitis occurs as an idiosyncratic reaction in approximately 1% of patients.

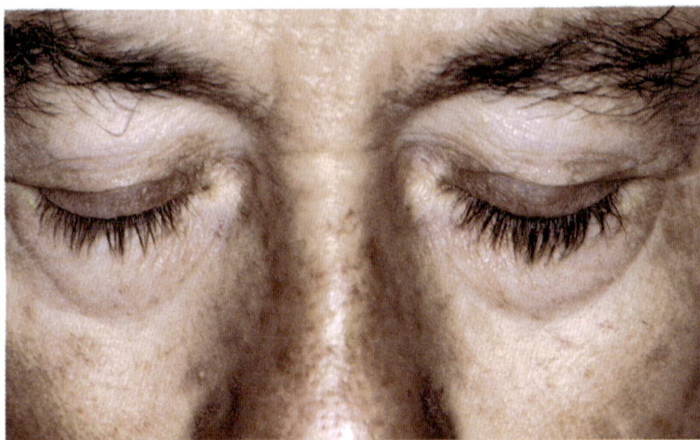

Figure 12-1 Hypertrichosis following use of latanoprost (left eye). *(Courtesy of F. Jane Durcan, MD.)*

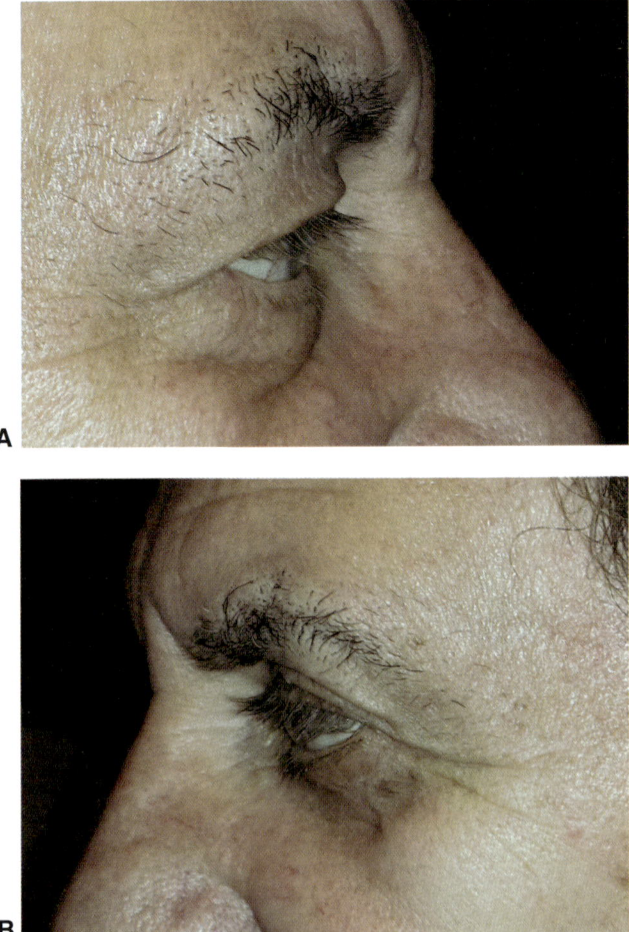

Figure 12-2 The right **(A)** and left **(B)** eyes of a patient receiving unilateral treatment with a topical prostaglandin analogue for the left eye. Left-sided periorbital skin hyperpigmentation, hypertrichosis, deepening of the superior eyelid sulcus, and loss of periorbital fat are evident. *(Courtesy of Chandrasekharan Krishnan, MD.)*

Camras CB, Alm A, Watson P, Stjernschantz J. Latanoprost, a prostaglandin analog, for glaucoma therapy. Efficacy and safety after 1 year of treatment in 198 patients. Latanoprost Study Groups. *Ophthalmology.* 1996;103(11):1916–1924.

Weinreb RN, Ong T, Scassellati Sforzolini B, et al. A randomised, controlled comparison of latanoprostene bunod and latanoprost 0.005% in the treatment of ocular hypertension and open angle glaucoma: the VOYAGER study. *Br J Ophthalmol.* 2015;99(6):738–745.

Sustained-Release Bimatoprost Implant

In 2020, the US Food and Drug Administration (FDA) approved an intracameral sustained-release biodegradable bimatoprost implant for 1-time use. The bimatoprost sustained-release implant contains a 10-μg dose of bimatoprost in a poly(D,L-lactide-co-glycolide) polymer matrix that slowly degrades after implantation in the anterior chamber.

The efficacy and safety of this implant (10 μg or 15 μg) compared with twice-daily topical timolol maleate were evaluated in a 20-month phase 3 clinical trial in which there was a 52-week active treatment period and an additional 8 months of extended follow-up. Participants in the bimatoprost implant groups underwent 3 administrations of the implant at 16-week intervals. Mean diurnal IOP lowering was similar with both the 10-μg and 15-μg implants, and neither was inferior to timolol. There was evidence of sustained IOP lowering with the bimatoprost implant; most subjects (69%) in the 10-μg bimatoprost implant group required no additional IOP-lowering treatment through month 20, a full year after the administration of the third implant.

The most concerning adverse effect observed in the clinical trial was a decrease in corneal endothelial cell density (CECD). At 20-month follow-up, a ≥20% decrease in CECD from baseline was seen in 10% and 22% of study eyes that received the 10-μg and 15-μg implants, respectively.

Adrenergic Drugs

β-Adrenergic Antagonists

Mechanism of action

Topical β-adrenergic antagonists, or *β-blockers,* lower IOP by inhibiting cyclic adenosine monophosphate (cAMP) production in the ciliary epithelium, thereby reducing aqueous humor secretion by 20%–50%, with a corresponding IOP reduction of 20%–30%. In healthy eyes, β-blocker administration reduces aqueous secretion and lowers IOP; interestingly, however, there is a compensatory reduction in aqueous outflow facility that dampens the magnitude of IOP reduction. The effect on aqueous production occurs within 1 hour of instillation and can last for up to 4 weeks after discontinuation of the medication. Because systemic absorption occurs, an IOP-lowering effect may also be observed in the untreated contralateral eye. β-Blockers have much less effect on aqueous production during sleep, as aqueous production is already reduced during the nocturnal period; thus, they are ineffective in lowering IOP during sleep.

Available agents

In the United States and Europe, 5 topical β-adrenergic antagonists are approved for the treatment of glaucoma: betaxolol, carteolol, levobunolol, metipranolol, and timolol. Betaxolol, the only topical β_1-selective antagonist, is less effective in lowering IOP than the others, which are nonselective β-adrenergic antagonists. Most β-blockers are approved for twice-daily therapy. In many cases, the nonselective agents can be used once daily. Generally, administration first thing in the morning is optimal to effectively blunt an early-morning pressure rise while minimizing the risk of systemic hypotension during sleep. Many nonselective β-blockers are available in more than 1 concentration. Clinical experience has shown that in many patients, timolol maleate 0.25% is as effective as timolol maleate 0.5% in lowering IOP.

In approximately 10%–20% of patients treated with topical β-blockers, IOP is not significantly lowered. Patients already taking a moderate or high dose of a systemic β-blocker may experience little additional IOP lowering from the addition of a topical ophthalmic β-blocker. Extended use of β-blockers may result in tachyphylaxis due to receptor upregulation. Physiologic changes in the trabecular meshwork may occur in response to decreased IOP and aqueous humor flow rate, resulting in decreased outflow facility. The underlying disease process responsible for decreased outflow facility and IOP elevation may also worsen during the course of therapy.

Adverse effects

Topical β-blockers are generally very well tolerated when administered to individuals without specific contraindications. Table 12-2 includes some of the more common ocular and systemic adverse effects of β-adrenergic antagonists. Plasma drug levels from topical medications can approach those achieved with systemic administration because of their absorption in the nasolacrimal drainage system and lack of first-pass hepatic metabolism. However, administering topical medications in a gel vehicle results in reduced systemic absorption and decreased plasma concentrations of β-blockers compared with the equivalent solution. Nasolacrimal occlusion also reduces systemic absorption.

Systemic adverse effects of β-adrenergic antagonists include bronchospasm, bradycardia, heart block, systemic hypotension, reduced exercise tolerance, and central nervous system (CNS) depression. Patients with diabetes may experience reduced glucose tolerance and masking of hypoglycemic signs and symptoms. In addition, abrupt withdrawal of ophthalmic β-blockers can exacerbate symptoms of hyperthyroidism.

Before a β-blocker is prescribed, the clinician should ask whether the patient has a history of asthma, because β-blockers may induce severe, life-threatening bronchospasm in susceptible patients. β_2-receptors are present in bronchial smooth muscle cells, and their inhibition results in bronchospasm in susceptible individuals. Because betaxolol is a β_1-selective antagonist, it is safer than the nonselective β-blockers for use in patients with asthma. In addition, betaxolol may be less likely to cause depression; however, β-blocker–related adverse effects can still occur with its use.

Ophthalmologists should consider the clinical impact of β-blockers on the patient's heart rate before initiating therapy. Baseline bradycardia or history of heart block may preclude the use of these agents. Use of topical β-blockers has been associated with the development of signs and symptoms of myasthenia gravis in patients without a preexisting diagnosis and can exacerbate the condition in patients with known disease. The mechanism by which this occurs is unclear.

Other adverse effects of β-blockers include lethargy, mood changes, depression, altered mentation, light-headedness, syncope, visual disturbance, corneal anesthesia, punctate keratitis, allergy, impotence, reduced libido, and alteration of serum lipids (reduction in high-density lipoprotein). In children, β-blockers should be used with caution, because of the relatively high systemic levels achieved. Because β-blockers decrease aqueous production, they may contribute to dry eye symptoms.

Adrenergic Agonists

α_2-Selective adrenergic agonists

Mechanism of action α_2-Selective agonists lower IOP primarily by reducing aqueous humor production. The α_2-adrenoceptor found on the ciliary epithelium is coupled to an inhibitory G protein. When this adrenoceptor is bound by catecholamines or pharmacologically active α_2-agonists, an intracellular cascade results in reduction in the activity of adenylate cyclase and the intracellular concentration of cAMP, with a resultant reduction in the rate of aqueous humor production. An alternate or possibly complementary mechanism by which aqueous humor production is reduced may be anterior segment vasoconstriction and reduced blood flow to the ciliary body. The α_2-selective adrenergic agonist brimonidine, but not apraclonidine, also results in increased uveoscleral outflow. How uveoscleral outflow may be increased with brimonidine is unclear, but evidence points to relaxation of ciliary smooth muscle cells. As with β-blockers, systemic absorption of α_2-selective agonists may lead to a crossover effect, although it appears to be small.

Available agents Brimonidine tartrate is the most commonly used α_2-adrenergic agonist. Apraclonidine hydrochloride (*para*-aminoclonidine), an α_2-adrenergic agonist and clonidine derivative, is used for long-term therapy only in rare instances because of the frequent occurrence of tachyphylaxis and a hypersensitivity reaction that can cause blepharoconjunctivitis. Use of apraclonidine is mostly limited to perioperative administration to blunt acute IOP spikes that may occur after laser peripheral iridotomy, laser trabeculoplasty, laser capsulotomy, and cataract extraction. Brimonidine is similarly effective when used perioperatively.

Tachyphylaxis is less profound with brimonidine than with apraclonidine. Brimonidine's peak IOP reduction is approximately 26% (2 hours post dose), which is comparable to the reduction achieved by a nonselective β-blocker and superior to that of the selective β-blocker betaxolol. At trough (12 hours post dose), the IOP reduction is only 14%–15%, or less than the reduction achieved with nonselective β-blockers. Studies have shown that brimonidine does not lower nocturnal IOP. Though approved for therapy 3 times daily in the United States, brimonidine is commonly used twice daily, particularly when used in combination with at least 1 other agent.

Adverse effects The incidence of ocular allergic reactions (eg, follicular conjunctivitis and contact blepharodermatitis; Fig 12-3) is common but lower with brimonidine than with apraclonidine. This ocular allergy is a delayed-type hypersensitivity reaction that is dose

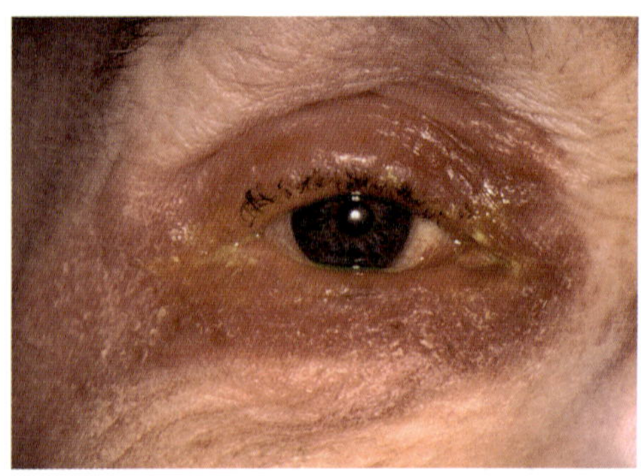

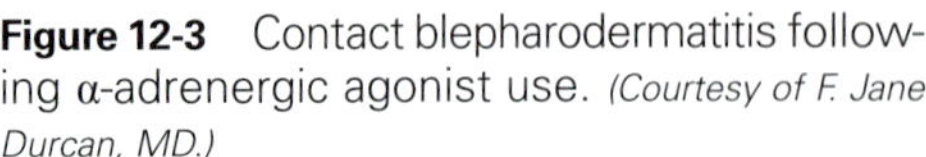

Figure 12-3 Contact blepharodermatitis following α-adrenergic agonist use. *(Courtesy of F. Jane Durcan, MD.)*

dependent, with a 1-year incidence of approximately 15% for brimonidine tartrate 0.2% preserved with benzalkonium chloride (BAK) and 10% for brimonidine tartrate 0.15% preserved with sodium chlorite (Purite). The incidence of allergy continues to increase beyond 1 year. Cross-sensitivity to brimonidine in patients with known hypersensitivity to apraclonidine is minimal. However, the incidence of long-term intolerance to brimonidine due to local adverse effects is high (>20%). Granulomatous anterior uveitis is rare but has been reported in association with the use of brimonidine.

α_2-Selective agonists have some α_1-binding activity. The ocular effects of α_1-adrenergic agonists include conjunctival vasoconstriction, pupillary dilation, and eyelid retraction. Apraclonidine has a much greater affinity for α_1-receptors than does brimonidine and is therefore more likely to produce these effects. In some patients, apraclonidine causes mydriasis, whereas brimonidine commonly causes miosis.

Systemic adverse effects of α_2-selective agonists include xerostomia (dry mouth) and lethargy, both mediated by their clonidine-like CNS activity. Patients taking these medications should be advised to perform nasolacrimal occlusion. Brimonidine should not be used in infants and young children because of the risk of CNS depression, apnea, bradycardia, and hypotension, due to a combination of the lower volume of distribution and the presumed increased CNS penetration of the drug.

Monoamine oxidase inhibitors and tricyclic antidepressants may interfere with metabolism of apraclonidine and brimonidine, resulting in a toxic effect on the patient.

Nonselective adrenergic agonists

The nonselective adrenergic agonists epinephrine (adrenaline) and dipivefrin (a prodrug of epinephrine) reduce aqueous humor production, increase uveoscleral outflow, and improve conventional outflow facility. Both drugs have been superseded by other classes of drugs and are now rarely used in glaucoma management because of the frequent occurrence of local adverse effects. Both are no longer available in the United States.

Carbonic Anhydrase Inhibitors

Mechanism of Action

Carbonic anhydrase inhibitors (CAIs) decrease aqueous humor production by inhibiting the activity of ciliary epithelial carbonic anhydrase. Systemic CAI therapy may further decrease aqueous humor formation because of the resultant renal metabolic acidosis, which may reduce the activity of Na^+,K^+-ATPase (also called *sodium-potassium pump*) in the ciliary epithelium. The enzyme carbonic anhydrase is present in many tissues, including corneal endothelium, iris, retinal pigment epithelium, red blood cells, epithelial cells lining the choroid plexus of the brain, and kidney. More than 90% of the ciliary epithelial enzyme activity must be inhibited to decrease aqueous production and lower IOP.

Available Agents

The topical CAI agents, dorzolamide and brinzolamide, are available for long-term treatment of elevated IOP and are associated with fewer systemic adverse effects than are the systemic CAIs. In the United States, these agents are currently approved for use 3 times daily, but most clinicians prescribe them for twice-daily use. Administration 3 times per day results in slightly greater IOP reduction. For patients taking an oral CAI at a full dose and the appropriate dosing frequency, there is no advantage to adding a topical CAI.

Systemic CAIs can be administered orally or intravenously and are most useful in patients who present with severely elevated IOP or as a temporizing measure until surgery can be performed. Oral CAIs begin to act within 1 hour of administration, with maximal effect within 2–4 hours, whereas intravenous CAIs begin to act within 15 minutes. Sustained-release acetazolamide can reach peak effect within 3–6 hours of administration. Because of the adverse effects of systemic CAIs, long-term therapy may be reserved for patients whose IOP is not controlled with topical therapy and who have refused surgery or in whom surgery would be inappropriate.

The most commonly used oral CAIs are acetazolamide and methazolamide. Compared with acetazolamide, methazolamide has a longer duration of action and is less bound to serum protein; however, it is also less effective. Methazolamide and sustained-release acetazolamide are the best tolerated of the systemic CAIs. Methazolamide is metabolized by the liver. Acetazolamide, which is not metabolized, is excreted by the kidney; it must be used with caution and at a reduced dose in patients with renal insufficiency.

Because oral CAIs are potent medications that are associated with considerable adverse effects, the lowest dose that reduces the IOP to an acceptable range should be used. Methazolamide is often effective in doses as low as 25–50 mg, given 2 or 3 times daily. Sustained-release formulations of acetazolamide may have fewer adverse effects than its standard formulation. The typical adult dosage of acetazolamide is 250 mg 4 times daily for the standard formulations or 500 mg twice daily for the sustained-release formulation.

Adverse Effects and Contraindications

Common adverse effects of topical CAIs include taste disturbance, blurred vision, burning upon instillation, and punctate keratopathy. Although many topical medications cause burning upon instillation, this is particularly common and more intense with dorzolamide, a solution formulated at a low pH due to the low solubility of the molecule at physiologic pH levels. Use of brinzolamide, a suspension, results in white deposits in the tear film. Eyes with compromised endothelial cell function may also be at risk of corneal decompensation with use of either of these drugs because of the dependence on carbonic anhydrase of the pumping function of endothelial cells.

Adverse effects of systemic CAI therapy are usually dose related and are driven primarily by the resultant metabolic acidosis. Many patients experience paresthesia of the fingers or toes and report loss of energy and anorexia. Weight loss is common. Severe mental depression, abdominal discomfort, diarrhea, loss of libido, impotence, and taste disturbance (especially with carbonated beverages) may also occur. Patients with sickle cell anemia are at risk of sickle cell crisis. There is an increased risk of formation of calcium oxalate and calcium phosphate renal calculi. Because methazolamide causes less acidosis, it may be less likely than acetazolamide to cause nephrolithiasis.

As the urine becomes more alkaline, ammonia excretion is reduced. Systemic CAIs are contraindicated in patients with hepatic cirrhosis, because either systemic agent can precipitate hepatic encephalopathy due to increased serum ammonia levels.

Historically, there has been concern about prescribing CAIs for patients with a known history of allergic reactions to sulfonamide antibiotics. However, there are important chemical differences between sulfonamide antibiotics and sulfonamide nonantibiotics. Only about 10% of patients with hypersensitivity to sulfonamide antibiotics experience allergic reactions when exposed to sulfonamide nonantibiotics such as CAIs. Such a response is thought to represent a predisposition to allergic reactions rather than true cross-reactivity, as the rate of reaction to penicillin antibiotics in those with an allergy to sulfonamide nonantibiotics is even higher.

Aplastic anemia and other blood dyscrasias, Stevens-Johnson syndrome, and hepatic necrosis are very rare but potentially fatal idiosyncratic reactions to CAIs. Although routine complete blood counts have been suggested, they are not predictive of blood dyscrasias and are not normally recommended. Hypokalemia is a potentially serious complication that is especially likely to occur when a patient uses an oral CAI concurrently with another drug that causes potassium loss (eg, a thiazide diuretic). Serum potassium should be monitored regularly in such patients.

Fraunfelder FT, Fraunfelder FW, Chambers WA. *Drug-Induced Ocular Side Effects.* 7th ed. Butterworth-Heinemann; 2014.

Shah TJ, Moshirfar M, Hoopes PC Sr. "Doctor, I have a sulfa allergy": clarifying the myths of cross-reactivity. *Ophthalmol Ther.* 2018;7(2):211–215. doi:10.1007/s40123-018-0136-8

Parasympathomimetic Agents

Parasympathomimetic agents, or *miotics,* have been used in the treatment of glaucoma for more than 100 years. Traditionally, they are divided into direct-acting cholinergic agonists and indirect-acting anticholinesterase agents.

The direct-acting agent pilocarpine continues to be employed in certain circumstances, although it is not commonly prescribed for long-term use. In patients with pigmentary glaucoma, pilocarpine is effective in blunting the IOP spike that can occur with jarring physical activities such as running. This drug is also useful in the management of elevated IOP in aphakic eyes and in patients whose drainage angles are persistently occludable despite laser peripheral iridotomy (plateau iris syndrome). Pilocarpine has been associated with poor patient adherence to the treatment regimen because of its adverse effect profile and because of its 3- or 4-times-daily dosing schedule; therefore, it is infrequently used. Lower concentrations and dosing frequencies may be acceptable for management of angles with persistent iridotrabecular contact with a patent peripheral iridotomy.

The indirect-acting agent echothiophate iodide fell out of favor because of its ocular and systemic adverse effects. Although rarely used, it can be very effective and well tolerated in aphakic eyes with glaucoma.

Mechanism of Action

Parasympathomimetic agents reduce IOP by causing contraction of the longitudinal ciliary muscle fibers that insert into the scleral spur, trabecular meshwork, and inner wall of Schlemm canal, which results in stretching of the trabecular meshwork and widening of the Schlemm canal, thereby improving outflow facility. Direct-acting agents affect the motor end plates in the same way as acetylcholine, which is transmitted at postganglionic parasympathetic junctions, as well as at other autonomic, somatic, and central synapses. Pilocarpine can reduce IOP by 15%–25%. Indirect-acting agents inhibit the enzyme acetylcholinesterase, thereby prolonging and enhancing the action of naturally secreted acetylcholine.

Adverse Effects

Miotic agents have been associated with numerous ocular adverse effects. Induced myopia resulting from ciliary muscle contraction is an adverse effect of all cholinergic agents; brow ache may accompany the ciliary spasm. The miosis interferes with vision in dim light conditions; in patients with significant lens opacities, vision is adversely affected in all ambient lighting conditions. Because miotic agents have been associated with retinal detachment, a peripheral retinal evaluation is suggested before the initiation of therapy. Miotics, particularly the indirect-acting agents, may be cataractogenic. In addition, the indirect-acting agents may induce formation of iris pigment epithelial cysts, may cause epiphora by both direct lacrimal stimulation and punctal stenosis, and may cause ocular surface changes that result in drug-induced ocular pseudopemphigoid.

Other potential ocular adverse effects include increased bleeding during surgery and increased inflammation and severe fibrinous iridocyclitis postoperatively. Because miotics can disrupt the blood–aqueous barrier, they should be avoided, if possible, in patients with uveitic glaucoma. Use of miotics occasionally induces paradoxical angle closure, particularly in eyes with phacomorphic narrow angles; contraction of the ciliary muscle leads to forward movement of the lens–iris interface and increased anteroposterior lens diameter, which may cause or exacerbate pupillary block in an eye with a large lens.

Systemic adverse effects, occurring mainly with indirect-acting medications, include diarrhea, abdominal cramps, increased salivation, bronchospasm, and enuresis. Depolarizing muscle relaxants such as succinylcholine cannot be used for 6 weeks after stopping indirect-acting agents.

Rho Kinase Inhibitors

Mechanism of Action

The Rho family of G proteins is activated by various cytokines and regulates cell morphology, cellular properties such as stiffness, and cellular processes such as adhesion and apoptosis, as well as smooth muscle cell contraction. The effectors of these G proteins are the

Rho kinases (ROCK1 and ROCK2). Activated Rho kinase phosphorylates various downstream proteins, including myosin light chain (MLC) phosphatase.

The net result of Rho kinase activity is increased phosphorylation and activation of MLC. Phosphorylated MLC interacts with actin, altering the physical characteristics of the cytoskeleton, thereby leading to increased cell stiffness and smooth muscle cell contraction. Rho kinase inhibitors lower IOP primarily by relaxing the cytoskeleton of outflow cells in the trabecular meshwork and Schlemm canal, increasing conventional (trabecular meshwork) outflow facility.

Available Agents

Ripasudil, a mixed ROCK1 and ROCK2 inhibitor, was the first Rho kinase inhibitor available for clinical use to lower IOP and has been approved in Japan. The only Rho kinase inhibitor approved for use in the United States is netarsudil, which was approved by the FDA in 2017. Like ripasudil, netarsudil is a mixed ROCK1 and ROCK2 inhibitor; however, it also is a norepinephrine transporter (NET) inhibitor. The NET inhibitor activity is thought to result in a reduction of episcleral venous pressure and may also decrease aqueous humor secretion, although the latter has not been demonstrated in humans. In clinical trials, the IOP-lowering efficacy of netarsudil was similar to or slightly lower than that of timolol. Some clinical trials were focused on eyes with fairly low baseline IOP because it was thought that the drug might be particularly effective in such eyes. In 2 clinical trials in which the mean baseline diurnal IOP was approximately 22 mm Hg, the IOP reduction achieved with once-daily netarsudil 0.02% was approximately 20%. The drug lowers IOP by an additional 1.3–2.5 mm Hg when combined with latanoprost. Although mean IOP lowering with netarsudil used as monotherapy or in combination with latanoprost in clinical trials appears to be modest, some patients respond very well, experiencing substantial IOP lowering.

Netarsudil is used once daily. The hyperemia that commonly occurs with this class of agents is most intense during the first few hours after instillation; therefore, nighttime dosing is preferable.

Kahook MY, Serle JB, Mah FS, et al. Long-term safety and ocular hypotensive efficacy evaluation of netarsudil ophthalmic solution: Rho Kinase Elevated IOP Treatment Trial (ROCKET-2). *Am J Ophthalmol.* 2019;200:130–137.

Tanna AP, Johnson M. Rho kinase inhibitors as a novel treatment for glaucoma and ocular hypertension. *Ophthalmology*. 2018;125(11):1741–1756.

Adverse Effects

The most common adverse event associated with the use of Rho kinase inhibitors is conjunctival hyperemia, which occurs in more than 50%–60% of patients and is thought to be a result of conjunctival vascular smooth muscle cell relaxation. In clinical trials of netarsudil, subconjunctival hemorrhages occurred in approximately 15%–20% of patients; eye pruritis, punctate keratitis, increased lacrimation, blepharitis, and decreased visual acuity were each reported in approximately 5%–10% of patients. Cornea verticillata was observed in approximately 15%–25% of patients after 1 year of use; it is similar in appearance to that observed

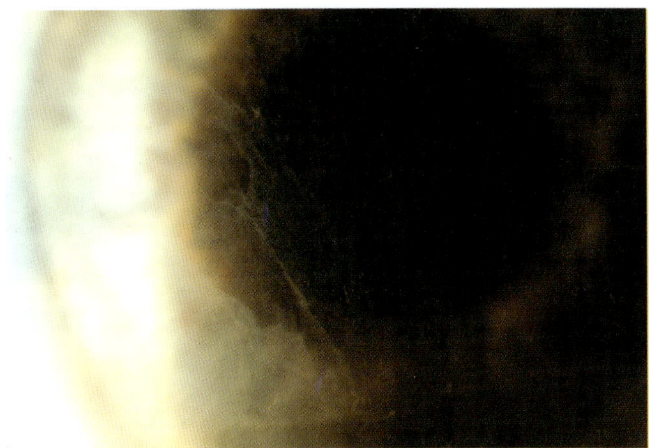

Figure 12-4 Cornea verticillata after use of netarsudil for 3 months. *(Courtesy of Angelo P. Tanna, MD.)*

after long-term use of amiodarone (Fig 12-4). Cornea verticillata does not seem to adversely affect visual function and resolves after a mean of approximately 1 year following discontinuation of the drug; it is believed to occur as a result of lysosomal accumulation of phospholipids within corneal epithelial cells. Reticular corneal edema is an adverse effect associated with netarsudil, although its frequency is not yet clear (Fig 12-5).

Combined Medications

Medications combined in a single bottle have the potential benefits of improved convenience and less exposure to preservatives. Fixed-combination medications consisting of timolol and another agent—a CAI (dorzolamide or brinzolamide), an α_2-adrenergic agonist (brimonidine), or a PG analogue (latanoprost, travoprost, or bimatoprost)—are available in many countries (see Table 12-2). In addition, fixed combinations of brimonidine and brinzolamide, and of latanoprost and netarsudil are available.

In general, the efficacy of fixed-combination formulations is similar to that of each of the components instilled separately. With fixed-combination agents that include timolol and are administered twice daily, the total amount of the β-blocker may be more than necessary, because nearly the full effect of a β-blocker can be achieved with once-daily dosing. The ocular adverse effects of fixed-combination medications are the same as for both drugs given individually. In general, except in the setting of an acutely elevated or dangerously high IOP, the clinician should make sure that each component of the fixed combination is effective in further lowering the IOP by adding the individual components sequentially.

Hyperosmotic Agents

Hyperosmotic agents are used to control acute episodes of severely elevated IOP. Common hyperosmotic agents include oral glycerol and intravenous mannitol.

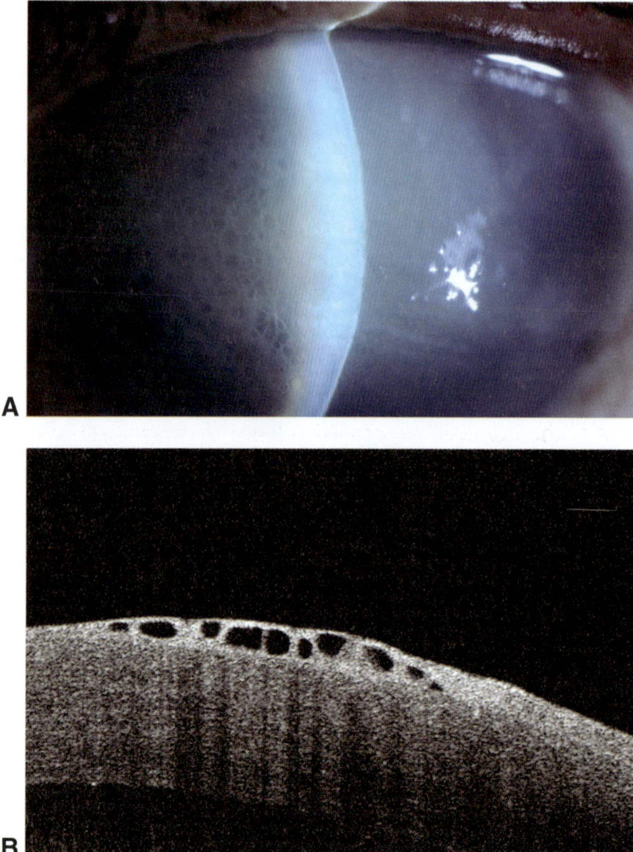

Figure 12-5 Corneal edema. **A,** Reticular corneal edema associated with use of topical netarsudil. **B,** Optical coherence tomography image showing the location of the cystic spaces in reticular cornea edema associated with netarsudil use. *(Part A courtesy of Michael Lin, MD; part B courtesy of Teresa C. Chen, MD, and Ashley Kim.)*

When given systemically, hyperosmotic agents increase blood osmolality, creating an osmotic gradient between the blood and the vitreous humor that draws water from the vitreous cavity and reduces IOP. Because of the increased gradient, the higher the dose administered and the more rapid the administration, the greater the subsequent IOP reduction will be.

Hyperosmotic agents are rarely administered for longer than a few hours because their effects are transient (a result of the rapid reequilibration of the osmotic gradient). They become less effective over time, and a rebound elevation in IOP may occur if the agent penetrates the eye and reverses the osmotic gradient.

Adverse effects of these drugs include headache, confusion, backache, acute congestive heart failure, and myocardial infarction. The rapid increase in extracellular volume and cardiac preload caused by hyperosmotic agents may precipitate or aggravate congestive heart failure. Intravenous administration is more likely to cause this problem than oral administration. In addition, subdural and subarachnoid hemorrhages have been reported after treatment with hyperosmotic agents. Glycerol can precipitate hyperglycemia or even ketoacidosis in patients with diabetes, because it is metabolized into glucose and ketone bodies.

Hyperosmotic agents are contraindicated in patients with renal failure. The patient's volume status should be closely monitored when receiving hyperosmotic agents.

General Approach to Medical Treatment

Long-Term Therapy

The ophthalmologist should tailor ocular hypotensive therapy to the individual needs of the patient, including consideration of a target IOP. IOP, though important, is only one of several factors to monitor. The effectiveness of the therapy can be determined only by careful, repeated scrutiny of the patient's optic nerve, retinal nerve fiber layer, and visual field status (see Chapters 5 and 6).

Characteristics of the medical agents available for the treatment of glaucoma are summarized in Table 12-2. When making management decisions, ophthalmologists should consider the efficacy, adverse effect profile, drug cost, patient preference, and likelihood of patient adherence to the drug regimen. Treatment is usually initiated with a single topical medication, unless the baseline IOP is extremely high, in which case 2 or more medications may be indicated. Collaborative decision-making between the physician and patient likely increases patient adherence to the prescribed regimen.

In most cases, laser trabeculoplasty is a reasonable choice as first-line therapy for open-angle glaucoma and ocular hypertension, as are PG analogues and β-blockers. PG analogues are the most commonly used first-line agents because of their superior efficacy, once-daily dosing, and favorable safety profile. Although the local adverse effects of β-blockers are minimal, these drugs have a greater potential for systemic adverse effects compared with PG analogues. Also, they lack nocturnal IOP-lowering efficacy. If PG analogues and β-blockers are contraindicated or ineffective, netarsudil (Rho kinase inhibitor), brimonidine (α_2-adrenergic agonist), or a topical CAI are all reasonable options.

If 1 agent is not adequate to reduce the IOP to the desired range, the initial agent may be discontinued and another tried, or a second agent can be added. Laser trabeculoplasty, if appropriate, may be considered at any point during the stepwise process of intensifying treatment, including as the initial treatment (see Chapter 13 for discussion of this procedure).

If a patient using a PG analogue requires a second agent, it is reasonable to add a β-blocker, α_2-adrenergic agonist, topical CAI, or Rho kinase inhibitor. All have similar additive mean diurnal IOP-lowering efficacies, although CAIs may have better nocturnal efficacy. The choice of drug should be based on each drug's adverse effect profile, dosing frequency, and possible contraindications, as well as patient preference. In some cases, it may be necessary to add a fourth or fifth agent; however, the clinician should keep in mind the diminishing returns of doing so.

Patients sometimes fail to associate systemic adverse effects with topical drugs and, consequently, seldom volunteer symptoms. The ophthalmologist must make sure to inquire about these symptoms. In addition, communicating with the primary care physician is important not only to provide information about the potential adverse effects of a glaucoma medication but also to discuss the effects that medications currently prescribed for systemic disease might have on the glaucomatous process. For example, modification of oral β-blocker therapy for systemic hypertension may affect IOP.

Glaucoma Medications and Ocular Surface Disease

In addition to the effect of the drugs themselves on the ocular surface, preservatives used in ophthalmic solutions can be toxic to the ocular surface after topical administration. Benzalkonium chloride (BAK), the most commonly used preservative in glaucoma medications, may cause an intense adverse reaction in some patients. Even in patients without a true allergy to BAK, frequent and prolonged exposure to this preservative often results in worsening ocular surface disease. Strategies to reduce the toxic effect of preservatives on the ocular surface include limiting the dosing frequency; combination agents may be helpful. A limited number of glaucoma medications are available without preservatives or with preservatives other than BAK (Table 12-3). In addition, compounding pharmacies, available in some areas of the country, may compound drugs tailored to the needs of an individual patient, for example, combining 2 or more drugs without preservatives. In considering this option, the physician should weigh the fact that there is less-robust knowledge about the safety and efficacy of compounded agents against the potential benefit to the ocular surface.

For rehabilitation of the ocular surface, it may be beneficial to stop all topical medications—if the level of glaucomatous damage permits—and have the patient use preservative-free artificial tears frequently. During this period, the temporary use of oral CAIs or an injectable medication such as the bimatoprost implant (Durysta; Allergan) may be helpful to lower IOP.

Therapy for Acute Intraocular Pressure Elevation

The goals of medical treatment of acute IOP elevation are to prevent further damage to the optic nerve; to clear corneal edema, if present; and to reduce intraocular inflammation. In eyes with severe IOP elevation, hyperosmotic agents and systemic CAIs may be required in order to lower IOP in preparation for definitive treatment. When IOP is severely elevated, ischemia of the pupillary constrictor muscle can interfere with the miotic action of pilocarpine and other parasympathomimetic agents. Therefore, in patients with acute primary angle closure, lowering the IOP also allows pupillary constriction before laser peripheral iridotomy is performed (see Chapter 9).

Table 12-3 Preservative-Free and Alternatively Preserved Ocular Hypotensive Agents

Medication	Preservative
Brimonidine 0.1%, 0.15% (Alphagan P)	Sodium chlorite (Purite)
Dorzolamide hydrochloride/timolol maleate 2%/0.5% (Cosopt PF)	Preservative-free unit dose vials
Latanoprost 0.005% (IYUZEH)	Preservative-free unit dose vials
Latanoprost 0.005% (Xelpros)	Potassium sorbate, borate, propylene glycol
Tafluprost 0.0015% (Zioptan)	Preservative-free unit dose vials
Timolol 0.25%, 0.5% (Timoptic in Ocudose)	Preservative-free unit dose vials
Timolol gel-forming solution 0.1%, 0.25%, 0.5% (Timoptic XE)	Benzododecinium bromide (a detergent closely related to BAK)
Travoprost 0.004% (Travatan Z)	Borate, sorbitol, propylene glycol, and zinc (SofZia)

BAK = benzalkonium chloride.

Administration of Ocular Medications

Patients, or their companions if applicable, should be taught how to properly instill eyedrops. Nearly 25% of people with glaucoma report having someone else administer their eyedrops. Thus, it is important to ask who will administer the drops and then ensure that this person can do so effectively. Conditions such as arthritis and tremor are common and may impair eyedrop instillation. Having patients (or their companions) demonstrate eyedrop administration may reveal these types of barriers and provides an excellent opportunity for personalized instruction. Ideally, one drop is instilled onto the globe or into the inferior fornix, followed by 1–3 minutes with the eyes closed to increase corneal penetration. Nasolacrimal occlusion can be performed during this time to limit systemic absorption and reduce the unpleasant taste associated with some agents. For patients instilling 2 or more agents concurrently, waiting at least 5 minutes after instillation of each drop should limit the washout of the first drug by the second.

Use of Glaucoma Medications During Pregnancy or While Breastfeeding

Often, IOP decreases during pregnancy, both in healthy individuals and in patients with glaucoma. However, glaucoma patients who are pregnant frequently continue to require ocular hypotensive medical therapy throughout the pregnancy. As mentioned previously, topical ocular hypotensive medications are systemically absorbed; they subsequently cross the placenta and enter the fetal circulation, or they can be secreted into breast milk. Unfortunately, there is little definitive information concerning the safety of glaucoma medication use during pregnancy or while breastfeeding.

The patient and obstetrician should collaborate in deciding whether to continue ocular hypotensive therapy during pregnancy and which agents to use. Ideally, these plans should be formulated and implemented before conception, if possible. The theoretical risk of teratogenicity and other adverse outcomes necessitates an assessment of the potential benefits of treatment and a careful evaluation of the treatment regimen.

With all topical ocular hypotensive medications, patients who are pregnant or breastfeeding should be advised to perform nasolacrimal occlusion during eyedrop instillation. In general, it is prudent to minimize the use of medications during pregnancy whenever possible. The lowest effective dose should be given. The clinician may want to consider laser trabeculoplasty or other surgical intervention in cases in which the benefits outweigh the potential risks. However, antifibrotic agents should be avoided because there is evidence of human fetal risk based on adverse reaction data.

Belkin A, Chen T, DeOliveria AR, Johnson SM, Ramulu PY, Buys YM; American Glaucoma Society and the Canadian Glaucoma Society. A practical guide to the pregnant and breastfeeding patient with glaucoma. *Ophthalmol Glaucoma.* 2020;3(2):79–89.

Prostaglandin analogues

Pregnancy Category C, a classification system that has been abandoned by the FDA, included drugs for which animal studies showed an adverse effect on the fetus but there were no adequate studies in humans. $PGF_{2\alpha}$ analogues, which were previously included in Category C, have been shown to be embryocidal in rodent studies when administered at high doses (15–97 times the human dose). Travoprost is teratogenic in rats at intravenous doses that correspond to exposure levels up to 250 times the human exposure at the maximum recommended human ocular dose. $PGF_{2\alpha}$, when given at much higher doses than those used in topical therapy, exerts abortifacient activity by increasing uterine contractility and may induce labor. It is unlikely that topically administered PG analogues place the fetus at significant risk during pregnancy.

β-Blockers

β-Blockers (formerly listed in Pregnancy Category C) are often used for the treatment of systemic hypertension during pregnancy. There have been reports of growth retardation, arrhythmia, bradycardia, and lethargy affecting the fetus or newborn exposed to systemically or topically administered β-adrenergic antagonists. These agents are concentrated in breast milk and are relatively contraindicated in breastfeeding patients because of their potential adverse effects on infants.

α_2-Adrenergic agonists

Previously listed in Pregnancy Category B (Category B included drugs for which animal studies failed to demonstrate a risk to the fetus, but there were no adequate and well-controlled studies in pregnant women), brimonidine is a preferred agent for use during pregnancy. Because brimonidine has been linked to apnea in infants, its use should be discontinued in pregnant patients prior to delivery to minimize the risk of this complication in the newborn. Brimonidine should also be avoided in patients who are breastfeeding. For more information about brimonidine use in infants and children, see Chapter 11.

Carbonic anhydrase inhibitors

The CAIs (formerly in Pregnancy Category C) are teratogenic in rodents, and there are case reports of forelimb deformities in infants whose mothers were using systemic CAIs during pregnancy. Systemic CAIs should be avoided for the treatment of glaucoma during pregnancy. When possible, it may be preferable to also avoid the use of topical CAIs in patients who are pregnant, particularly during the first trimester.

Rho kinase inhibitors

No clear teratogenic effects were observed in animal studies of Rho kinase inhibitors. However, because of the potential for adverse fetal events due to inhibition of downstream targets of the enzyme rho kinase, caution about use of these agents during pregnancy or while breastfeeding is warranted.

Generic Medications

Many glaucoma medications are available as generic drugs. Although the generic agents are required to be chemically or biologically equivalent to the brand-name product, in some cases there may be differences in formulation that could potentially alter a drug's effect. Brimonidine and bimatoprost, for example, are available in generic formulations that differ in concentration of the active ingredients from the brand-name products. The use of lower-cost generic medications has been shown to improve patient adherence to medication regimens. Cost is a very important consideration given the lifelong nature of glaucoma treatment in most cases.

Patient Adherence to a Medication Regimen

Proper adherence to a medication regimen includes obtaining the medication(s), using it on schedule each day, and successfully instilling eyedrops. Unfortunately, multiple studies show that patient adherence to the prescribed medication regimen for glaucoma is often poor. However, there is ample evidence that physicians can positively influence adherence.

The physician can increase the likelihood that the patient will adhere to the medication regimen by

- providing clear communication about the nature of the disease and the need for treatment
- engaging in collaborative decision-making with the patient
- prescribing a medication regimen that is acceptable for the patient in regard to dosing schedule, side effects, and cost

Strategies for clear health communication include assessing the patient's health literacy level. Fortunately, patient education materials designed for various literacy levels, with dense text used sparingly and with clear graphics, are available from multiple sources. See BCSC Section 1, *Update on General Medicine,* for discussion of social determinants of health.

In general, the lowest number of medication bottles and the least-frequent dosing are preferable. Generic medications are usually the most cost-effective for long-term treatment.

The barrier to medication adherence that is cited most often by patients is forgetfulness. To help patients take their medications every day at the correct time, physicians can provide a dosing chart, encourage use of telephone or reminder apps, or work with companions and caregivers to develop a feasible schedule. It is useful to pair glaucoma medication dosing with another routine activity, such as taking an oral medication, brushing teeth, or eating breakfast. PG analogues are often prescribed for bedtime dosing due to hyperemia, but morning dosing may be easier to remember for patients who have an irregular bedtime routine.

Eyedrop aids may improve adherence by helping patients overcome specific challenges, such as squeezing or aiming the medication bottle. By watching the patient (or companion, if responsible for drug administration) instill eyedrops, the clinician can determine which eyedrop aid would be useful and provide instruction on proper instillation technique if needed.

Because a patient's physical condition, cognitive abilities, and living situation are likely to change over the course of treatment, discussions about medication adherence should be ongoing.

Medeiros FA, Walters TR, Kolko M, et al; ARTEMIS 1 Study Group. Phase 3, Randomized, 20-Month Study of Bimatoprost Implant in Open-Angle Glaucoma and Ocular Hypertension (ARTEMIS 1). *Ophthalmology.* 2020;127(12):1627–1641. doi:10.1016/j.ophtha.2020.06.018

CHAPTER 13

Surgical Therapy for Glaucoma

This chapter includes related videos. Go to aao.org/bcscvideo_section10 or scan the QR codes in the text to access this content.

Highlights

- Laser trabeculoplasty is an effective primary or adjunctive treatment for open-angle glaucoma and ocular hypertension.
- Laser peripheral iridotomy is beneficial only for pupillary block–induced forms of angle closure.
- The number of surgical options for patients with glaucoma has greatly expanded in the past decade; comparative effectiveness studies are needed to guide selection for a particular patient.
- Tube shunt surgery and trabeculectomy continue to have important roles in glaucoma management.
- Cataract surgery can be effective in the management of angle-closure disease.

Introduction

Surgical treatments for glaucoma are designed to lower intraocular pressure (IOP) by reducing resistance to aqueous humor outflow or—in cyclodestructive procedures—by reducing aqueous production. Aqueous outflow can be improved by enhancing the physiologic aqueous outflow pathways or by creating alternative pathways. *Laser surgery* is performed as a primary or adjunctive treatment. *Incisional surgery* is usually performed when there is documented progressive glaucomatous damage or a high risk of further damage despite maximally tolerated medical therapy. Other reasons for surgery include situations in which medical treatment is inappropriate, not tolerated, or not properly used by a particular patient.

Incisional surgery is the first-line treatment for primary congenital glaucoma (see Chapter 11). For most other types of glaucoma, medication or laser surgery (or both) is typically used as initial therapy. The clinician should exercise caution when recommending incisional surgery, because potential adverse effects (infection, hypotony, and cataracts) can result in vision loss. The results of early studies involving trabeculectomy as initial therapy for glaucoma (conducted before the introduction of many contemporary glaucoma medications) suggested that trabeculectomy had some advantages, including better control of IOP, a reduced number of patient follow-up visits, and the potential for better visual field preservation. The results of the Collaborative Initial Glaucoma Treatment Study (CIGTS; see Chapter 7) confirmed that, for open-angle glaucoma (OAG), initial surgical therapy provided better IOP control compared with initial medical therapy; however, this control generally did *not* lead to better visual field stabilization. In both the surgical and medication groups, the incidence of visual field progression was low. The 9-year follow-up data suggested that initial surgery resulted in less visual field progression compared with initial medical therapy among patients who had advanced visual field loss at baseline. Based on the results of this study and current practice, most clinicians defer incisional surgery for OAG unless medical and laser therapies have failed. Earlier surgical treatment can be considered in patients with advanced visual field loss at presentation.

Although conventional surgeries (trabeculectomy and tube shunt surgery) are quite effective in lowering IOP, they are associated with additional risk. Thus, over the past several years, there has been a strong effort to develop safer and reasonably effective alternative approaches. These "microinvasive" procedures differ from traditional surgeries in that they utilize physiologic aqueous outflow pathways. In contrast, trabeculectomy and tube shunt surgeries involve the creation of a new pathway into the subconjunctival space.

When surgery is indicated, various factors guide selection of the appropriate procedure. The proliferation of microinvasive glaucoma surgery devices and procedures has provided surgeons with a range of options. Each type of surgery has distinct indications and contraindications. However, there is considerable overlap, and few comparative studies are available; thus, it is difficult to customize a procedure to meet the needs of a particular patient. Figure 13-1 presents the procedures discussed in this chapter according to their mechanism of action, pathway, and use of an implant.

Boland MV, Ervin AM, Friedman DS, et al. Comparative effectiveness of treatments for open-angle glaucoma: a systematic review for the U.S. Preventive Services Task Force. *Ann Intern Med.* 2013;158(4):271–279.

Musch DC, Gillespie BW, Lichter PR, Niziol LM, Janz NK; CIGTS Study Investigators. Visual field progression in the Collaborative Initial Glaucoma Treatment Study: the impact of treatment and other baseline factors. *Ophthalmology.* 2009;116(2):200–207.

Laser Trabeculoplasty

In *laser trabeculoplasty (LTP),* spots of laser energy are applied to the trabecular meshwork (TM), usually covering 180° to 360° of the TM per treatment. LTP is intended to reduce IOP by increasing outflow facility. Various laser wavelengths and delivery systems can be used. In current clinical practice, the most commonly utilized methods are selective laser trabeculoplasty, argon laser trabeculoplasty, and micropulse laser trabeculoplasty. Note that the term *argon laser trabeculoplasty* is based on the historical use of argon laser technology; most green lasers currently used in ophthalmology are diode-pumped solid-state (eg, frequency-doubled Nd:YAG or Nd:YLF) lasers.

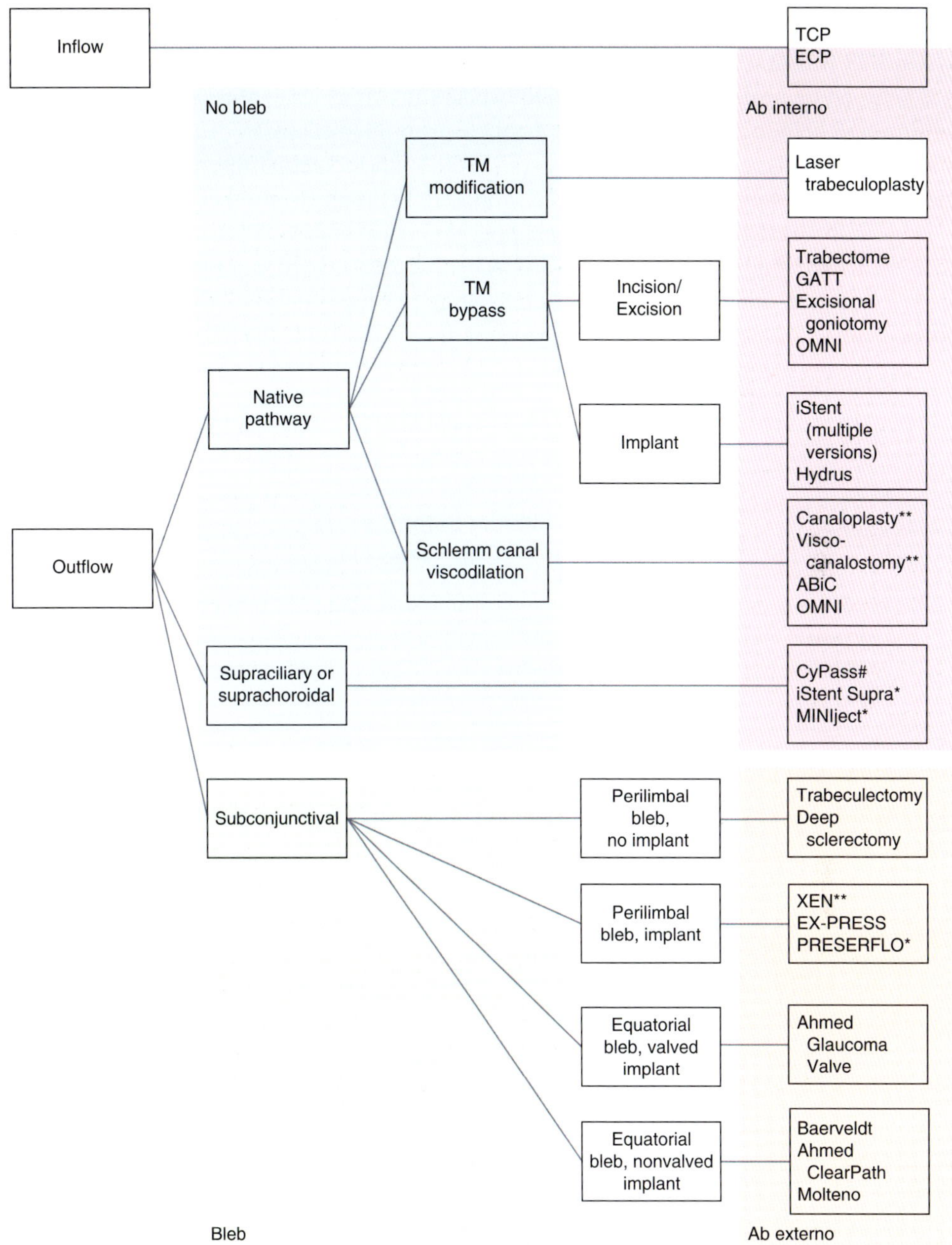

Figure 13-1 Diagram showing different types of microinvasive and traditional glaucoma surgeries. ABiC = ab interno canaloplasty; ECP = endoscopic cyclophotocoagulation; GATT = gonioscopy-assisted transluminal trabeculotomy; TCP = transscleral cyclophotocoagulation; TM = trabecular meshwork. * Not approved by US Food and Drug Administration; ** can be inserted ab interno or ab externo; # withdrawn from market. *(Diagram developed by Michael V. Boland, MD, PhD, and JoAnn A. Giaconi, MD.)*

Mechanism of Action

When LTP was first attempted in the 1970s, the application of thermal energy to the TM was believed to create holes, which would bypass the primary site of resistance to aqueous outflow and help to reduce IOP. Subsequent electron microscopy studies showed that this putative mechanism of action was incorrect. Although the actual mechanism of LTP remains unclear, several theories have been proposed. In argon laser trabeculoplasty, thermal damage to the treated TM causes collagen fiber shrinkage, thereby stretching and widening adjacent areas of the uveoscleral TM. This mechanism may help to improve aqueous outflow facility; however, other lasers are as effective while causing little or no damage to collagen fibers. In all forms of LTP, possible mechanisms of action include the following:

- stimulation of cell division
- cytokine release from treated TM cells, leading to alterations in the extracellular matrix of the TM or biomechanical changes in the Schlemm canal endothelial cells
- monocyte and macrophage recruitment to the TM
- increased phagocytic activity among cells in the TM

Alvarado JA, Alvarado RG, Yeh RF, Franse-Carman L, Marcellino GR, Brownstein MJ. A new insight into the cellular regulation of aqueous outflow: how trabecular meshwork endothelial cells drive a mechanism that regulates the permeability of Schlemm's canal endothelial cells. *Br J Ophthalmol.* 2005;89(11):1500–1505.

Indications and Contraindications

Laser trabeculoplasty is indicated for IOP reduction in patients with OAG or ocular hypertension. Historically, LTP was reserved for patients in whom maximally tolerated medical therapy was unsuccessful. However, it has been shown to be more effective when performed earlier and is cost-effective compared with medical therapy. Accordingly, many surgeons now use LTP as a first-line treatment option. Patients with difficulty applying topical medications, poor adherence to treatment, or clinically significant ocular surface disease are good candidates for trabeculoplasty.

LTP should only be performed in patients with an open angle. In a patient with advanced glaucoma and significantly elevated IOP, other treatment options should be considered. Despite the lack of extensive studies, LTP should generally be avoided in eyes with anterior uveitis because there are risks of increased inflammation and formation of peripheral anterior synechiae (PAS); however, the technique has potential benefit when inflammation is well-controlled and the IOP elevation is presumably steroid-induced. LTP is ineffective in eyes with iridocorneal endothelial syndrome, angle neovascularization, or extensive PAS.

Technique

A goniolens designed for laser treatment is placed on the eye with a coupling agent, allowing the surgeon to visualize anatomical landmarks; this facilitates TM recognition. Care is needed to identify the Schwalbe line, which can be mistaken for pigmented TM in some patients (ie, the Sampaolesi line). Because individuals with a heavily pigmented TM have a higher risk of acute postoperative IOP elevation (ie, spikes), lower energy settings are used for these patients.

Laser-specific techniques

In *argon laser trabeculoplasty (ALT),* a beam is focused on the junction of the anterior nonpigmented and posterior pigmented edge of the TM (Fig 13-2). The power setting should be titrated to achieve TM blanching or small bubble formation. The formation of a large bubble indicates a need for power reduction and titration to achieve the desired endpoint. Approximately 40–50 spots are applied over 180° of the TM. Usually, only half of the TM is treated; this reduces the risk of postoperative IOP spikes and permits future treatment (if necessary).

Selective laser trabeculoplasty (SLT) targets intracellular melanin. A frequency-doubled (532-nm) Q-switched Nd:YAG laser with a fixed 400-µm spot size and 3-nanosecond pulse is applied to the TM (see Fig 13-2), with laser energy titrated to the appearance of cavitation bubbles or a level immediately below that. Most surgeons treat 360° in 1 session. Typically, 80–120 spots are applied over 360° of the TM.

Micropulse laser trabeculoplasty (MLT) comprises application of energy to the TM, using the same wavelength involved in SLT. Unlike SLT, MLT uses a substantially longer thermal laser application, but the energy is only delivered for 15% of the application time. This approach allows the tissue to cool during the application of individual laser spots and may reduce thermal injury to the target and adjacent tissues. Approximately 120–140 confluent spots are applied over 360° of the TM.

Postoperative Care

For ALT, there is evidence that postoperative steroids or nonsteroidal anti-inflammatory drugs (NSAIDs) can improve patient comfort. In a small randomized controlled trial of SLT,

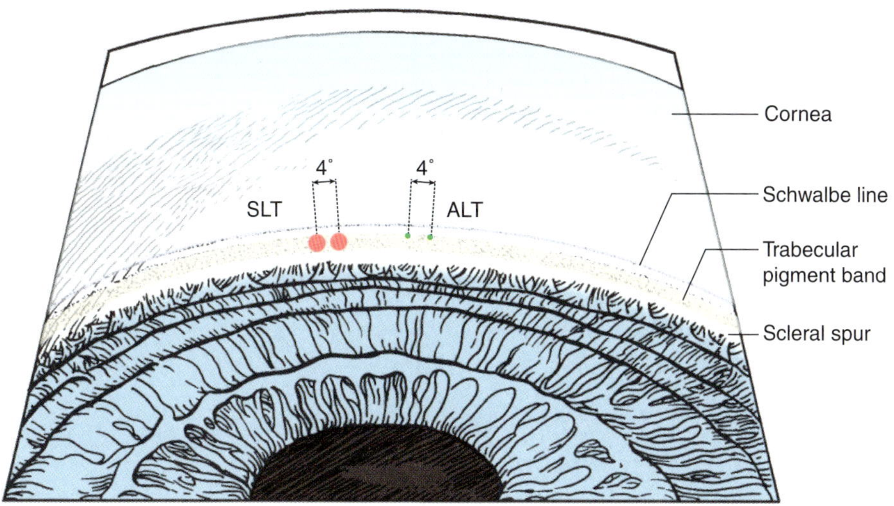

Figure 13-2 Illustration showing the positions of laser spots on the trabecular meshwork for argon laser trabeculoplasty (ALT) and selective laser trabeculoplasty (SLT).

the results suggested that the use of steroids or NSAIDs might improve IOP outcomes; but in the large Laser in Glaucoma and Ocular Hypertension (LiGHT) Trial (see efficacy section), no postoperative drops were used, and SLT was successful in a majority of eyes. There have been no studies regarding postoperative medications after MLT; however, no medications are specifically indicated. Because laser-induced changes in the TM occur over time, patients are usually examined between 4 and 6 weeks after treatment to determine whether an adequate IOP response has occurred.

Complications

Complications of LTP include corneal abrasion, inflammation, acute IOP elevation, and pain. IOP elevation is particularly concerning in patients with advanced glaucoma; it is usually evident within the first hour after surgery. The pre-laser use of topical apraclonidine or brimonidine has been shown to blunt postoperative IOP elevation. Other medications that minimize acute IOP elevation include β-blockers and pilocarpine. Hyperosmotic agents and oral carbonic anhydrase inhibitors may be helpful in eyes with IOP elevation that is not responsive to topical medications. In rare cases, patients exhibit prolonged, intractable IOP elevation requiring incisional surgery. Treatment of 180° can decrease the risk of postoperative IOP spikes, especially when the treatment involves ALT.

In ALT, PAS can form if the laser is applied too posteriorly. Low-grade anterior segment inflammation can occur after treatment with any LTP method. Other complications include hyphema and herpes simplex virus reactivation. In rare cases, keratitis can develop, leading to irregular astigmatism.

Efficacy

Selective laser trabeculoplasty and ALT have similar efficacy in terms of IOP reduction. Approximately 80% of patients with medically uncontrolled OAG experience a decrease in IOP for at least 6 months after LTP. Among patients with an initial response, 50% maintain significantly lower IOP for 3–5 years after treatment. The success rate at 10 years is approximately 30%. Success rates are higher in older patients with primary open-angle glaucoma (POAG) and pseudoexfoliation glaucoma.

SLT and MLT treatments can be repeated, although success rates seem to decline with each subsequent treatment. Because the initial ALT treatment is usually applied to only 180° of the TM, the laser can be applied to the untreated half of the TM later, if needed. However, in previously treated areas, multiple ALT treatments may be less effective and carry an increased risk of IOP elevation. SLT can be performed in areas previously treated with ALT; the results are similar to those in eyes that have undergone multiple SLT treatments. LTP is less effective in patients with angle-recession glaucoma, inflammatory glaucoma, or abnormal angle structures.

The Glaucoma Laser Trial (GLT) was a multicenter randomized clinical trial that assessed the efficacy and safety of ALT as an alternative to topical medical therapy in patients with newly diagnosed, previously untreated POAG. As initial therapy, ALT appeared to be at least as effective as medication in reducing IOP, preventing visual field loss, and slowing the increase in cup–disc ratio. However, the study was flawed in that 1 eye was assigned to ALT, whereas the fellow eye was assigned to timolol treatment; the fellow eye treatment may have confounded the results because timolol can have an IOP-lowering effect on the contralateral eye. More than half of the eyes treated initially with laser required the addition of 1 or more medications to control IOP during the study.

The LiGHT Trial was a prospective randomized study that compared SLT with medical treatment for the initial management of ocular hypertension and glaucoma. At 36 months, IOP control was similar between the 2 groups, but SLT was more cost-effective. Patients who underwent SLT demonstrated similar or better scores on quality-of-life measures, compared with patients using medication. At the 6-year follow-up, long-term disease control was better with SLT; there was a reduced need for incisional glaucoma and cataract surgery.

Gazzard G, Konstantakopoulou E, Garway-Heath D, et al; LiGHT Trial Study Group. Selective laser trabeculoplasty versus eye drops for first-line treatment of ocular hypertension and glaucoma (LiGHT): a multicentre randomised controlled trial. *Lancet*. 2019;393(10180):1505–1516.

Glaucoma Laser Trial Research Group. The Glaucoma Laser Trial (GLT) and glaucoma laser trial follow-up study: 7. Results. *Am J Ophthalmol*. 1995;120(6):718–731.

Cyclophotocoagulation

Mechanism of Action

In the past, cyclodestruction techniques involved heat, freezing, and ultrasound. These approaches were destructive to ocular tissues other than the intended target tissue and resulted in high complication rates; accordingly, they have been replaced by laser energy. Cyclophotocoagulation procedures are intended to reduce aqueous production by damaging or destroying the nonpigmented ciliary epithelium; in addition, because these procedures (specifically, external approaches) affect the ciliary muscle, they may increase uveoscleral outflow. Laser energy can be applied internally or externally. Internal delivery permits a more targeted approach with less collateral tissue destruction; however, it involves entry into the eye, which

KEY POINTS 13-1

Laser trabeculoplasty The following are essential points for the ophthalmologist to remember about this procedure.

- Patients who are good candidates for laser trabeculoplasty (LTP) need initial therapy, have difficulty applying topical medications, are poorly adherent to treatment, or have clinically significant ocular surface disease.
- Approximately 80% of patients with medically uncontrolled open-angle glaucoma experience a decrease in intraocular pressure for at least 6 months after LTP.
- The success rate at 10 years after LTP is approximately 30%.

introduces a risk of infection and requires the use of an operating room. External delivery can be performed in the office when the patient can tolerate a block without anesthesia support.

Pantcheva MB, Kahook MY, Schuman JS, Noecker RJ. Comparison of acute structural and histopathological changes in human autopsy eyes after endoscopic cyclophotocoagulation and trans-scleral cyclophotocoagulation. *Br J Ophthalmol.* 2007;91(2):248–252.

Indications and Contraindications

Historically, cyclophotocoagulation procedures were reserved for patients with poor visual potential because the procedures were assumed to have a high risk of postoperative visual decline. For prior cyclodestructive procedures, this perspective may have been deserved. However, experience has shown that patients who undergo cyclophotocoagulation procedures often have acceptable visual outcomes. The procedures are useful for most types of glaucoma, especially for older adult patients who refuse or cannot tolerate other glaucoma surgeries (eg, because of poor health). They are also useful for patients who cannot discontinue antiplatelet and/or anticoagulation therapy and thus have a greater risk of suprachoroidal hemorrhage during incisional glaucoma surgery. In addition, in patients with eye pain and poor visual potential, cyclophotocoagulation procedures can be performed to provide some comfort through IOP reduction. However, such procedures carry a small risk of sympathetic ophthalmia.

Technique

Cyclophotocoagulation is painful, so local anesthesia (retrobulbar, peribulbar, or sub-Tenon) is administered before the procedure. If the patient can tolerate a periocular injection without sedation, the procedure can be performed in the office. If a block is not possible, a short course of general anesthesia can be administered in the operating room. In eyes with abnormal anatomy (ie, extremely long or short eyes), a transilluminating device can help to identify the ciliary body prior to treatment.

Transscleral cyclophotocoagulation

There are 2 ways to externally deliver laser energy (Video 13-1): discrete treatment spots (16–22 spots) or broad, continuous application (so-called micropulse). Although discrete delivery is easier to perform, it may be associated with greater collateral tissue damage. Both discrete and continuous techniques use a fiber-optic probe, which is placed posterior to the limbus to target the underlying ciliary processes (Fig 13-3); both techniques also deliver 810-nm diode laser energy. In the continuous technique, the laser cycles on and off; the energy is "on" for 31.3% of the application time and "off" for the remainder. When first introduced, the continuous technique delivered less total energy; however, the duration of treatment has steadily increased to reach an energy level similar to that of the discrete technique. The continuous technique is more challenging in patients with tight orbits. In both techniques, avoidance of the 3 and 9 o'clock positions is needed to prevent damage to the long posterior ciliary nerves.

VIDEO 13-1 Transscleral cyclophotocoagulation.
Courtesy of Lauren Bierman, MD.
Available at: aao.org/bcscvideo_section10

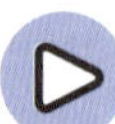

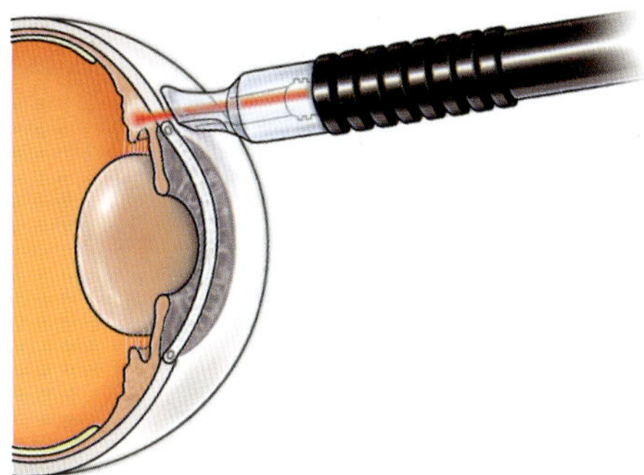

Figure 13-3 Depiction of diode cyclophotocoagulation laser handpiece (example of 1 manufacturer) aligned with the limbus and ready to treat. *(Figure developed by Angelo P. Tanna, MD, and illustrated by Wendy Hiller Gee.)*

Endoscopic cyclophotocoagulation

When performing endoscopic cyclophotocoagulation (ECP; also referred to as *endocyclophotocoagulation*), the surgeon views the ciliary epithelium with an endoscopic probe placed in the ciliary sulcus, posterior to the iris. Laser energy is directly delivered to the target tissue over a range of 270° to 360°. The endpoint is whitening and shrinkage of the ciliary processes without tissue rupture. This procedure is performed in the operating room, often in combination with cataract surgery.

Postoperative Care

After surgery, topical and/or subconjunctival steroids are used to control inflammation. Cycloplegics mitigate postoperative pain by paralyzing the ciliary muscles, which are often inflamed after treatment. Medical ocular hypotensive therapy is continued in the immediate postoperative period and tapered as appropriate. Oral analgesics, including narcotics, may be required for pain control.

Complications

Cyclophotocoagulation procedures may result in prolonged hypotony, pain, inflammation, cystoid macular edema, hemorrhage, retinal detachment, and phthisis bulbi. Sympathetic ophthalmia is a rare but serious complication. The endoscopic approach carries a risk of endophthalmitis.

Souissi S, Le Mer Y, Metge F, et al. An update on continuous-wave cyclophotocoagulation (CW-CPC) and micropulse transscleral cyclophotocoagulation treatment (MP-TLT) for adult and pediatric refractory glaucoma. *Acta Ophthalmol.* 2021;99(5):e621–e653. doi:10.1111/aos.14661

Efficacy

All forms of cyclophotocoagulation have been shown to reduce IOP. A randomized study comparing continuous and discrete external cyclophotocoagulation showed similar reductions in IOP, number of glaucoma medications, and re-treatment rates at 18 months.

No prospective randomized study has shown that cataract surgery combined with ECP is more effective than cataract surgery alone. These procedures often need to be repeated because their IOP-lowering effect diminishes over time.

Aquino MC, Barton K, Tan AM, et al. Micropulse versus continuous wave transscleral diode cyclophotocoagulation in refractory glaucoma: a randomized exploratory study. *Clin Exp Ophthalmol.* 2015;43(1):40–46.

Laser Peripheral Iridotomy

In laser peripheral iridotomy (LPI), laser energy is used to create a hole in the peripheral iris, which provides an alternative pathway for aqueous to enter the anterior chamber, bypassing the channel between the lens and iris.

Mechanism of Action

As described in Chapter 9, primary angle closure (PAC) occurs as a result of a relative increase in resistance to aqueous flow through the pupil to the anterior chamber (ie, *pupillary block*) and increases pressure posterior to the iris, causing it to bow anteriorly against the TM. These events lead to narrowing of the anterior chamber angle. LPI provides an alternative pathway for aqueous to enter the anterior chamber (Fig 13-4), relieving the pupillary block; this allows the iris to fall back and subsequently widen the angle.

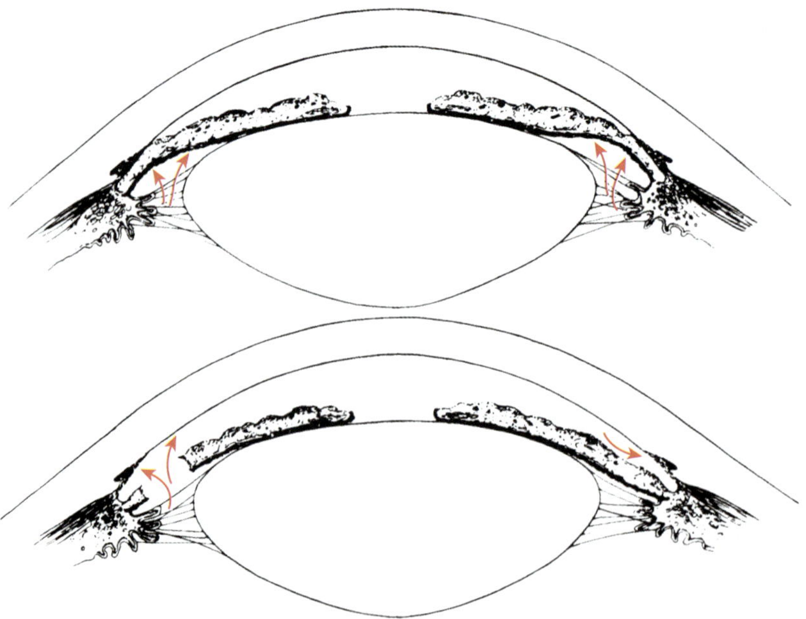

Figure 13-4 Illustration of an eye with angle closure *(top)*. Laser peripheral iridotomy or surgical iridectomy disrupts the pupillary block and results in opening of the entire peripheral angle *(bottom)* if no permanent peripheral anterior synechiae are present. *(Modified with permission from Kolker AE, Hetherington J, eds.* Becker-Shaffer's Diagnosis and Therapy of the Glaucomas. *5th ed. Mosby; 1983.)*

Indications and Contraindications

Laser peripheral iridotomy is performed when pupillary block is the suspected cause of iris–trabecular meshwork contact. Patients with acute primary angle closure (APAC), PAC, and primary angle-closure glaucoma (PACG) all benefit from iridotomy. In addition, LPI is often performed in PAC suspects, although it is unclear whether LPI is beneficial for these patients (see the section Efficacy for further discussion). Eyes with pupillary block–induced secondary angle closure also benefit from iridotomy. Multiple and/or larger iridotomies may be indicated for patients with substantial posterior synechiae.

In patients with a very shallow or flat peripheral anterior chamber, LPI can cause damage to the corneal endothelium. In patients who have angle closure without pupillary block (eg, neovascular glaucoma or iridocorneal endothelial syndrome), iridotomy is ineffective. Eyes with 360° of synechial angle closure (caused by chronic iridotrabecular contact) do not benefit from iridotomy.

Technique

Laser peripheral iridotomy requires a cooperative patient and an adequate view of the iris. To achieve these conditions in patients with APAC, medical IOP reduction is helpful because it reduces corneal edema and alleviates pain. Any form of ocular hypotensive medication can be used. IOP reduction can also be achieved via careful paracentesis.

When a prophylactic iridotomy is performed, a topical hypotensive agent is administered before the procedure to prevent postoperative IOP elevation. Pilocarpine may be instilled to constrict the pupil, which then stretches the iris and facilitates iris penetration by the laser. Pilocarpine may be ineffective in patients with ischemia of the iris sphincter muscle caused by prolonged APAC.

An iridotomy lens with a viscous coupling agent is used for visualization. The surgeon should evaluate the iris to determine iridotomy placement; the most peripheral location possible is preferred. A smaller amount of energy is required when the iridotomy is placed in an area of thinner iris (eg, an iris crypt). Nd:YAG or photothermal lasers (argon green or diode) can be used for iridotomy creation. For patients with thicker and darker irides, some surgeons suggest pretreatment with a photothermal laser to thin the iris, then using the Nd:YAG laser to penetrate the iris. Because pretreatment coagulates underlying blood vessels, it may also be beneficial for patients with a high risk of prolonged bleeding (ie, patients taking blood thinners). Laser settings vary widely according to surgeon preference and laser type. When the laser penetrates the iris, fluid and pigment are usually released into the anterior chamber. Although transillumination is useful for locating the iridotomy, it does not signify patency. The iridotomy should be of sufficient size. There is evidence that the creation of a larger iridotomy in eyes with small iridotomies can help to deepen the anterior chamber.

Postoperative Care

Intraocular pressure is checked 30 minutes to 1 hour after the procedure to monitor for potential acute pressure elevations. If necessary, steroids can be prescribed for approximately 1 week to treat postoperative inflammation associated with tissue disruption and bleeding. Topical hypotensive agents can also be used (when needed) for IOP control. The patient is examined 1–6 weeks after LPI to confirm iridotomy patency, determine whether the angle has deepened on gonioscopic examination, and evaluate the fundus. If the angle remains narrow after iridotomy, further evaluation can be considered (see Chapter 9).

Complications

Complications of iridotomy include hyphema, persistent postoperative inflammation, accelerated cataract formation, pupil distortion, and lens damage. Retinal tears, postoperative acute IOP elevation, and corneal endothelial damage can also occur. Visual dysphotopsias (glare, streaks, lines, and/or halos) may be present; they are suspected to result from iridotomy proximity to the tear meniscus, which acts as a prism and bends incident light through the iridotomy. Thus, some surgeons suggest temporal placement of the iridotomy, with precautions to ensure it remains distant from the tear meniscus. However, there is mixed evidence concerning whether iridotomy location (superior or temporal) affects the likelihood of dysphotopsias.

Srinivasan K, Zebardast N, Krishnamurthy P, et al. Comparison of new visual disturbances after superior versus nasal/temporal laser peripheral iridotomy: a prospective randomized trial. *Ophthalmology*. 2018;125(3):345–351.

Vera V, Naqi A, Belovay GW, Varma DK, Ahmed II. Dysphotopsia after temporal versus superior laser peripheral iridotomy: a prospective randomized paired eye trial. *Am J Ophthalmol.* 2014;157(5):929–935.

Efficacy

Laser peripheral iridotomy is effective in deepening the angle in pupillary block–induced forms of angle closure. However, some patients exhibit persistent angle closure despite a patent iridotomy; this situation requires further evaluation. LPI can be useful for controlling IOP in patients with PAC; however, long-term medical or surgical treatment is required in approximately 40%–60% of patients with PAC who undergo LPI. Iridotomy is also useful in the immediate management of APAC. However, it is less effective than phacoemulsification for long-term IOP control. One study showed that approximately 50% of patients who underwent LPI for APAC had IOP elevation >21 mm Hg at 18 months, compared with 3% in the phacoemulsification group. Most PACG eyes require additional IOP treatment despite iridotomy. The rate of conversion from PAC to PACG despite iridotomy is low, but the rate of conversion from APAC to PACG despite iridotomy is high.

The Zhongshan Angle-Closure Prevention (ZAP) trial prospectively enrolled 889 patients with suspected PAC. For each patient, management comprised LPI treatment in one eye and observation in the other eye. At 6 years, angle-closure disease was more likely to develop in control eyes (36 eyes vs 19 eyes; $P = .004$), most commonly on the basis of PAS formation. However, both groups had a very low rate of conversion overall, and there were no significant differences in acute angle-closure events or IOP elevation >24 mm Hg (see Chapter 9, Treatment Controversies sidebar).

Table 13-1 summarizes the main points of the preceding subsections on LPI.

Table 13-1 Iris Laser Procedures: Key Points

Laser Peripheral Iridotomy	Laser Iridoplasty
Patients with APAC, PAC, and PACG may benefit from LPI. In patients who have either angle closure without pupillary block or 360° of synechial angle closure, LPI is ineffective. Photothermal laser pretreatment may be beneficial for patients with a high risk of bleeding or with thick irises. There is mixed evidence concerning whether iridotomy location affects the likelihood of dysphotopsias. The rate of conversion from PAC to PACG despite iridotomy is low, but the rate of conversion from APAC to PACG despite iridotomy is high.	Laser parameters differ from those for LPI in that energy is lower, spot size is larger, and duration is longer. For patients with APAC who are not candidates for iridotomy, laser iridoplasty has efficacy similar to medical management in terms of short-term IOP reduction. The effectiveness of laser iridoplasty in preventing PAC or PACG is unclear.

APAC = acute primary angle closure; IOP = intraocular pressure; LPI = laser peripheral iridotomy; PAC = primary angle closure; PACG = primary angle closure-glaucoma.

He M, Jiang Y, Huang S, et al. Laser peripheral iridotomy for the prevention of angle closure: a single-centre, randomised controlled trial. *Lancet.* 2019;393(10181):1609–1618.

Radhakrishnan S, Chen PP, Junk AK, Nouri-Mahdavi K, Chen TC. Laser peripheral iridotomy in primary angle closure: a report by the American Academy of Ophthalmology. *Ophthalmology.* 2018;125(7):1110–1120.

Laser Iridoplasty

Mechanism of Action

Laser iridoplasty (also called *laser peripheral iridoplasty* or *gonioplasty*) is performed by using a thermal laser (argon green or diode) to treat the peripheral iris stroma. This treatment causes contraction of collagen fibers and thinning of the peripheral iris, pulling it away from the angle recess. For a summary of the main points made in the following subsections on laser iridoplasty, see Table 13-1.

Indications and Contraindications

Laser iridoplasty is performed to prevent the development of PAC and PACG in eyes that have narrow angles despite a patent peripheral iridotomy. Occasionally, iridoplasty is used to disrupt episodes of acute angle closure in eyes with an anterior chamber too shallow to allow iridotomy. Although there is controversy and minimal evidence, laser iridoplasty may be beneficial in patients with plateau iris syndrome, phacomorphic angle closure, or nanophthalmos if iridotomy cannot adequately open the angle.

Technique

Pilocarpine is instilled to induce miosis and stretch the iris; a topical aqueous suppressant is administered to prevent acute postoperative IOP elevation. Approximately 16–20 evenly spaced laser burns are placed on the peripheral iris using a laser lens. Laser parameters differ from those for LPI in that energy is lower, spot size is larger, and duration is longer (ie, burns are long and slow). The energy level and duration of laser treatment are adjusted according to iris color and tissue response (see Chapter 9, Video 9-2).

Postoperative Care

Intraocular pressure is measured approximately 1 hour after treatment to detect acute IOP elevation. A corticosteroid is used to control postoperative inflammation and pain.

Complications

Complications include anisocoria, pupil distortion, persistent postoperative inflammation, PAS, and localized iris discoloration.

Efficacy

For patients with APAC who are not candidates for iridotomy, laser iridoplasty has efficacy similar to medical management in terms of short-term IOP reduction. The effectiveness of laser iridoplasty in preventing PAC or PACG is unclear. A randomized prospective trial comparing iridotomy alone with iridotomy plus iridoplasty showed no difference in IOP reduction between the 2 groups at 1 year; however, there was less PAS formation at 1 year in the iridoplasty plus iridotomy group. A randomized prospective study comparing peripheral iridoplasty with prostaglandin analogue therapy showed that prostaglandin analogue therapy was significantly more effective in terms of IOP control at 1 year. A retrospective review of iridoplasty in plateau iris revealed that the angle recess was wider at the 6-year follow-up, which could help to slow the development of PAC (see Chapter 9, Treatment Controversies sidebar).

Narayanaswamy A, Baskaran M, Perera SA, et al. Argon laser peripheral iridoplasty for primary angle-closure glaucoma: a randomized controlled trial. *Ophthalmology.* 2016;123(3):514–521.

Sun X, Liang YB, Wang NL, et al. Laser peripheral iridotomy with and without iridoplasty for primary angle-closure glaucoma: 1-year results of a randomized pilot study. *Am J Ophthalmol.* 2010;150(1):68–73.

Trabeculectomy

Mechanism of Action

Trabeculectomy is an incisional procedure in which a fistula is created between the anterior chamber and the subconjunctival space, bypassing the normal aqueous outflow pathway. This category of procedure was initially performed as a full-thickness ("unguarded") procedure with a direct path from the anterior chamber to the subconjunctival space. High complication rates related to hypotony led to a major evolution in the surgical technique, such that the fistula is now created under a partial-thickness scleral flap ("guarding" the flow of aqueous) to provide some resistance to aqueous flow through the fistula; this approach reduces the risk of postoperative hypotony.

Indications and Contraindications

Trabeculectomy may be appropriate in multiple clinical scenarios, including—but not limited to—when medical and laser treatments have proven inadequate, when there is severe damage at presentation, and when the target IOP is low (see the Treatment Decisions and Data sidebar titled "Trabeculectomy or Tube Shunt Surgery?" at the end of the Trabeculectomy section).

Because of the potential complications of trabeculectomy, it is unlikely to be an appropriate choice in eyes with ocular hypertension and a low risk of functional loss. However, in less clear situations, such as when 1 eye has sustained considerable glaucomatous damage and IOP in the fellow eye remains high despite maximally tolerated therapy, some ophthalmologists recommend trabeculectomy prior to unequivocal evidence of damage. In eyes with severely elevated, uncontrollable IOP, surgery may be appropriate if glaucomatous damage has not occurred. In the absence of documented progression, the decision to proceed with trabeculectomy is based on clinical judgment that the IOP elevation is excessive for the current stage of disease.

The absence of light perception is a contraindication for incisional glaucoma surgery. It is important to consider the risk of sympathetic ophthalmia when planning any procedure in a blind eye or an eye with poor vision potential. Relative contraindications include conditions that increase the risk of trabeculectomy failure, such as active anterior segment neovascularization or active anterior uveitis. If possible, the underlying problem should be addressed first, or a surgical alternative such as tube shunt surgery considered. It may be difficult to successfully perform trabeculectomy in an eye with extensive conjunctival injury (eg, from previous surgery or trauma). The likelihood of complications is greater in patients with an extremely thin or abnormal sclera (eg, from surgery, scleritis, or degenerative myopia).

Trabeculectomy has a lower success rate in patients with diabetes; younger patients; patients with African, Asian, or Hispanic ancestry; aphakic or pseudophakic patients who previously underwent cataract extraction through a scleral tunnel incision; and eyes inflamed from long-term topical therapy. The risk of trabeculectomy failure is higher in patients with certain types of secondary glaucoma, predisposition to an aggressive postoperative inflammatory response, or prior failed trabeculectomy. Preoperative use of topical steroids can reduce the need for postoperative interventions and the need for long-term postoperative glaucoma medications. Patients who are unwilling or unable to comply with postoperative care may be poor candidates for trabeculectomy.

The EX-PRESS Glaucoma Filtration Device (Alcon) is a shunt used in a variation of trabeculectomy. It was initially designed to function as a standalone subconjunctival device inserted at the limbus. However, the surgical approach was modified to reduce the incidence of postoperative hypotony and avoid erosion of the device through the conjunctiva. Several retrospective and prospective randomized trials comparing EX-PRESS device–based trabeculectomy with standard trabeculectomy have revealed similar long-term IOP results, although vision recovery may be faster with the shunt than with trabeculectomy alone. Complications are similar. EX-PRESS devices are safe for magnetic resonance imaging (up to an intensity of 3 tesla).

Technique

There are multiple trabeculectomy techniques (Video 13-2). Exposure of the superior sclera is important (Fig 13-5). The initial conjunctival flap can be fornix-based (Fig 13-6A, B; Video 13-3), where the conjunctiva is incised adjacent or slightly posterior to the limbus, or limbus-based (Fig 13-6C, D), where the conjunctiva is incised 8–12 mm posterior to the limbus. Fornix-based trabeculectomies offer the advantages of better exposure, whereas limbus-based flaps reduce the risk of early wound leak because the incision is distant from the scleral flap. Fornix-based flaps are associated with more diffuse blebs (Fig 13-7).

VIDEO 13-2 Trabeculectomy fundamentals.
Courtesy of Joseph Caprioli, MD.
Available at: aao.org/bcscvideo_section10

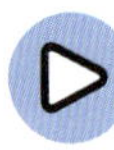

VIDEO 13-3 Fornix-based trabeculectomy with running closure.
Courtesy of James A. Savage, MD.
Available at: aao.org/bcscvideo_section10

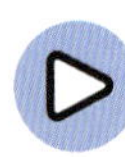

A partial-thickness scleral flap is created in the superior sclera, hinged at the limbus (Fig 13-8), and preferably adjacent to the 12 o'clock position; this placement helps to prevent postoperative bleb exposure and dysesthesia. The flap can be triangular, rectangular, or trapezoidal. A block of corneoscleral tissue is removed from under this flap (Fig 13-9A–C), either in a freehand manner or using a trephining device, thereby providing a new route for aqueous humor outflow from the anterior chamber. A peripheral iridectomy can be performed to prevent the iris from occluding the fistula (Fig 13-9D); however, some surgeons attempt to

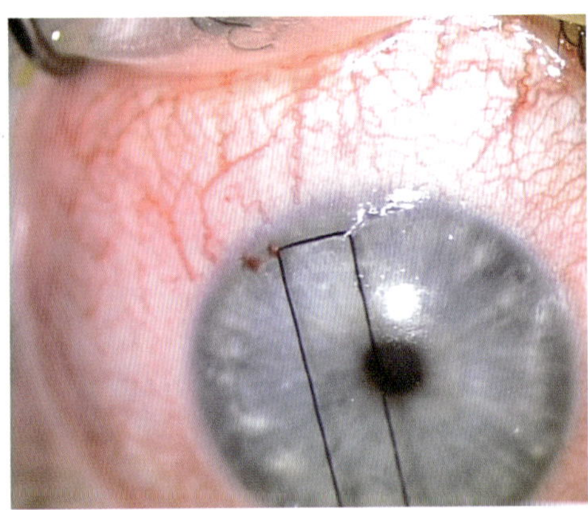

Figure 13-5 Exposure of superior quadrant using a corneal traction suture, prior to trabeculectomy. *(Courtesy of Keith Barton, MD. Reproduced with permission from Moorfields Eye Hospital.)*

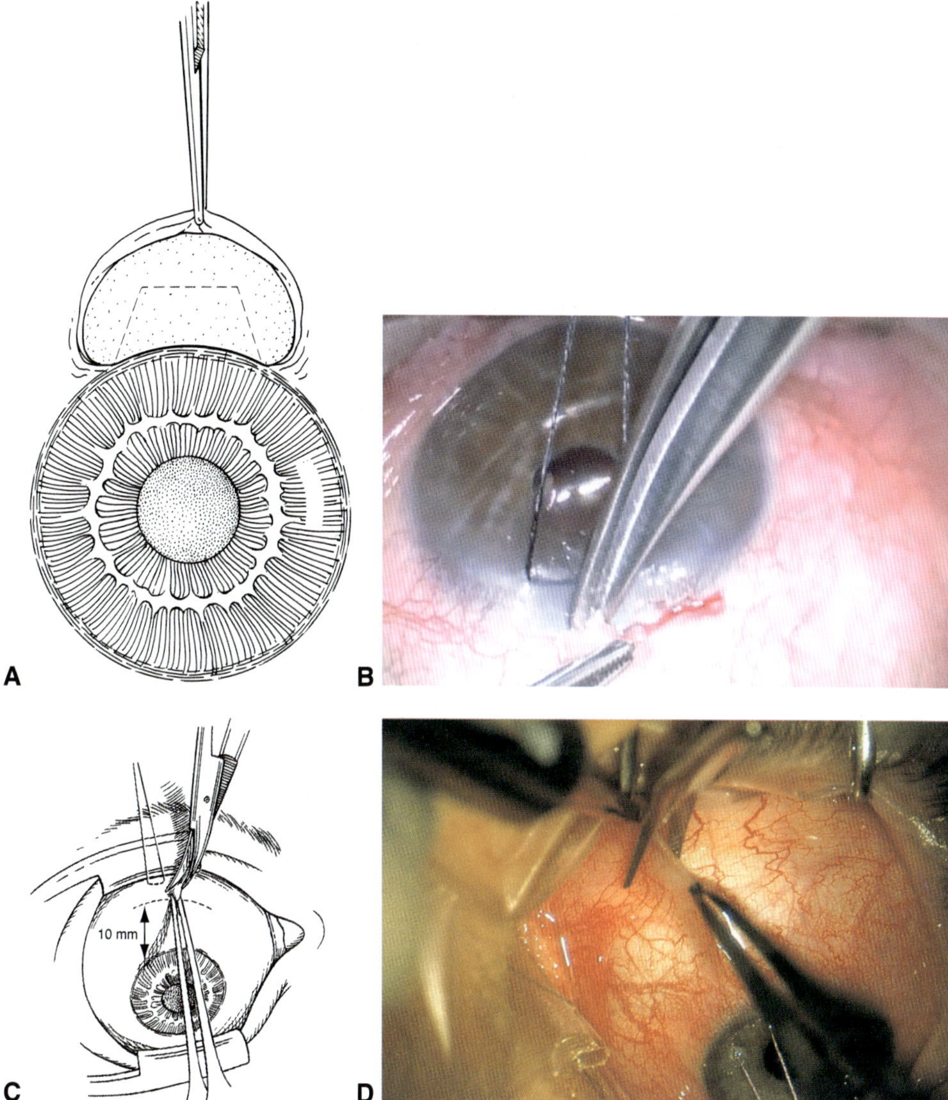

Figure 13-6 Comparison of fornix-based and limbus-based conjunctival flaps. **A,** Diagram showing complete incision through the conjunctiva at the limbus and the insertion of the Tenon capsule (*dashed line* indicates future scleral flap). The arc length of the initial incision is approximately 6–8 mm. **B,** Clinical photograph (corresponding to part A) showing the location of the initial incision for creation of a fornix-based flap. **C,** Diagram showing the initial incision through the conjunctiva and Tenon capsule, 10 mm posterior to the limbus with an anticipated arc length of 8–10 mm. **D,** Clinical photograph (corresponding to part C) showing the location of the initial incision for creation of a limbus-based conjunctival flap. *(Parts A and C modified with permission from Weinreb RN, Mills RP, eds.* Glaucoma Surgery: Principles and Techniques. *2nd ed. Ophthalmology Monographs 4. American Academy of Ophthalmology; 1998. Part B courtesy of JoAnn A. Giaconi, MD; part D courtesy of Robert D. Fechtner, MD.)*

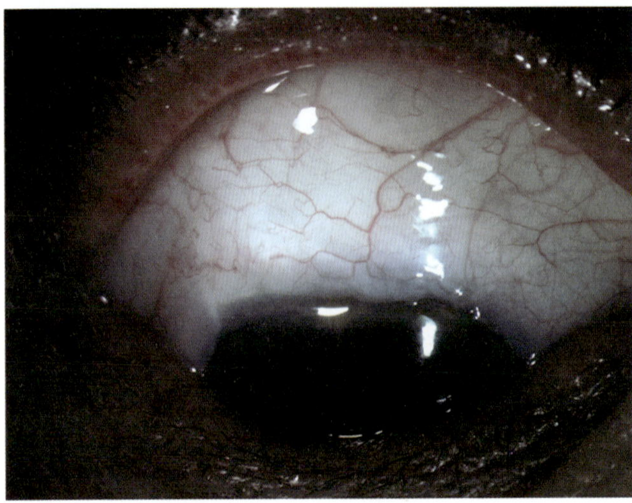

Figure 13-7 Clinical photograph showing a diffuse conjunctival bleb. Although it is difficult to distinguish the bleb, its location can be determined by the irregular conjunctival border at the limbus and scarring at the 10 and 2 o'clock positions, where sutures were placed during surgery. Careful slit-lamp examination reveals that the bleb is elevated from the sclera. *(Courtesy of JoAnn A. Giaconi, MD.)*

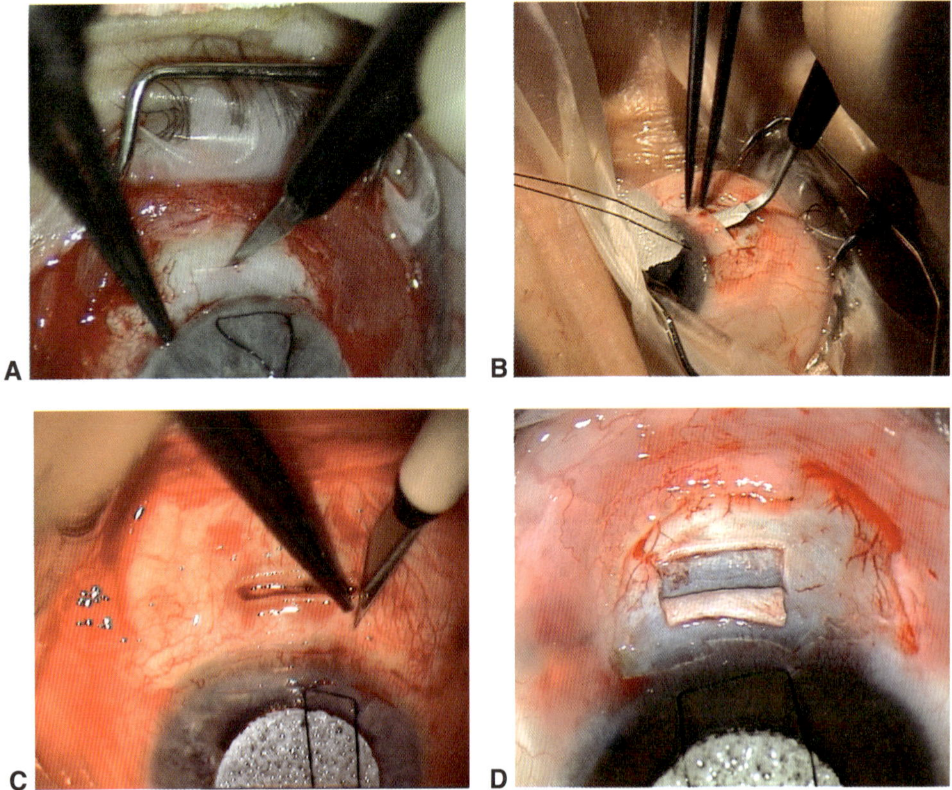

Figure 13-8 Creation of a scleral flap (4 mm wide and 2.0–2.5 mm long at 50%–75% scleral depth). **A,** Posterior margin is dissected with a fine blade. **B,** Crescent knife is used to dissect a partial-thickness scleral tunnel. **C,** Sides of the tunnel are opened to create a flap. **D,** Final appearance. *(Courtesy of Keith Barton, MD. Reproduced with permission from Moorfields Eye Hospital.)*

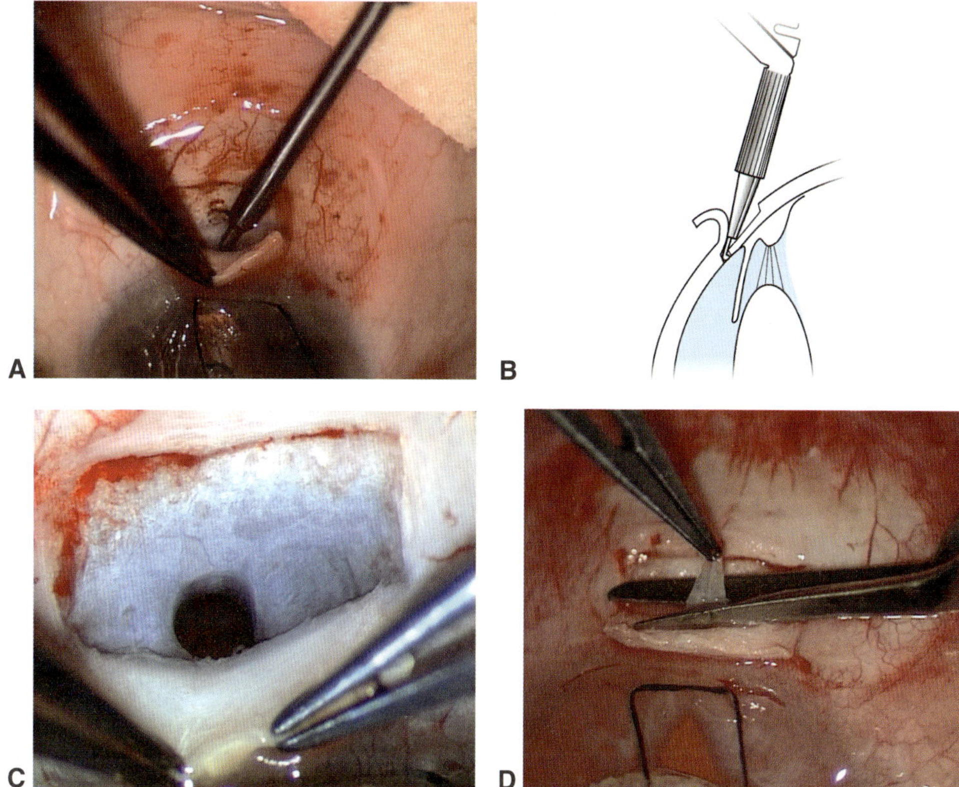

Figure 13-9 The surgeon can create a fistula by inserting a punch under the scleral flap **(A),** snaring the posterior lip of the anterior chamber entry site **(B),** and removing a punch (0.75–1.0 mm) of peripheral posterior cornea **(C).** A peripheral iridectomy is then created (shown here in an albino eye) using iridectomy scissors **(D).** *(Clinical photographs courtesy of Keith Barton, MD; illustration based on original drawing by Alan Lacey. All parts reproduced with permission from Moorfields Eye Hospital.)*

lower the risk of hyphema by avoiding iridectomy in pseudophakic patients. The flap is then reapproximated to its bed via nylon suture tightening to provide resistance to aqueous outflow. These sutures can be cut with a laser if there is insufficient outflow in the postoperative period. If a laser is not readily available, it is possible to use releasable sutures (Fig 13-10) that are externalized through the peripheral cornea (Video 13-4). The final conjunctival closure must be watertight to prevent postoperative complications and maximize surgical success. For a limbus-based flap, the Tenon capsule and conjunctiva are closed separately or together. For a fornix-based trabeculectomy, the conjunctiva can be closed with various techniques.

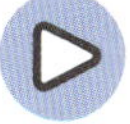

VIDEO 13-4 Placement of a releasable suture for flap closure.
Courtesy of Marlene Moster, MD.
Available at: aao.org/bcscvideo_section10

The current technique for implantation of an EX-PRESS device (Fig 13-11) follows steps similar to those used in the trabeculectomy procedure. The main difference is that the surgeon inserts the device under the partial-thickness scleral flap, rather than removing a

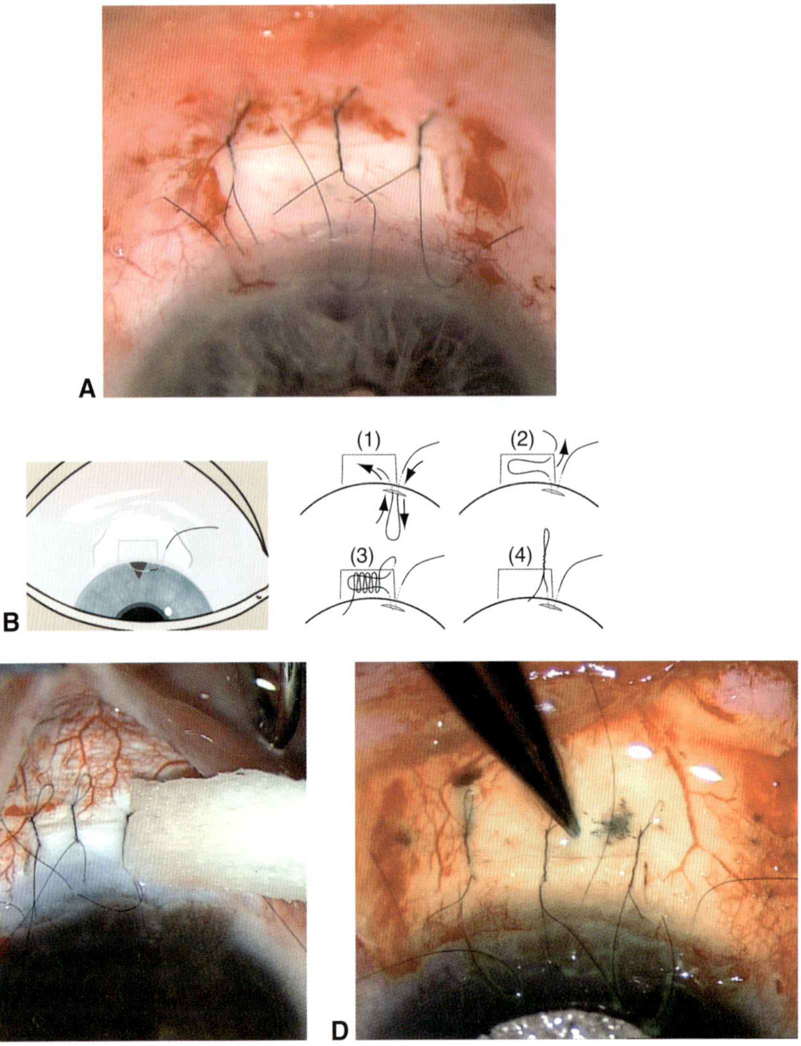

Figure 13-10 During trabeculectomy with mitomycin C, the scleral flap is closed relatively tightly to minimize spontaneous drainage. Closure may be performed with releasable sutures **(A, B)** that can subsequently be removed under slit-lamp view to increase flow, or with interrupted sutures that can be cut after surgery using a laser. Part **B** shows the sequence of movements for placing 1 type of releasable suture. After scleral closure, the surgeon should assess flow using a sponge **(C)** or fluorescein **(D).** *(Clinical photographs courtesy of Keith Barton, MD; illustration courtesy of Alan Lacey. All parts reproduced with permission from Moorfields Eye Hospital.)*

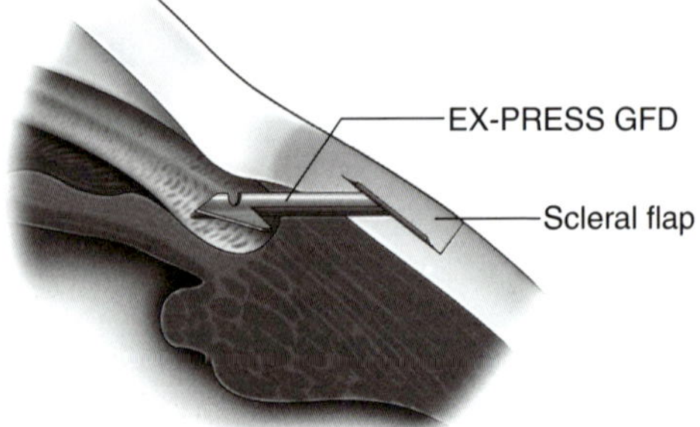

Figure 13-11 Schematic illustration of an EX-PRESS device placed under a scleral flap. GFD = glaucoma filtration device. *(© 2023 American Academy of Ophthalmology.)*

block of corneoscleral tissue. In addition, no peripheral iridectomy is performed with the EX-PRESS device.

Antifibrotic Agents in Trabeculectomy

The use of mitomycin C and 5-fluorouracil during trabeculectomy (immediately before or after scleral flap creation) has improved the rate of surgical success, especially in patients with risk factors for failure. Although the use of these antifibrotic agents has also led to higher rates of bleb leak, infection, and hypotony, the increases in these complications are related to the longer trabeculectomy survival attained with these agents.

5-Fluorouracil (5-FU) is a pyrimidine analogue that inhibits DNA synthesis by acting on thymidylate synthetase, thereby interfering with fibroblast proliferation. This agent can be used both intraoperatively and postoperatively (via subconjunctival injection) to increase the rate of trabeculectomy success. Because 5-FU can be highly toxic to the corneal epithelium it should be used with caution in patients with ocular surface disease.

Mitomycin C (MMC) is a naturally occurring compound with antineoplastic and antibiotic activities. As an alkylating agent, MMC crosslinks DNA, thus inhibiting DNA replication and inducing apoptosis. Because it is cytotoxic to fibroblasts and vascular endothelial cells, MMC modulates the fibroproliferative and angiogenic steps of wound healing. It is administered by application of soaked sponges or subconjunctival injection. Both techniques produce similar IOP outcomes. MMC is highly toxic, and intracameral exposure should be avoided.

A Cochrane review of the literature revealed that IOP was significantly lower with adjunctive MMC than with 5-FU at 1 year after trabeculectomy. Visual outcomes were similar between the treatment groups.

Cabourne E, Clarke JC, Schlottmann PG, Evans JR. Mitomycin C versus 5-fluorouracil for wound healing in glaucoma surgery. *Cochrane Database Syst Rev.* 2015;11:CD006259. doi:10.1002/14651858.CD006259.pub2

Esfandiari H, Pakravan M, Yazdani S, Doozandeh A, Yaseri M, Conner IP. Treatment outcomes of mitomycin C-augmented trabeculectomy, sub-Tenon injection versus soaked sponges, after 3 years of follow-up: a randomized clinical trial. *Ophthalmol Glaucoma.* 2018;1(1): 66–74.

Postoperative Complications and Management

Although meticulous surgical technique is important, the success of an incisional glaucoma procedure greatly depends on careful postoperative management (Fig 13-12). Many complications can arise during the early and late postoperative period, with the potential to compromise surgical success, vision, and ocular health (Table 13-2). Thus, timely identification of potential complications is essential.

Overfiltration

Overfiltration occurs when there is insufficient resistance to aqueous flow from the anterior chamber into the subconjunctival space. It is usually caused by inadequate tightening

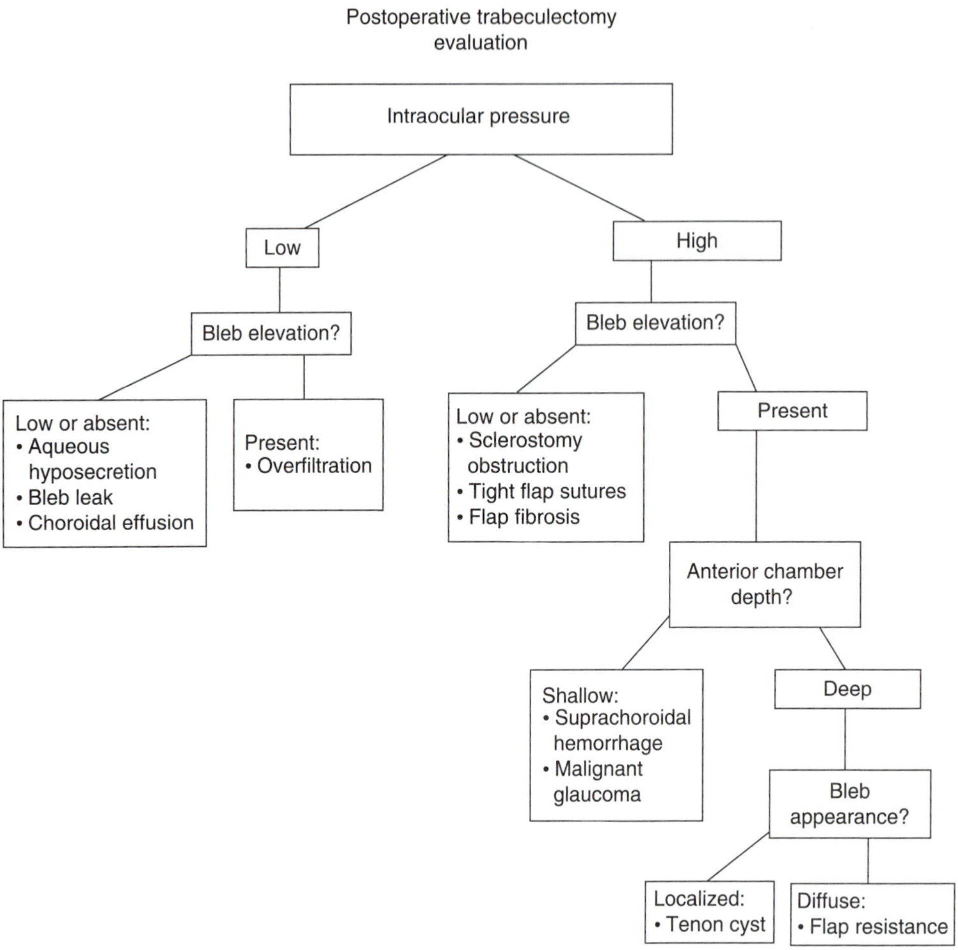

Postoperative trabeculectomy evaluation

Intraocular pressure

Low

Bleb elevation?

Low or absent:
• Aqueous hyposecretion
• Bleb leak
• Choroidal effusion

Present:
• Overfiltration

High

Bleb elevation?

Low or absent:
• Sclerostomy obstruction
• Tight flap sutures
• Flap fibrosis

Present

Anterior chamber depth?

Shallow:
• Suprachoroidal hemorrhage
• Malignant glaucoma

Deep

Bleb appearance?

Localized:
• Tenon cyst

Diffuse:
• Flap resistance

Figure 13-12 Algorithm depicting suggested evaluation approach after trabeculectomy. *(Courtesy of Chandrasekharan Krishnan, MD.)*

of scleral flap sutures. Other causes include a thin scleral flap, irregularities in the shape of the flap or flap bed, holes in the flap, and fistula proximity to the flap edge. Overfiltration may be associated with a large, diffuse bleb (in the absence of a bleb leak) and a shallow anterior chamber.

Treatment options include the reduction of topical steroids (to allow development of subconjunctival fibrosis) and placement of additional scleral flap sutures (Video 13-5). Intervention is indicated if decreased vision develops secondary to hypotony from a shallow anterior chamber or maculopathy (optic nerve and/or retinal edema and macular folds).

VIDEO 13-5 Transconjunctival scleral flap suturing at the slit lamp.
Courtesy of Susan Liang, MD.
Available at: aao.org/bcscvideo_section10

Table 13-2 Complications of Trabeculectomy

Early Complications	Late Complications
Cataract progression	Bleb migration onto cornea
Choroidal effusion	Blebitis
Cystoid macular edema	Cataract
Dellen	Endophthalmitis
Endophthalmitis	EX-PRESS extrusion/erosion
Fibrosis/scarring	Eyelid retraction
Hyphema	Fibrosis/scarring
Hypotony leading to decreased vision	Filtering bleb leakage or failure
Loss of vision	Hypotony leading to decreased vision
Malignant glaucoma	Ptosis
Persistent uveitis	Symptomatic bleb (dysesthetic bleb)
Sclerostomy obstruction	
Shallow or flat anterior chamber	
Suprachoroidal hemorrhage	
Transient intraocular pressure elevation	
Wound or bleb leak	

Bleb leaks

Bleb leaks can occur at any point in the postoperative period. In the early postoperative period, leaks most commonly occur at the incision site. Leaks can also result from unrecognized buttonholes and flap suture erosion through the conjunctiva. Bleb leaks are often symptomatic (patients report excessive tearing) and can be identified using the Seidel test (Video 13-6; see also Chapter 4). In addition to hypotony, patients with leaks may have a shallow or normal anterior chamber depth and a low-lying bleb. Untreated leaks can lead to early bleb fibrosis and infection.

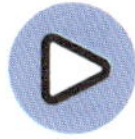

VIDEO 13-6 Identifying a bleb leak.
Courtesy of Chandrasekharan Krishnan, MD.
Available at: aao.org/bcscvideo_section10

There are several treatment options for bleb leaks. Decreasing topical steroids can promote fibrosis and healing. Aqueous suppressants diminish flow through the defect, allowing epithelialization to seal the leak. The placement of an oversized contact lens can provide a scaffold for re-epithelialization and may help to stop the leak. If conservative measures fail, the site of the leak may require suturing.

Choroidal effusions

Choroidal effusions can also occur at any point in the postoperative period when the IOP is low, regardless of bleb size; however, they are most frequently seen with early postoperative hypotony. In older adult patients with low IOP, choroidal effusions rather than hypotony maculopathy are more likely to develop (perhaps because of greater scleral rigidity). The anterior chamber becomes shallow, particularly in peripheral regions. Fundus examination shows characteristic grayish dome-shaped effusions anchored in the region of the vortex veins.

Treatment includes the use of cycloplegics to deepen the anterior chamber. If the effusions have resulted from overfiltration or a bleb leak, healing and fibrosis may be promoted by decreasing steroids. Conversely, if the effusions have resulted from ciliary body inflammation (and aqueous hyposecretion), increasing steroids may be beneficial. If conservative management fails, effusions can be drained in the operating room via posterior sclerotomies. The scleral flap is often reinforced at the same time to increase resistance to outflow (Video 13-7).

VIDEO 13-7 Scleral flap resuturing and choroidal drainage.
Courtesy of Lauren Blieden, MD.
Available at: aao.org/bcscvideo_section10

Sclerostomy obstruction

Sclerostomy obstruction can occur at any time but is most frequent in the early postoperative period (Fig 13-13). The condition is characterized by a low or flat bleb, deep chamber,

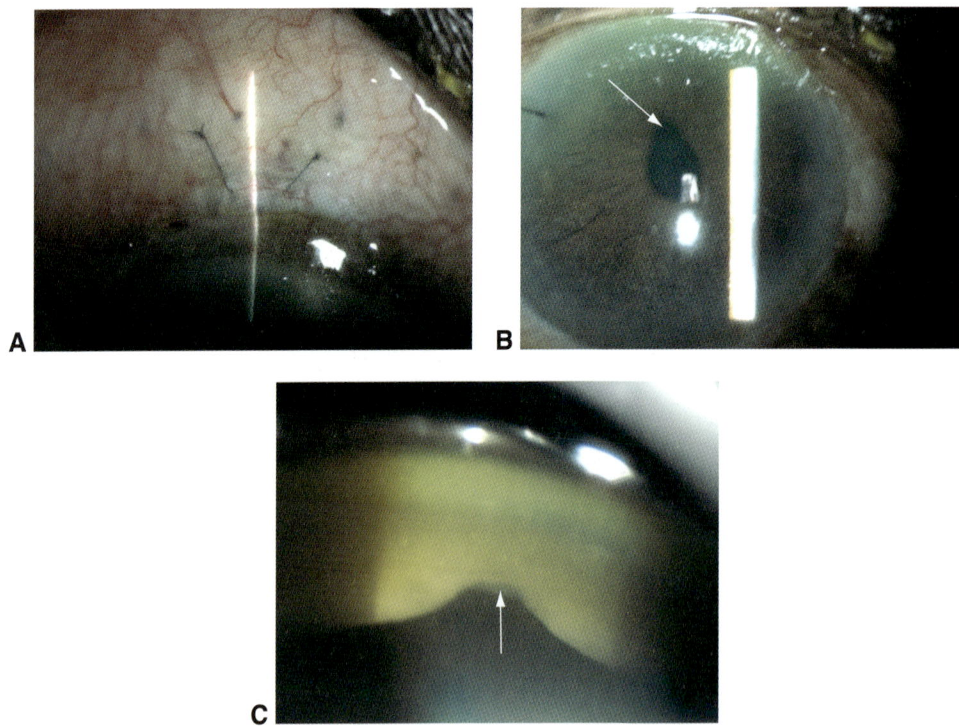

Figure 13-13 Sclerostomy obstruction. **A,** Patients with iris occlusion of the trabeculectomy fistula will display elevated intraocular pressure and a flat bleb. **B,** A peaked pupil *(arrow)* should alert the physician to this possibility. **C,** Gonioscopic photograph reveals iris within the fistula *(arrow)*. *(Courtesy of Chandrasekharan Krishnan, MD.)*

and elevated IOP. The sclerostomy may be blocked by a blood clot, fibrin, vitreous, or iris; gonioscopy is crucial to determine the cause of the obstruction.

Laser iridoplasty or LPI can be used to manage iris tissue that is incarcerated in the sclerostomy. If necessary, tissue plasminogen activator can be used to rapidly dissolve a blood clot.

Tight scleral flap sutures

Tight scleral flap sutures impair the egress of aqueous humor, resulting in a low bleb, deep anterior chamber, and higher-than-desired IOP (Fig 13-14A). Moderate to firm digital ocular massage forces fluid through the flap, thereby elevating the bleb and lowering the IOP. It can be difficult to determine the optimal time to cut flap sutures (Fig 13-14B, C). If the sutures are cut too soon, overfiltration may occur; if they are cut too late, fibrosis under the flap (from lack of flow) may result in inadequate long-term control of IOP.

Malignant glaucoma and suprachoroidal hemorrhage

Malignant glaucoma (also known as *aqueous misdirection*) and *suprachoroidal hemorrhage* can have very similar findings: shallow chamber, variable bleb extent (none to extensive), and normal or high IOP (Fig 13-15). The central anterior chamber is very shallow. Fundus evaluation (or B-scan ultrasonography if the view of the posterior segment is poor) is usually

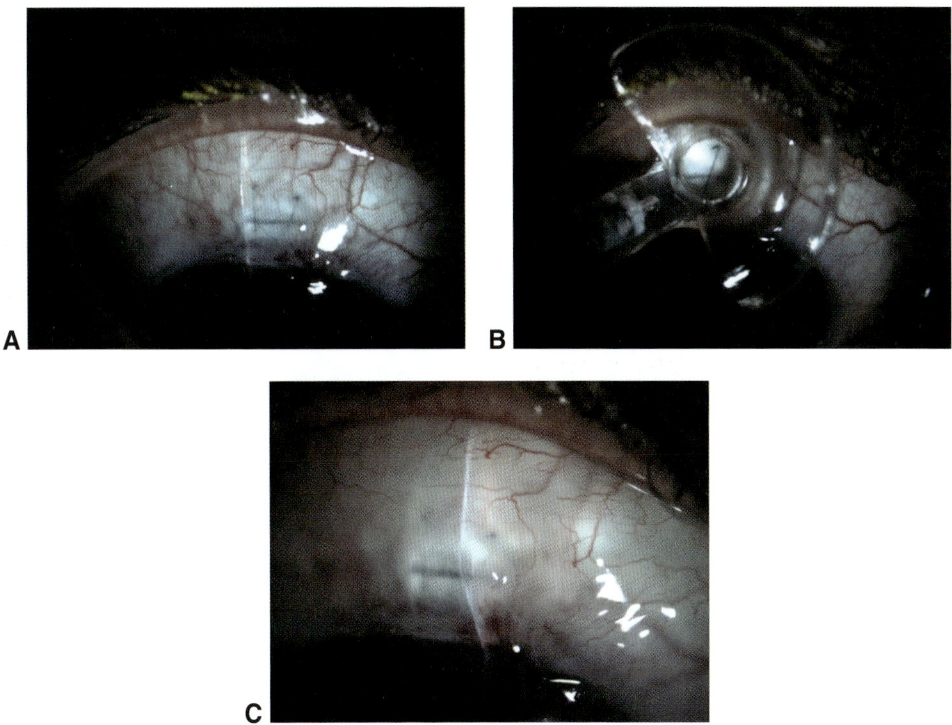

Figure 13-14 Tight scleral flap sutures. **A,** Tight flap sutures can cause a low bleb after surgery. **B,** A laser suture lysis lens can be used to visualize the suture. **C,** After the suture is cut with a laser, the bleb should elevate. *(Courtesy of Chandrasekharan Krishnan, MD.)*

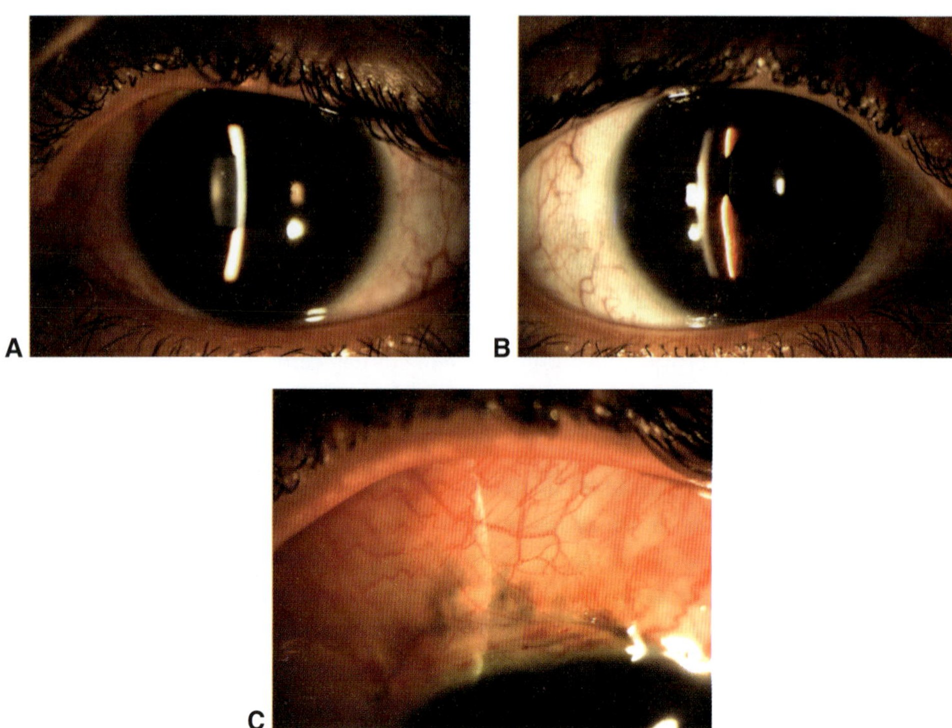

Figure 13-15 Malignant glaucoma after trabeculectomy. **A,** Early postoperative period. Note that the central anterior chamber is flat. B-scan ultrasonography did not reveal posterior abnormalities. **B,** The shallow depth of the anterior chamber in the unaffected eye increases the risk of postoperative malignant glaucoma. **C,** Pressure in the surgically treated eye is not significantly elevated because the filtering bleb is functioning appropriately. *(Courtesy of Chandrasekharan Krishnan, MD.)*

required to determine the cause of these findings. Treatment of suprachoroidal hemorrhage involves pain control and temporizing medical management of IOP. Anticoagulant and antiplatelet therapy should be stopped if possible. Choroidal drainage should be delayed unless corneolenticular touch or "kissing choroidals" are present or the patient has intractable pain.

Malignant glaucoma is treated with cycloplegics and medical management of IOP. Disruption of the vitreous face with an Nd:YAG laser (through the pupil in a pseudophakic patient or through a peripheral iridotomy in a phakic patient) can be attempted. If these approaches are unsuccessful, creation of a unicameral eye via vitrectomy, zonulectomy, and iridectomy is warranted, with particular attention to disruption of the anterior hyaloid.

Fibrosis

Fibrosis most commonly occurs in the subconjunctival space but can also occur at the level of the scleral flap. In the early postoperative period, adequate flow through the scleral flap and into the subconjunctival space is important for long-term surgical success. Accordingly, there is a need to control fibrosis. *Conjunctival hyperemia* in the postoperative period is an indication of subsequent fibrosis and requires management with additional corticosteroids and/or antifibrotic therapy (MMC, 5-FU). Scleral flap sutures can be cut or removed to increase flow and mitigate fibrosis. Transconjunctival needle revision (*bleb needling;* Video 13-8) can help to disrupt fibrosis. In this procedure, a sharp-tipped instrument is introduced under the conjunctiva to disrupt fibrotic tissue, allowing the formation of a more diffuse bleb.

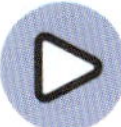

VIDEO 13-8 Bleb needling.
Courtesy of Cynthia Mattox, MD.
Available at: aao.org/bcscvideo_section10

Infection

Bleb-related infection (Fig 13-16), a potentially vision-threatening complication after trabeculectomy, occurs in 1.5%–6.0% of patients. Patients typically present with tearing, irritation, pain, and/or blurry vision. Risk factors for infection include untreated blepharitis, as well as the presence of an inferior bleb, bleb leak, and/or thin-walled blebs; there is a tendency for thin-walled blebs (Fig 13-17) to occur with localized blebs. The use of MMC and 5-FU is also a risk factor; these agents are associated with higher incidences of thin-walled blebs and bleb leaks. Fornix-based trabeculectomies and diffuse application of antifibrotic agents can mitigate the formation of thin-walled blebs and bleb leaks.

One proposed classification scheme divides bleb-related infection into 3 stages, although these stages represent a continuum of infection:

- *stage 1:* erythema around the bleb, bleb infiltrate
- *stage 2:* anterior chamber inflammation
- *stage 3:* hypopyon and/or intravitreal involvement

Stages 1 and 2 bleb-related infection *(blebitis)* can be treated with topical antibiotics or fortified topical and subconjunctival antibiotics, as needed. Stage 3, indicated by the presence of a hypopyon or intravitreal involvement *(bleb-related endophthalmitis),* requires either vitreous tap with antibiotic injection or vitrectomy. In late-onset bleb-related endophthalmitis, more

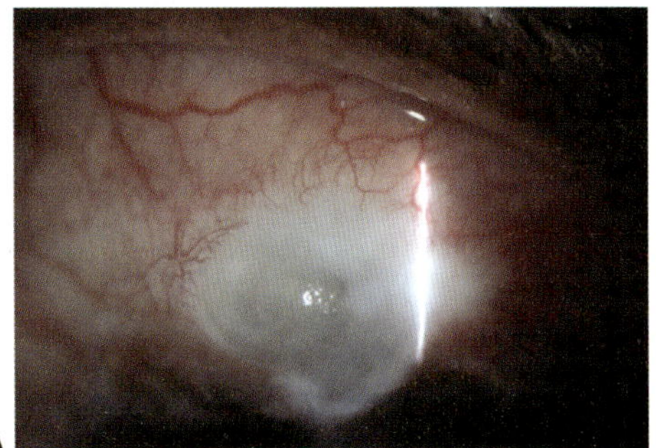

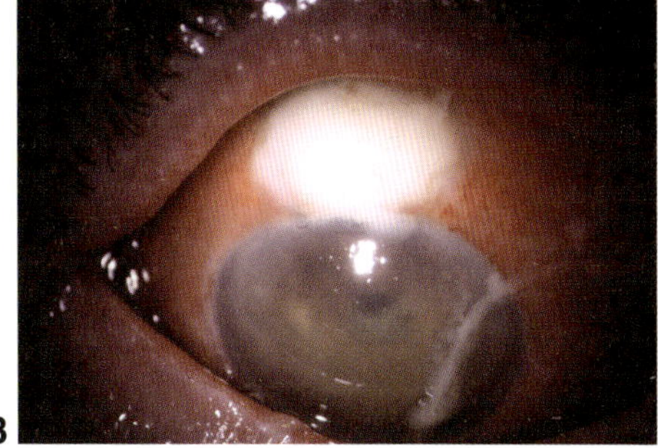

Figure 13-16 Bleb-related infection. **A,** Patients may present with blebitis, which is characterized by mucopurulent infiltrate within the bleb, localized conjunctival hyperemia, and minimal intraocular inflammation. **B,** Bleb-related endophthalmitis is characterized by diffuse bulbar conjunctival hyperemia, purulent material within the bleb, and anterior chamber cellular reaction; it is occasionally characterized by hypopyon formation and marked vitritis. *(Part A courtesy of Chandrasekharan Krishnan, MD; part B courtesy of Keith Barton, MD. Part B is reproduced with permission from Moorfields Eye Hospital.)*

virulent organisms (*Streptococcus* and gram-negative species) are involved. The Endophthalmitis Vitrectomy Study (EVS) results may not be applicable in this context because the EVS investigated acute endophthalmitis after cataract surgery, which typically involves different species. There is a trend toward immediate vitrectomy with intravitreal antibiotic injection for severe stage 3 infections. Patients with stages 1 and 2 bleb-related infection tend to have a good prognosis, whereas patients with stage 3 bleb-related infection tend to have poor visual outcomes.

See Table 13-3, which summarizes the main points made in the preceding subsections on trabeculectomy.

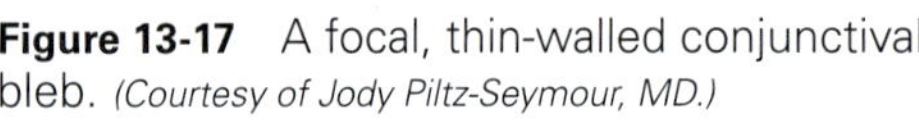

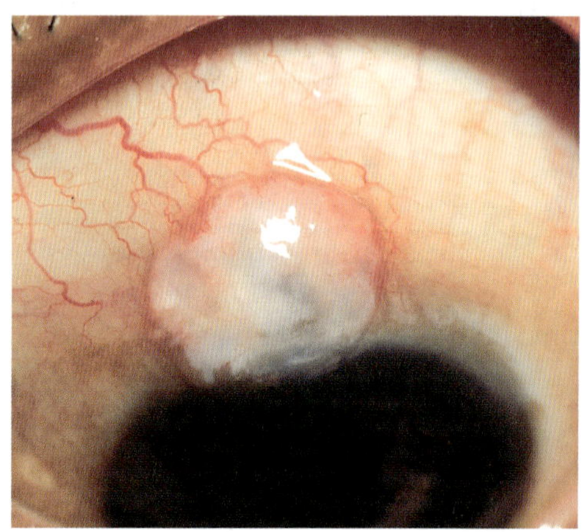

Figure 13-17 A focal, thin-walled conjunctival bleb. *(Courtesy of Jody Piltz-Seymour, MD.)*

Table 13-3 Filtering Surgery: Key Points

Trabeculectomy	Plate-Based Tube Shunt Surgery
Trabeculectomy may be appropriate when medical and laser treatments have proven inadequate, when there is severe damage at presentation, and when the target IOP is low.	The indications and preoperative considerations are similar for plate-based tube implants and trabeculectomy.
Trabeculectomy has a lower success rate in patients with diabetes; younger patients; patients with African, Asian, or Hispanic ancestry; aphakic or pseudophakic patients who previously underwent cataract extraction through a scleral tunnel incision; and eyes inflamed from long-term topical therapy.	A valved tube typically provides more immediate IOP control, whereas a nonvalved tube with a large plate size often requires less medication.
A literature review revealed that IOP was significantly lower with adjunctive mitomycin C than with 5-FU at 1 year after trabeculectomy, but visual outcomes were similar between treatment groups.	Compared with trabeculectomy, plate-based tube implants tend to require fewer interventions in the postoperative period.
There are many possible complications after trabeculectomy, including overfiltration, leaks, obstruction, malignant glaucoma, fibrosis, and infection.	For primary tube implants, the number of medications needed is higher and the rate of complete success is lower than for a primary trabeculectomy.
	The risk of endophthalmitis within 5 years after tube shunt surgery is approximately 0.5%.

Yassin SA. Bleb-related infection revisited: a literature review. *Acta Ophthalmol.* 2016;94(2): 122–134.

Clinical pearl Patients with a bleb have lifelong risks of blebitis and endophthalmitis. They should be educated to immediately report new redness, tearing, vision loss, and/or pain.

TREATMENT DECISIONS AND DATA

Trabeculectomy or Tube Shunt Surgery?

In the Tube Versus Trabeculectomy (TVT) Study, 212 eyes with uncontrolled glaucoma that had previously undergone trabeculectomy or cataract surgery were randomly assigned to 2 treatment groups. One group underwent trabeculectomy with mitomycin C (MMC) (0.4 mg/mL for 4 minutes); the other group underwent Baerveldt tube shunt surgery (350 mm^2).

At 5 years, the mean intraocular pressure (IOP) and number of glaucoma medications were similar between the groups. However, the failure rate (which was defined as IOP >21 mm Hg, <20% decrease in IOP, persistent IOP <5 mm Hg, or loss of light perception) was significantly higher in the trabeculectomy group; more reoperations were required in that group. The "complete success" rate (achievement of successful IOP control without medication) and quality-of-life measures were similar between the 2 groups. In the trabeculectomy group, the most common postoperative complications were shallow/flat anterior chamber, wound leak, and choroidal effusions. In contrast, the most common postoperative complications in the tube shunt group were shallow/flat anterior chamber, persistent corneal edema, and choroidal effusions. Furthermore, more postoperative clinic interventions were required in the trabeculectomy group. The rate of reoperation for complications was similar between the 2 groups. Importantly, >40% of patients overall lost 2 or more lines of Snellen visual acuity during the 5-year follow-up period. This visual acuity loss did not significantly differ between the trabeculectomy and tube shunt groups; it was most commonly caused by cataract progression and persistent corneal edema.

The Primary Tube Versus Trabeculectomy Study was a subsequent trial with a design similar to that of the TVT Study, except the participants had no prior intraocular surgery. At 5 years, the mean IOP was similar between the 2 groups, but the number of glaucoma medications was significantly lower in the trabeculectomy group. The rate of complete success (ie, no requirement for glaucoma medication) was significantly higher with trabeculectomy. There was no difference in the rate of surgical failure between groups; inadequate IOP reduction was the most common cause of failure in both treatment groups. In addition, there were no significant differences between groups in terms of complications or vision

(Continued on next page)

(continued)

loss. An intriguing finding was that patients with lower preoperative IOP (<21 mm Hg) experienced the greatest benefit from primary trabeculectomy with MMC, while patients with higher IOPs (>25 mm Hg) experienced the greatest benefit from tube shunt surgery.

Gedde SJ, Feuer WJ, Lim KS, et al; Primary Tube versus Trabeculectomy Study Group. Treatment outcomes in the Primary Tube versus Trabeculectomy Study after 5 years of follow-up. *Ophthalmology.* 2022;129(12):1344–1356.

Gedde SJ, Schiffman JC, Feuer WJ, Herndon LW, Brandt JD, Budenz DL; Tube versus Trabeculectomy Study Group. Treatment outcomes in the Tube Versus Trabeculectomy (TVT) study after five years of follow-up. *Am J Ophthalmol.* 2012;153(5):789–803.

Plate-Based Tube Shunt Surgery

For a summary of the main points made in the following subsections on plate-based tube shunt surgery, see Table 13-3 in the previous section.

Mechanism of Action

Plate-based tube implants are designed to shunt aqueous from the anterior chamber to a space-maintaining plate in the equatorial subconjunctival space. Generally, plate-based tube implants can be divided into *valved* and *nonvalved* types. The *Ahmed Glaucoma Valve* (New World Medical; Video 13-9) has 2 leaflets in the plate that are designed to separate when the IOP exceeds a specific threshold (approximately 8–12 mm Hg). When the IOP is below this threshold, the leaflets come together to prevent flow through the tube. The nonvalved *Baerveldt* (Johnson & Johnson Vision Care, Inc; Video 13-10), nonvalved *Ahmed ClearPath* (New World Medical), and *Molteno* (Molteno Ophthalmic Limited) implants do not restrict flow from the tube to the plate and rely on encapsulation of the plate by fibrosis to limit flow.

VIDEO 13-9 Ahmed valve implantation.
Courtesy of Simon K. Law, MD, PharmD.
Available at: aao.org/bcscvideo_section10

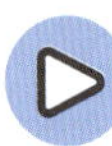

VIDEO 13-10 Baerveldt tube shunt implantation.
Courtesy of JoAnn A. Giaconi, MD.
Available at: aao.org/bcscvideo_section10

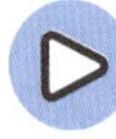

Indications and Contraindications

The indications and preoperative considerations for plate-based tube implants are similar to those for trabeculectomy. In the past, these implants were used in eyes with multiple prior failed trabeculectomies, eyes with active inflammation or neovascularization, and eyes with severe conjunctival scarring. There has been a gradual expansion of the indications for plate-based tube implants; they are increasingly utilized as first-line surgical treatment for glaucoma.

The Tube Versus Trabeculectomy Study (see the Treatment Decisions and Data sidebar titled "Trabeculectomy or Tube Shunt Surgery?" earlier in the chapter) demonstrated that tube shunt surgery success rates were better in eyes with previous incisional surgery (trabeculectomy or cataract surgery). The Primary Tube Versus Trabeculectomy Study compared the 2 surgeries as the initial intervention in patients without prior incisional surgery; at 5 years, the rate of complete success (ie, no requirement for glaucoma medication) was significantly higher in the trabeculectomy group, but there were no differences in terms of surgical failure rate or IOP. Plate-based tube implants can cause corneal endothelial cell loss and corneal decompensation over time. Posterior placement of the tube may reduce the rate of corneal endothelial cell loss.

The choice between a valved or nonvalved plate-based tube implant can be guided by the findings from 2 trials (see the Treatment Decisions and Data sidebar titled "Valved Versus Nonvalved Plate-Based Tube Implants"). Generally, a valved tube provides more immediate IOP control, whereas a nonvalved tube with a large plate size requires less medication. There is a need for caution in eyes with neovascular glaucoma, where valved tubes have been found to be safer in terms of vision loss, and in eyes with uveitis, where smaller plate sizes have been found to be beneficial in terms of preventing hypotony.

TREATMENT DECISIONS AND DATA

Valved Versus Nonvalved Plate-Based Tube Implants

The Ahmed Baerveldt Comparison (ABC) Study and Ahmed Versus Baerveldt (AVB) Study both compared the efficacies of the Ahmed FP7 and Baerveldt 350 implants over 5 years. Analysis of the pooled data showed that, at 5 years, the Baerveldt group had lower mean IOP (13.2±4.8 mm Hg vs 15.8±5.2 mm Hg) and was taking fewer glaucoma medications (1.5±1.4 vs 1.9±1.5), compared with the Ahmed group. Visual acuity loss of 2 or more Snellen lines was similar between the groups (47% in the Ahmed group and 46% in the Baerveldt group). At 5 years, the rate of failure (defined as IOP <6 mm Hg or >18 mm Hg, IOP reduction <20% below baseline at 2 consecutive visits after 3 months, requirement for additional glaucoma procedures, or loss of light perception) was higher in the Ahmed group than in the Baerveldt group (49% vs 37%). The most common reason for failure in both groups was elevated IOP. The number of patients with serious complications (defined as a complication requiring reoperation or a visual acuity loss of 2 or more lines) was higher in the Baerveldt group than in the Ahmed group. Notably, hypotony-related failure occurred in 4% of patients in the Baerveldt group.

Budenz DL, Feuer WJ, Barton K, et al; Ahmed Baerveldt Comparison Study Group. Postoperative complications in the Ahmed Baerveldt Comparison Study during five years of follow-up. *Am J Ophthalmol.* 2016;163:75–82.e3.

Christakis PG, Zhang D, Budenz DL, Barton K, Tsai JC, Ahmed IIK; ABC-AVB Study Groups. Five-year pooled data analysis of the Ahmed Baerveldt Comparison Study and the Ahmed Versus Baerveldt Study. *Am J Ophthalmol.* 2017;176:118–126.

Technique

Similar to trabeculectomy, there are various techniques for the implantation of plate-based tubes. The first plate-based tube shunt in an eye is typically implanted in the superotemporal quadrant. The placement of a second implant (if necessary) depends on implant type and surgeon preference. A conjunctival incision can be made either at the limbus *(fornix-based flap)* or 5–6 mm posterior to the limbus *(limbus-based flap)*. Typically, dissection of approximately 90° is performed to provide ample space for plate implantation. To reduce the risk of erosion, the plate is sutured to the sclera approximately 8 mm posterior to the limbus; this distance also keeps the posterior plate edge a safe distance from the optic nerve. Care must be taken to avoid globe perforation with scleral sutures, as the sclera is relatively thin in this area. When a Baerveldt implant is used, the rectus muscles may be isolated and lifted to place the plate wings under them. The tube can be placed into the anterior chamber, sulcus, or—if the eye is completely vitrectomized—pars plana.

Valved devices require priming to separate valve leaflets; nonvalved devices require modification to prevent hypotony in the immediate postoperative period (Video 13-11). A dissolvable suture (or *ligature*) is tied around the tube near the tube–plate junction to restrict aqueous flow through the tube; this allows a capsule to form around the plate before suture dissolution. When the suture loosens (approximately 5–10 weeks postoperatively, depending on suture size), the capsule surrounding the plate creates resistance to flow and—usually—prevents hypotony. A monofilament suture *(ripcord)* can be placed in or adjacent to the lumen of the tube and carried subconjunctivally. If necessary, this ripcord can be pulled within the first 6 weeks to reduce the IOP. Venting slits can be created between the ligature and the point of tube entry into the eye to allow aqueous flow during the early postoperative period.

VIDEO 13-11 Intraoperative tube adjustments.
Courtesy of Chandrasekharan Krishnan, MD.
Available at: aao.org/bcscvideo_section10

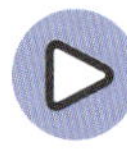

Tube coverage under the conjunctiva is important for erosion prevention. Several different types of human donor materials (eg, cornea, pericardium, or sclera) can be utilized; alternatively, the tube can be implanted through a long scleral tunnel or under a scleral flap (Video 13-12). Subsequently, the conjunctiva is closed to cover the entire device and patch graft.

VIDEO 13-12 Tube coverage.
Courtesy of Chandrasekharan Krishnan, MD.
Available at: aao.org/bcscvideo_section10

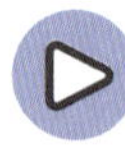

Postoperative Management

Compared with trabeculectomy, plate-based tube implants tend to require fewer interventions in the postoperative period. However, complications can occur (Table 13-4).

Table 13-4 Complications of Tube Shunt Surgery and Options for Prevention or Management

Complication	Prevention or Management
Tube–cornea touch	Insert the tube in the anterior chamber parallel to the iris plane. Use a tube occlusion technique to avoid flat chambers with nonvalved shunts. Minimize this complication by pars plana or ciliary sulcus insertion.
Shallow or flat chamber and hypotony	Valved devices decrease overfiltration, leading to these complications—it may be beneficial to retain a small amount of anterior chamber viscoelastic at the end of the procedure. For nonvalved devices, early hypotony can be minimized by tube occlusion via ligature or ripcord suture placement within the tube. Use viscoelastic agents if a flat chamber develops. Ensure that the tube entry site is watertight (ie, carefully select the needle size for scleral track creation). Correct overdrainage early. Consider drainage of choroidal effusions. Cycloplegics and corticosteroids can help deepen a shallow (but not flat) chamber. A flat chamber resulting from a complication such as suprachoroidal hemorrhage requires management based on the clinical context.
Valve malfunction	Test valves for patency before tube insertion. Several valve-clearing techniques have been described.
IOP elevation in early postoperative period	Treat with hypotensive agents, as needed.
Malignant glaucoma (aqueous misdirection)	Perform cycloplegia to prevent postoperative complications. If malignant glaucoma develops, treat with cycloplegia, laser hyloidectomy, or surgical irido-zonulo-hyloidectomy.
Tube occlusion	Bevel the tube away from uveal tissue (iris) or vitreous: upward for anterior chamber placement and downward for sulcus placement. Perform a generous vitrectomy, if needed. A YAG laser can be used to clear an occlusion; however, surgical intervention is often required.
Severe inflammation after tube opening	Steroid treatment
Suprachoroidal hemorrhage	Avoid hypotony. Instruct the patient to avoid vigorous activity if the eye is hypotonous.
Plate migration or tube retraction	Secure the plate to the sclera with nonabsorbable sutures. If the plate migrates, the intraocular tube may become longer or retract. Plate migration toward the limbus requires repositioning of the plate in the equatorial subconjunctival space. The extent of plate migration away from the limbus is rarely sufficiently severe to require repositioning, but a tube extender may be necessary if the tube retracts from the anterior chamber.

(Continued)

Table 13-4 *(continued)*

Complication	Prevention or Management
Tube or plate exposure or erosion	Tube or plate exposure can be resolved by removing any protruding sutures that have precipitated the erosion, securing the tube tightly to the sclera, covering the tube with reinforcing material (eg, sclera, cornea, or pericardium), and mobilizing the conjunctiva.
	Patch graft requires adequate conjunctiva coverage to prevent further erosion.
	If adequate conjunctiva coverage is not available, conjunctival autograft or amniotic membrane may be used.
	Exposure increases the risk of endophthalmitis. In some contexts, tube removal is necessary if adequate coverage cannot be achieved.
	Consider re-routing the tube.
Corneal decompensation	Avoid tube entry anterior to Schwalbe line (ie, in the cornea).
	If cornea is decompensating, move the tube posteriorly.
	This complication may be unavoidable in some eyes; refer for keratoplasty, as needed.
Diplopia	Prisms may resolve diplopia.
	Strabismus surgery may be required for intractable diplopia.
	Tube removal may be necessary in some cases.

Elevated IOP in the early postoperative period can have various causes. The *hypertensive phase* is marked by sudden elevation of IOP after a period of good IOP control, usually between 3 weeks and 3 months after surgery. The hypertensive phase is caused by a decrease in permeability of the capsule that forms around the end plate. This phase may gradually resolve as the capsule reorganizes and becomes more permeable to aqueous. Thus, management involves medical treatment to ensure reasonably low IOP during capsule reorganization. The incidence of this complication is higher with the Ahmed implant than with the Baerveldt implant, perhaps because the capsule is exposed to aqueous in the early postoperative period with the Ahmed device. The use of aqueous suppression early in postoperative management (ie, when the IOP reaches approximately 10–12 mm Hg) is associated with a decrease in hypertensive phase incidence and improved long-term outcomes. Conversely, when Baerveldt implants are used, the ligature delays capsule exposure to aqueous. Existing evidence does not support the use of intraoperative or postoperative adjunctive MMC or 5-FU with tube shunt surgery.

Other causes of elevated IOP in the postoperative period include valve defects, *occlusion, suprachoroidal hemorrhage,* and *aqueous misdirection.* Tubes can become occluded with fibrin, blood, vitreous, or iris tissue. LPI can remedy iris occlusion; fibrin and heme usually clear over time without intervention. Elevated IOP in ligated Baerveldt shunts can be managed by applying a green or diode laser to the ligature, using settings similar to those used for the nylon suture lysis method. If a ripcord has been placed, it can be pulled. However, if these procedures are performed too early, hypotony may occur. Fenestrations can

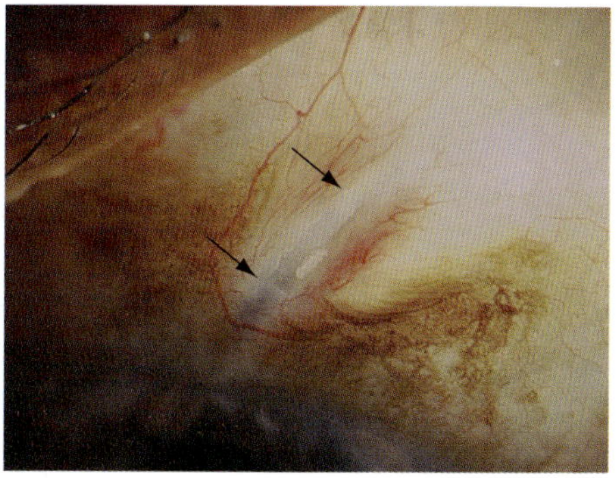

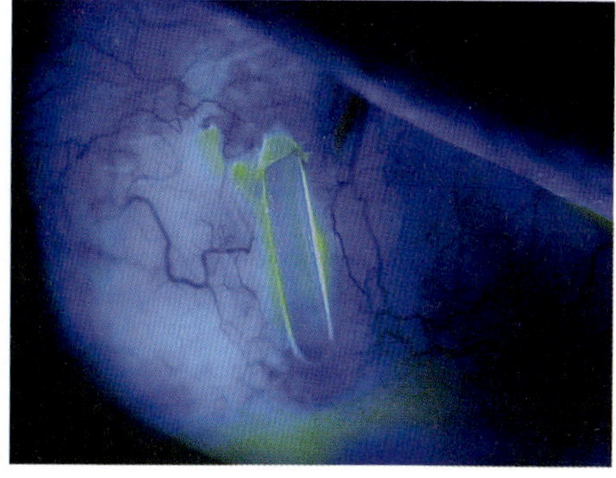

Figure 13-18 Tube exposure increases the risk of endophthalmitis and requires prompt repair. **A,** Photograph of conjunctiva erosion over the tube that begins 1–2 mm from the site of tube entry into the sclera. *Arrows* indicate the extent of the erosion. Note the mild hypervascularity around the exposed tube section. **B,** The exposed section of the tube is labeled with fluorescein. *(Courtesy of Kelly Walton Muir, MD, MHSc.)*

also be created under slit-lamp view or during the original procedure to provide temporary IOP relief prior to ligature dissolution.

The causes of a *shallow* or *flat anterior chamber* after plate-based tube shunt surgery are similar to the causative factors after trabeculectomy. *Choroidal effusions* and *malignant glaucoma* are managed in a similar manner, as described earlier (see the discussion of these topics under the section Postoperative Complications and Management). *Overfiltration* may require a return to the operating room for tube ligation or suture placement in the tube lumen to restrict aqueous outflow.

Tube erosion occurs in 1%–8% of plate-based tube implant surgeries (Fig 13-18). The causes include mechanical factors, immune response, and fragile conjunctiva overlying the tube. Tube erosion requires urgent surgical correction because patients with this complication have a high risk of infection. Repair may involve the placement of a new allograft, movement of the tube to a different location, or removal of the tube (Video 13-13). The risk of endophthalmitis within 5 years after tube shunt surgery is approximately 0.5%. Management of endophthalmitis often requires tube removal.

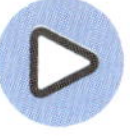

VIDEO 13-13 Tube revision.
Courtesy of Chandrasekharan Krishnan, MD.
Available at: aao.org/bcscvideo_section10

Diplopia occurs in approximately 5% of patients, often because of limited motility due to a large bleb, injury, or extraocular muscle impingement. Management with prisms is usually successful. If the deviation precludes the use of prisms, strabismus surgery or tube removal may be indicated.

Bains U, Hoguet A. Aqueous drainage device erosion: a review of rates, risks, prevention, and repair. *Semin Ophthalmol.* 2018;33(1):1–10.

Pakravan M, Rad SS, Yazdani S, Ghahari E, Yaseri M. Effect of early treatment with aqueous suppressants on Ahmed glaucoma valve implantation outcomes. *Ophthalmology.* 2014;121(9): 1693–1698.

Yazdani S, Doozandeh A, Pakravan M, Ownagh V, Yaseri M. Adjunctive triamcinolone acetonide for Ahmed glaucoma valve implantation: a randomized clinical trial. *Eur J Ophthalmol.* 2017;27(4):411–416.

Zheng CX, Moster MR, Khan MA, et al. Infectious endophthalmitis after glaucoma drainage implant surgery: clinical features, microbial spectrum, and outcomes. *Retina.* 2017;37(6):1160–1167.

Cataract Surgery in Patients With Glaucoma

After cataract extraction, patients with ocular hypertension or glaucoma may experience IOP reduction. This reduction most commonly occurs in eyes with higher preoperative pressures.

Ocular Hypertension

In the Ocular Hypertension Treatment Study (see Chapter 7), 42 patients underwent cataract surgery while assigned to the study's control arm. These patients were compared with patients in the control arm who did not undergo cataract surgery. At 36 months, the mean IOP reduction in cataract surgery patients was 17%. Moreover, 40% of eyes that underwent cataract surgery had a ≥20% reduction in IOP at 36 months. Conversely, the mean IOP in eyes that did not undergo cataract surgery was unchanged at 36 months.

Mansberger SL, Gordon MO, Jampel H, et al; Ocular Hypertension Treatment Study Group. Reduction in intraocular pressure after cataract extraction: the Ocular Hypertension Treatment Study. *Ophthalmology.* 2012;119(9):1826–1831.

Primary Open-Angle Glaucoma

Many retrospective and prospective studies have shown that cataract surgery reduces IOP in patients with POAG. This reduction is attributed to an increase in outflow facility. Hypothesized mechanisms for this effect include the following:

- anatomical changes in the eye because of lens removal
- surgery-induced biochemical changes
- TM irrigation

Two meta-analyses revealed a mean IOP reduction of 2–3 mm Hg after cataract surgery in eyes with POAG, although the IOP reduction appears to diminish over time. However, cataract surgery has been associated with acute and persistent IOP elevation in some patients. There is no evidence to support the removal of cataracts that are *not* visually significant in the management of OAG.

Chen PP, Lin SC, Junk AK, Radhakrishnan S, Singh K, Chen TC. The effect of phacoemulsification on intraocular pressure in glaucoma patients: a report by the American Academy of Ophthalmology. *Ophthalmology.* 2015;122(7):1294–1307.

Masis M, Mineault PJ, Phan E, Lin SC. The role of phacoemulsification in glaucoma therapy: a systematic review and meta-analysis. *Surv Ophthalmol.* 2018;63(5):700–710.

Angle-Closure Glaucoma

During normal aging, the anteroposterior diameter of the lens increases, leading to relative pupillary block. This process can cause PAC in susceptible eyes. Because an intraocular lens is substantially thinner than the crystalline lens, cataract surgery can alleviate pupillary block and thus be effective in the management of all stages of angle-closure disease.

The Effectiveness of Early Lens Extraction for the Treatment of Primary Angle-Closure Glaucoma (EAGLE) study compared cataract surgery in eyes with clear lenses or non–visually significant cataracts with LPI plus medical therapy in a prospective randomized controlled trial that involved patients with either PAC (defined unconventionally in this study as the presence of ≥180° of synechial or appositional iridotrabecular contact, along with IOP ≥30 mm Hg) or PACG. At 3 years, the clear lens extraction group had lower IOP, used fewer medications, and required fewer additional interventions to control IOP (see also Chapter 9, Treatment Controversies sidebar).

In patients with PAS, goniosynechialysis may reduce IOP (Video 13-14). After cataract removal, the adherent iris is detached from the TM using a blunt instrument, viscoelastic, and/or forceps. Goniosynechialysis is more effective when performed in combination with cataract surgery and when PAS formation is more recent.

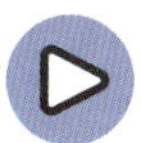

VIDEO 13-14 Goniosynechialysis.
Courtesy of Chandrasekharan Krishnan, MD.
Available at: aao.org/bcscvideo_section10

Azuara-Blanco A, Burr J, Ramsay C, et al; EAGLE study group. Effectiveness of early lens extraction for the treatment of primary angle-closure glaucoma (EAGLE): a randomised controlled trial. *Lancet*. 2016;388(10052):1389–1397.

Rodrigues IA, Alaghband P, Beltran Agullo L, et al. Aqueous outflow facility after phacoemulsification with or without goniosynechialysis in primary angle closure: a randomised controlled study. *Br J Ophthalmol*. 2017;101(7):879–885.

Cataract Surgery in Combination With Glaucoma Surgery

Patients with cataract may benefit from a glaucoma procedure to lessen their medication burden or to increase the likelihood of lower IOP after cataract surgery. In this context, a microinvasive glaucoma surgery procedure can be offered (see the section Microinvasive Glaucoma Surgeries). In addition, some patients with cataract require a much lower IOP than can be achieved via medication; trabeculectomy or plate-based tube shunt surgery is advised for these patients. If appropriate, cataract surgery prior to tube shunt surgery or trabeculectomy is indicated to minimize postoperative inflammation during tube implantation or trabeculectomy; such inflammation can hinder success in these glaucoma surgeries. When glaucoma surgery is urgent, the surgeon may determine that the best approach involves cataract removal during glaucoma surgery, especially because cataract progression increases after glaucoma surgery.

AGIS (Advanced Glaucoma Intervention Study) Investigators. The Advanced Glaucoma Intervention Study: 8. Risk of cataract formation after trabeculectomy. *Arch Ophthalmol*. 2001;119(12):1771–1779.

Cataract surgery and trabeculectomy

When cataract removal is performed in combination with trabeculectomy, the surgeon can use a single-site surgery method (insertion of the phacoemulsification handpiece under the trabeculectomy flap) or a 2-site surgery method (creation of a corneal incision separate from the trabeculectomy flap). The outcomes are considered similar.

Studies evaluating the outcomes of cataract surgery after trabeculectomy have had mixed results: some studies have shown no effect on IOP, whereas other studies have demonstrated a slight rise in IOP or an increase in the number of medications needed for IOP control. When the surgical treatment plan comprises trabeculectomy and subsequent cataract surgery, a 6–12-month delay prior to cataract surgery may improve long-term trabeculectomy survival and IOP control.

Cataract surgery and plate-based tube shunt implants

For patients with glaucoma who have visually significant cataracts, particularly with a narrow angle, consideration should be given to removing the cataract during tube shunt implantation. Anterior chamber deepening via cataract extraction allows for more posterior tube placement in the anterior chamber or the possibility of implantation in the ciliary sulcus, thereby reducing the risk of corneal decompensation.

Husain R, Liang S, Foster PJ, et al. Cataract surgery after trabeculectomy: the effect on trabeculectomy function. *Arch Ophthalmol.* 2012;130(2):165–170.

Other Glaucoma Surgeries

Microinvasive Glaucoma Surgeries

Microinvasive glaucoma surgery (MIGS), also known as *minimally invasive* or *microincisional glaucoma surgery,* refers to a group of procedures that are intended to reduce IOP with less tissue disruption and less risk compared with traditional procedures. A number of MIGS procedures enhance preexisting pathways with approaches that include bypassing TM resistance to aqueous flow, improving aqueous flow through the Schlemm canal, and/or creating a low-resistance pathway for aqueous flow between the anterior chamber and the suprachoroidal space. Other procedures considered to be in the MIGS category bypass the natural outflow pathways or reduce inflow but generally do so with smaller incisions than are used in traditional surgeries. Despite the name, MIGS procedures are incisional and invasive surgeries that carry risk. However, significant complications occur less frequently with MIGS procedures than with conventional glaucoma surgeries.

Because MIGS procedures are intended to increase flow through preexisting pathways, their efficacies (except for procedures that shunt aqueous to the suprachoroidal space) are limited by episcleral venous pressure and distal outflow resistance. In most patients, the episcleral venous pressure is 6–9 mm Hg. Typically, MIGS procedures result in average IOPs in the mid to high teens.

MIGS procedures can be classified into the following general categories (see Figure 13-1 earlier in the chapter):

- outflow augmentation (without bleb)
  - disruption of TM (goniotomy with blade or electrocautery)

  - bypass of TM with stent
  - viscodilation of the Schlemm canal
  - stent placement in the supraciliary or suprachoroidal space
- outflow augmentation (with bleb)
  - stent placement in the subconjunctival space
- inflow reduction
  - endoscopic cyclophotocoagulation
  - transscleral cyclophotocoagulation

Indications and contraindications

Angle-based, ab interno MIGS procedures require a gonioscopic view of the anterior chamber angle during surgery. Therefore, preoperative gonioscopy (particularly involving the nasal angle) is important to confirm the presence of an open angle. A functionally significant cataract must be present for some MIGS procedures, which were only evaluated in trials in combination with cataract surgery.

Postoperative management involves the use of steroids and antibiotics. For procedures requiring TM disruption, pilocarpine may also be used to help prevent PAS formation. Complications include hyphema, acute postoperative IOP elevations (spikes), prolonged postoperative inflammation, obstruction of the device or incision by iris tissue, improper insertion of the device, cyclodialysis, iridodialysis, corneal decompensation, and hypotony.

Patient selection

There is limited evidence to guide the use of MIGS procedures in advanced glaucoma, and they are not appropriate for eyes that require a very low target IOP. MIGS procedures are often performed in combination with cataract surgery. Patients for whom MIGS is indicated include

- those with mild to moderate glaucoma requiring additional IOP reduction, including beyond that expected from cataract extraction
- those expected to benefit from a reduction in topical medications

Trabecular bypass devices

Trabecular bypass devices are designed to create a low-resistance pathway between the anterior chamber and the Schlemm canal. Multiple devices with various designs are available; all are preloaded in a specific injector/inserter. Each device pierces the TM to enter the Schlemm canal; some devices facilitate partial stenting of the Schlemm canal. A small section of the device resides in the anterior chamber to allow aqueous entry. A 1-mm section of the canal is stented open by the first-generation *iStent* (Glaukos) (Fig 13-19A). The second-generation *iStent Inject* device (Glaukos) is placed in the Schlemm canal without any appreciable stenting (Fig 13-19B). Multiple iStent Inject devices can be placed in a single eye. An 8-mm section of the canal is stented open by the *Hydrus Microstent* (Alcon) (Fig 13-20).

Technique Successful surgery requires proper positioning of the patient's head and the operating microscope. It is important to visualize angle structures en face, rather than at an angle. An incision is made in the temporal cornea, and the eye is filled with viscoelastic. The nasal angle is visualized with a direct goniolens. Subsequently, the injector/inserter delivers

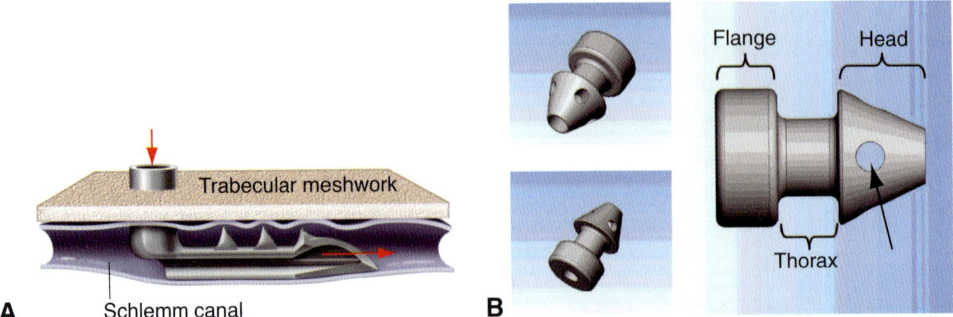

Figure 13-19 Illustrations of iStent devices. **A,** In the first-generation iStent device, the tip pierces the trabecular meshwork, allowing the device to enter the Schlemm canal. Retention rings subsequently immobilize the device. The snorkel is open to the anterior chamber, allowing aqueous to flow through the device into the Schlemm canal. *Arrows* indicate aqueous flow and also the opening of the snorkel portion of the device. **B,** In the second-generation iStent Inject device, the head contains 4 equally sized and evenly spaced ports for fluid passage *(arrow)*. The head is connected to a narrow thorax, which is attached to a wider flange region. An inlet port spans the entire length of the iStent Inject device. *(Part A illustration courtesy of Mark Miller. Part B reproduced with permission from Bahler CK, Hann CR, Fjield T, Haffner D, Heitzmann H, Fautsch MP. Second-generation trabecular meshwork bypass stent (iStent inject) increases outflow facility in cultured human anterior segments.* Am J Ophthalmol. *2012;153(6):1206–1213.)*

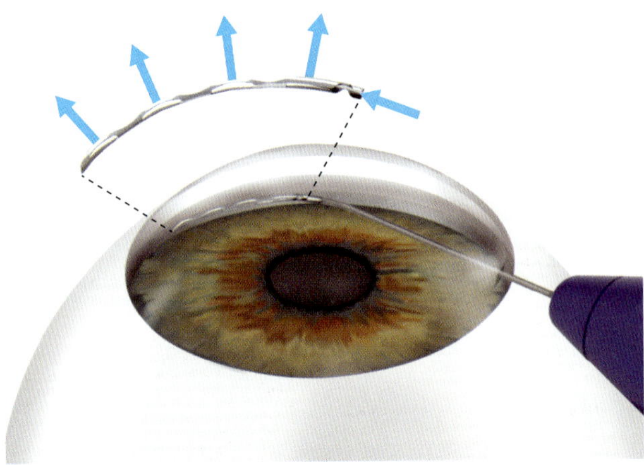

Figure 13-20 Illustration of the Hydrus Microstent (Alcon). The 8-mm-long stent has multiple windows that are visible through lightly pigmented trabecular meshwork and a neck that is placed in the anterior chamber, where it directs aqueous to the Schlemm canal. *(Illustration by Cyndie C. H. Wooley. Redrawn based on image available at https://www.willseye.org/hydrus-implant/.)*

the device through the TM into the Schlemm canal. Videos 13-15 and 13-16 demonstrate delivery of the iStent Inject and Hydrus Microstent, respectively.

VIDEO 13-15 iStent Inject.
Courtesy of Wayne Tie, MD.
Available at: aao.org/bcscvideo_section10

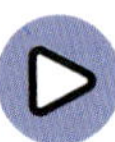

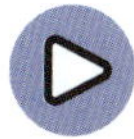

VIDEO 13-16 Hydrus Microstent.
Courtesy of Iqbal "Ike" Ahmed, MD.
Available at: aao.org/bcscvideo_section10

Effectiveness The use of trabecular bypass devices for the treatment of mild to moderate glaucoma with high IOP (21–36 mm Hg) is supported by the results of industry-sponsored randomized controlled trials comparing cataract extraction alone with cataract extraction plus TM bypass device placement. These studies showed that, compared with eyes treated with cataract surgery alone, eyes receiving a TM bypass device were more likely to achieve a 20% reduction in IOP without medication from unmedicated baseline (approximately 60% versus approximately 75%); they were also more likely to reduce their medication burden by 1–1.5 medications. The mean decrease in unmedicated IOP was approximately 7–7.5 mm Hg in eyes receiving a TM bypass device, compared with 5 mm Hg in eyes treated with cataract surgery alone. Five-year data from the Hydrus Microstent randomized controlled trial suggested less visual field progression in eyes that underwent cataract surgery plus microstent placement compared with eyes that underwent cataract surgery alone.

Ahmed IIK, Fea A, Au L, et al; COMPARE Investigators. A prospective randomized trial comparing Hydrus and iStent microinvasive glaucoma surgery implants for standalone treatment of open-angle glaucoma: the COMPARE Study. *Ophthalmology.* 2020;127(1):52–61.

Samuelson TW, Chang DF, Marquis R, et al; HORIZON Investigators. A Schlemm canal microstent for intraocular pressure reduction in primary open-angle glaucoma and cataract: the HORIZON study. *Ophthalmology*. 2019;126(1):29–37.

Samuelson TW, Sarkisian SR Jr, Lubeck DM, et al; iStent inject Study Group. Prospective, randomized, controlled pivotal trial of ab interno implanted trabecular micro-bypass in primary open-angle glaucoma and cataract: two-year results. *Ophthalmology.* 2019;126(6):811–821.

Trabecular meshwork disruption and Schlemm canal viscodilation

Some MIGS procedures are designed to disrupt or remove the inner wall of the Schlemm canal and TM, thereby opening the canal and directly exposing downstream collector channels to aqueous outflow. The TM can be removed with a bent 27-gauge needle or blades specifically designed for this purpose (Video 13-17), or ablated using an instrument that simultaneously irrigates and aspirates fluid (Video 13-18). Although MIGS procedures typically disrupt or remove 90°–180° of the TM, some procedures attempt to disrupt 360° of the TM. An example is gonioscopy-assisted transluminal trabeculotomy (GATT), in which either a microcatheter or a suture is threaded into the Schlemm canal using an ab interno approach (Video 13-19). The microcatheter can perform both Schlemm canal viscodilation and TM disruption. GATT is also known as *360° ab interno suture trabeculotomy*; this is distinct from the ab externo trabeculotomy procedure often performed in children.

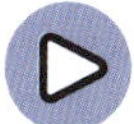

VIDEO 13-17 Excisional goniotomy.
Courtesy of Iqbal "Ike" Ahmed, MD.
Available at: aao.org/bcscvideo_section10

VIDEO 13-18 Trabectome: setup and procedure.
Courtesy of Sameh Mosaed, MD.
Available at: aao.org/bcscvideo_section10

VIDEO 13-19 GATT and ab interno canaloplasty.
Courtesy of Iqbal "Ike" Ahmed, MD.
Available at: aao.org/bcscvideo_section10

Technique Microscope and patient positioning are critical considerations (see Video 13-18). A clear corneal incision and a gonioprism are used in all angle-based surgeries. Some instruments only remove the nasal TM and the inner wall of the Schlemm canal; the surgeon directly incises and removes tissue. Other instruments (eg, the OMNI Surgical System; Sight Sciences Inc) cannulate and disrupt the angle (180° or 360°) (Video 13-20). Immediately before trabeculotomy, viscocanaloplasty (ie, injection of viscoelastic for viscodilation of the canal and—possibly—downstream collector channels) can be performed with specific devices: a lighted microcatheter that injects viscoelastic or a curved needle–like device containing viscoelastic and a suture.

VIDEO 13-20 OMNI canaloplasty and trabeculotomy.
Courtesy of JoAnn A. Giaconi, MD.
Available at: aao.org/bcscvideo_section10

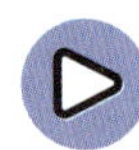

Effectiveness Thus far, no prospective randomized trials have compared the efficacy of TM removal or TM disruption with the efficacy of cataract surgery alone, which is known to reduce IOP. As standalone procedures, TM removal and TM disruption have been shown to reduce pressure and medication burden in retrospective studies with relatively short follow-up. Some eyes may be more responsive to TM removal or TM disruption, such as eyes with secondary OAG in which the pathology primarily involves the TM.

Aqueous shunting into the suprachoroidal space

There are currently no devices approved by the US Food and Drug Administration (FDA) for aqueous shunting into the suprachoroidal space. In the past, the *CyPass Micro-Stent* (Alcon) was available; this tube-shaped device was placed in the anterior chamber angle to create a conduit from the anterior chamber to the suprachoroidal space. The device was recalled by the FDA in 2018 because increased corneal endothelial cell loss was observed during long-term observation of patients in the pivotal clinical trial.

Short Aqueous Stent Placement in the Subconjunctival Space

The *XEN Gel Stent* (Allergan) is a device that shunts aqueous humor to the subconjunctival space. In contrast to conventional plate-based tube implants, this device does not feature a plate attached to the subconjunctival portion of the tube. The XEN Gel Stent was originally designed for ab interno implantation through a clear corneal incision using an injector (Video 13-21), but many surgeons have chosen to perform ab externo implantation with or without conjunctival peritomy, similar to trabeculectomy (Video 13-22). Postoperative fibrosis, the main cause of failure, is minimized through the use of MMC.

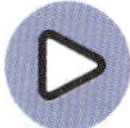

VIDEO 13-21 XEN implantation, ab interno approach.
Courtesy of Wayne Tie, MD.
Available at: aao.org/bcscvideo_section10

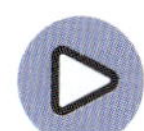

VIDEO 13-22 XEN implantation, ab externo open conjunctiva.
Courtesy of Leon Herndon, MD.
Available at: aao.org/bcscvideo_section10

Generally, use of the XEN Gel Stent results in mean pressures in the mid to high teens. Among patients in the pivotal clinical trial, 75% had ≥20% reduction of IOP at 12 months, 32% required postoperative transconjunctival needle revision, and 25% had transient hypotony. Similar to trabeculectomy and tube shunt surgery, the complications included choroidal effusion, tube erosion, prolonged hypotony, and infection. Notably, the trial did not involve a comparator arm. In several retrospective studies, final IOPs were higher after XEN Gel Stent implantation than after trabeculectomy. Also, visual recovery was faster after XEN Gel Stent implantation than trabeculectomy. A similar device (PRESERFLO; Glaukos) is approved for use in multiple countries but not the United States.

Fili S, Kontopoulou K, Vastardis I, Perdikakis G, Kohlhaas M. PreserFlo microshunt versus trabeculectomy in patients with moderate to advanced open-angle glaucoma: 12-month follow-up of a single-center prospective study. *Cureus.* 2022;14(8):e28288. doi:10.7759/cureus.28288

Grover DS, Flynn WJ, Bashford KP, et al. Performance and safety of a new ab interno gelatin stent in refractory glaucoma at 12 months. *Am J Ophthalmol.* 2017;183:25–36.

Nonpenetrating Glaucoma Surgery

Nonpenetrating glaucoma procedures are incisional glaucoma surgeries that do not involve anterior chamber entry; they are intended to reduce IOP while avoiding some complications of trabeculectomy. These procedures include *deep sclerectomy, viscocanalostomy,* and *canaloplasty* (Video 13-23). In both viscocanalostomy and canaloplasty, deep sclerectomy is performed to open the external wall of the Schlemm canal. In viscocanalostomy, a cannula is used to inject viscoelastic into a limited portion of the Schlemm canal. In canaloplasty, a flexible illuminated catheter is utilized to inject viscoelastic into the full 360° of the Schlemm canal, then pass a suture through the canal; subsequently, the suture is tied under moderate tension, leaving the canal stretched. For these 3 procedures, the surgeon creates a fornix-based conjunctival incision, followed by a superficial scleral flap. The removal of deeper sclera from under the flap results in a thin layer of sclera and Descemet membrane. This approach allows aqueous to percolate through the Descemet membrane into a scleral lake formed by removal of the deep scleral flap.

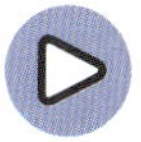

VIDEO 13-23 Canaloplasty.
Courtesy of Steven Vold, MD.
Available at: aao.org/bcscvideo_section10

Nonpenetrating glaucoma procedures are indicated for OAG. Thus far, there are limited long-term data from prospective randomized trials in which these newer procedures are compared with trabeculectomy. Although nonpenetrating procedures may avoid some complications associated with trabeculectomy, they are technically challenging; most results suggest that these procedures result in less IOP reduction, compared with trabeculectomy. They also cause conjunctival scarring, which can limit future surgical options. In addition, intraoperative conversion to trabeculectomy might be required. Postoperative YAG laser goniopuncture of the Descemet membrane may be necessary to increase aqueous flow. Complications include Descemet detachment and infection.

Gilmour DF, Manners TD, Devonport H, Varga Z, Solebo AL, Miles J. Viscocanalostomy versus trabeculectomy for primary open angle glaucoma: 4-year prospective randomized clinical trial. *Eye (Lond)*. 2009;23(9):1802–1807.

Special Patient Considerations

When deciding whether a patient is a candidate for surgical treatment, it is important for the surgeon to consider the whole patient, with particular attention to age, terminal illness, and any other major health problems. Key considerations include glaucoma severity, risk of functional vision loss in the patient's lifetime, and the presence of any major systemic disease that could affect the outcome. Many conditions may interfere with healing, such as heritable connective tissue disorders (also called *collagen vascular diseases*), autoimmune diseases, and diabetes. Another key consideration is whether the patient can adhere to medical therapy. For example, a patient who has poor preoperative medication adherence (because

KEY POINTS 13-2

MIGS and other glaucoma surgeries The following are essential points for the ophthalmologist to remember about microinvasive glaucoma surgery (MIGS), short aqueous stent placement, and nonpenetrating glaucoma surgery.

- Typically, MIGS results in intraocular pressures (IOPs) in the mid to high teens.
- Compared with cataract surgery alone, cataract surgery plus trabecular meshwork bypass device placement facilitates greater reduction in IOP without medication, and greater likelihood of reduced medication burden.
- Short-term retrospective studies have shown that trabecular meshwork removal and trabecular meshwork disruption reduce pressure and medication burden.
- Retrospective analyses have revealed faster visual recovery after short aqueous stent placement in the subconjunctival space, compared with trabeculectomy.
- Although nonpenetrating procedures can avoid some complications associated with trabeculectomy, they may result in comparatively less IOP reduction.

of memory loss, poor vision, tremor, or arthritis) is likely to also display poor postoperative adherence, which could jeopardize the outcome of surgical treatment. Social determinants of health, such as socioeconomic constraints, may also jeopardize surgical outcomes if patients cannot attend all planned postoperative appointments.

After the decision has been made to proceed with surgery, the surgeon should recommend to the patient the procedure that is most likely to successfully reduce IOP with the fewest possible complications. This selection involves considering the patient's ability to return for multiple follow-up visits. If a patient is not mobile or lacks easy transportation options, a nonpenetrating, MIGS, or cyclodestructive procedure may be preferred; these types of procedures require fewer postoperative visits, compared with trabeculectomy or tube shunt surgery. If trabeculectomy is selected, it may be beneficial to use a limbus-based conjunctival flap because it is less likely to leak, compared with a fornix-based flap. Another key consideration is the patient's use of anticoagulants and antiplatelet medications; although these drugs increase the risk of serious intraocular hemorrhage–related complications, discontinuation is associated with a risk of vascular events. The final consideration is the need for caution regarding the use of antifibrotics in older adult patients; compared with younger patients, older patients display diminished healing capacity and fragile tissues that tend to be thinner.

Sustainability and Glaucoma Surgery

As with surgery in general, ophthalmic surgery generates significant waste, particularly in resource-rich countries. There is increased awareness of the need to make surgery a sustainable enterprise both in terms of waste and carbon emissions. To achieve this, ophthalmology organizations from around the world are collaborating by sharing knowledge and resources.

EyeSustain. Sustainability Resources for Ophthalmology. Accessed January 29, 2024. https://eyesustain.org/

Sherry B, Lee S, Ramos Cadena MLA, et al. How ophthalmologists can decarbonize eye care: a review of existing sustainability strategies and steps ophthalmologists can take. *Ophthalmology.* 2023;130(7):702–714.

Additional Materials and Resources

Related Academy Materials

The American Academy of Ophthalmology is dedicated to providing a wealth of high-quality clinical education resources for ophthalmologists.

Print Publications and Electronic Products

For a complete listing of Academy clinical education products, including the BCSC Self-Assessment Program, visit our online store at aao.org/store. Or call Customer Service at 866.561.8558 (toll free, US only) or +1 415.561.8540, Monday through Friday, between 8:00 AM and 5:00 PM (PST).

Online Resources

Visit the David E. I. Pyott Glaucoma Education Center on the **Ophthalmic News and Education (ONE®) Network** (aao.org/glaucoma) to find relevant videos, podcasts, webinars, online courses, journal articles, practice guidelines, self-assessment quizzes, images, and more. The ONE Network is a free Academy-member benefit.

The **Residents page** on the ONE Network (aao.org/residents) offers resident-specific content, including courses, videos, flash cards, and OKAP and Board Exam study tools.

The **Resident Knowledge Exchange** (resident-exchange.aao.org) provides peer-generated study materials, including flash cards, mnemonics, and presentations that offer unique perspectives on complex concepts.

Find comprehensive **resources for diversity, equity, inclusion, and accessibility** in ophthalmology on the ONE Network at aao.org/diversity-equity-and-inclusion.

Access free, trusted articles and content with the Academy's collaborative online encyclopedia, **EyeWiki,** at aao.org/eyewiki.

Get mobile access to *The Wills Eye Manual* and *EyeWiki,* watch the latest 1-minute videos and podcast episodes, challenge yourself with weekly Diagnose This activities, and set up alerts for clinical updates relevant to you with the free **AAO Ophthalmic Education app.** Download today: search for "AAO Ophthalmic Education" in the Apple app store or in Google Play.

Basic Texts and Additional Resources

Allingham RR, Moroi SE, Shields MB, et al. *Shields' Textbook of Glaucoma.* 7th ed. Lippincott Williams & Wilkins; 2020.

Kahook MY, Schuman JS, eds. *Chandler and Grant's Glaucoma.* 6th ed. Slack Incorporated; 2020.

Levin LA, Nilsson SFE, Ver Hoeve J, Wu SM, Kaufman PL, Alm A. *Adler's Physiology of the Eye: Clinical Application.* 11th ed. Saunders/Elsevier; 2011.

Schacknow PN, Samples JR, eds. *The Glaucoma Book: A Practical, Evidence-Based Approach to Patient Care.* Springer-Verlag New York; 2010.

Stamper RL, Lieberman MF, Drake MV, eds. *Becker-Shaffer's Diagnosis and Therapy of the Glaucomas.* 8th ed. Mosby; 2009.

Weinreb RN, Mills RP, eds. *Glaucoma Surgery: Principles and Techniques.* 2nd ed. Ophthalmology Monographs 4. American Academy of Ophthalmology; 1998.

Requesting Continuing Medical Education Credit

The American Academy of Ophthalmology is accredited by the Accreditation Council for Continuing Medical Education (ACCME) to provide continuing medical education for physicians.

The American Academy of Ophthalmology designates this enduring material for a maximum of 10 *AMA PRA Category 1 Credits*™. Physicians should claim only the credit commensurate with the extent of their participation in the activity.

To claim *AMA PRA Category 1 Credits*™ upon completion of this activity, learners must demonstrate appropriate knowledge and participation in the activity by taking the posttest for Section 10 and achieving a score of 80% or higher.

To take the posttest and request CME credit online:

1. Go to aao.org/cme-central and log in.
2. Click on "Claim CME Credit and View My CME Transcript" and then "Report AAO Credits."
3. Select the appropriate media type and then the Academy activity. You will be directed to the posttest.
4. Once you have passed the test with a score of 80% or higher, you will be directed to your transcript. *If you are not an Academy member, you will be able to print out a certificate of participation once you have passed the test.*

CME expiration date: June 1, 2027. *AMA PRA Category 1 Credits*™ may be claimed only once between June 1, 2024 (original release date), and the expiration date.

For assistance, contact the Academy's Customer Service department at 866.561.8558 (US only) or +1 415.561.8540 between 8:00 AM and 5:00 PM (PST), Monday through Friday, or send an e-mail to customer_service@aao.org.

Study Questions

Please note that these questions are not part of your CME reporting process. They are provided here for your own educational use and for identification of any professional practice gaps. The required CME posttest is available online (see "Requesting Continuing Medical Education Credit"). Following the questions are answers with discussions. Although a concerted effort has been made to avoid ambiguity and redundancy in these questions, the authors recognize that differences of opinion may occur regarding the "best" answer. The discussions are provided to demonstrate the rationale used to derive the answer. They may also be helpful in confirming that your approach to the problem was correct or, if necessary, in fixing the principle in your memory. The Section 10 faculty thanks the Resident Self-Assessment Committee for developing these self-assessment questions and the discussions that follow.

1. From where is the arterial blood supply of the anterior optic nerve primarily derived?
   a. central retinal artery
   b. circle of Zinn-Haller
   c. pial arteries
   d. short posterior ciliary arteries

2. According to the Goldmann equation, what is the ratio of the increase in intraocular pressure (IOP) to the increase in episcleral venous pressure in millimeters of mercury (mm Hg)?
   a. 1:0.5
   b. 1:1
   c. 1:1.5
   d. 1:2

3. What type of tonometer is based on the Imbert-Fick principle for measurement of IOP?
   a. Perkins tonometer
   b. pneumotonometer
   c. rebound tonometer
   d. Schiøtz tonometer

4. Which parameter of the modified Goldmann equation cannot be directly measured clinically and must be calculated from the Goldmann equation after determination of the other parameters?
   a. aqueous humor production rate
   b. episcleral venous pressure
   c. outflow facility
   d. uveoscleral outflow rate

5. When the biomechanical properties of the cornea and glaucoma are considered, what instrument can measure corneal hysteresis?
   a. corneal pachymeter
   b. dynamic contour tonometer
   c. iCare tonometer
   d. Ocular Response Analyzer

6. While on call, an ophthalmologist managing a patient with acutely elevated IOP of 58 mm Hg considers administering oral acetazolamide to this patient in the clinic. A review of the patient's allergies reveals a documented "sulfa" allergy. The patient reports having had a "rash" after taking trimethoprim-sulfamethoxazole as a child. What is the approximate chance of an allergic reaction to acetazolamide in this scenario?
   a. 10%
   b. 30%
   c. 50%
   d. 70%

7. A patient presents with narrow angles and findings suggestive of iris and/or ciliary body cysts. What is the best imaging modality for further investigation?
   a. anterior segment optical coherence tomography
   b. anterior segment ultrasound biomicroscopy
   c. B-scan ultrasonography
   d. computed tomography scan of the orbits

8. An ophthalmologist examines a patient's optic nerve head at the slit lamp using indirect biomicroscopy. The patient's cup–disc ratio is asymmetric, with a difference of approximately 0.3 between the 2 eyes. What percentage of individuals without glaucoma would be expected to have this amount of asymmetry?
   a. less than 20%
   b. less than 10%
   c. less than 5%
   d. less than 1%

9. What optic nerve head characteristic is most specific for glaucoma?
   a. exposed lamina cribrosa
   b. focal notching of the neuroretinal rim
   c. nasal displacement of vessels
   d. peripapillary atrophy

10. A glaucoma suspect patient demonstrates superior and inferior defects in the left eye on perimetry with a reliable baseline visual field test (Swedish Interactive Threshold Algorithm Standard 24-2). What is the most appropriate next step?
    a. Begin medical therapy with a prostaglandin analogue.
    b. Obtain imaging of the optic nerve head.
    c. Order neuroimaging.
    d. Repeat visual field testing.

11. When is a false-positive error recorded in perimetry?
    a. when, on retesting, the patient does not respond to a stimulus that was previously seen
    b. when the patient falsely responds to a stimulus presented in the blind spot
    c. when the patient moves their eyes from the central fixation point
    d. when the patient responds even though no stimulus was presented

12. In the Collaborative Normal-Tension Glaucoma Study (CNTGS), what was the IOP reduction target?
    a. 10%
    b. 20%
    c. 30%
    d. 40%

13. What percentage of patients with primary open-angle glaucoma (POAG) present with an IOP below 22 mm Hg?
    a. 0%–25%
    b. 30%–50%
    c. 50%–75%
    d. 75%–100%

14. What was the finding of the Baltimore Eye Survey regarding the impact of aging on glaucoma?
    a. The impact of perfusion pressure on glaucoma increases with age.
    b. The prevalence of glaucoma increases with age.
    c. The rate of conversion from ocular hypertension to POAG increases with age.
    d. The rate of glaucoma progression increases with age.

15. A patient with a history of 2 piggyback intraocular lenses in the left eye, both placed within the capsular bag, is referred by a local optometrist for evaluation of elevated IOP in that eye. Endothelial pigment deposition is noted on slit-lamp examination. What gonioscopic finding might be expected in this scenario?
    a. peripheral anterior synechiae
    b. posterior embryotoxon
    c. Sampaolesi line
    d. widened ciliary body band

16. An 89-year-old woman presents with pain in her right eye. She reports that the vision in her right eye has been poor for years, owing to complications from a retinal detachment. On examination, the IOP in the right eye is 40 mm Hg. Her examination is significant for a white cataract with a wrinkled anterior capsule. On gonioscopy, ciliary body is visible in all quadrants. Cell and flare is noted in the anterior chamber, but no keratic precipitates are observed. What is the most likely diagnosis?
    a. lens particle glaucoma
    b. phacoantigenic glaucoma
    c. phacolytic glaucoma
    d. phacomorphic glaucoma

17. Which category of topical medication should be avoided in patients with uveitic glaucoma?
    a. α-agonists
    b. β-blockers
    c. carbonic anhydrase inhibitors
    d. miotic agents

18. Steroid administration is associated with secondary increases in IOP in approximately what percentage of individuals without glaucoma?
    a. 10%
    b. 25%
    c. 33%
    d. 45%

19. What is the most common cause of glaucoma associated with primary or metastatic tumors of the ciliary body?
    a. angle closure resulting from rotation of the ciliary body
    b. deposition of tumor cells and inflammatory cells in the trabecular meshwork
    c. direct invasion of the anterior chamber angle
    d. neovascularization of the anterior chamber angle

20. A patient reports seeing halos and having blurred vision, with mild pain in the left eye, for 2 days. The IOP is 14 mm Hg in the right eye and 46 mm Hg in the left eye. There is no conjunctival hyperemia. There are a few inferior keratic precipitates, and the anterior chamber is deep with occasional circulating cells. Eight months previously, the patient had a similar episode that resolved within days of using timolol eyedrops. What is the most likely diagnosis?
    a. primary angle-closure glaucoma
    b. Fuchs uveitis syndrome
    c. herpetic keratouveitis
    d. glaucomatocyclitic crisis

21. What is the most common cause of blindness related to glaucoma in the Chinese population?
    a. POAG
    b. secondary open-angle glaucoma
    c. primary angle-closure glaucoma
    d. secondary angle-closure glaucoma

22. What were the findings of the Zhongshan Angle-Closure Prevention (ZAP) trial?
    a. Laser peripheral iridotomy (LPI) had no impact on the course of progression of any type of angle closure.
    b. LPI significantly reduced the incidence of the development of acute angle closure.
    c. LPI significantly reduced the incidence of the development of primary angle closure.
    d. LPI significantly reduced the incidence of the development of POAG.

23. What surgical vitreoretinal procedure can result in non–pupillary block angle closure?
    a. scleral buckle placement
    b. pars plana vitrectomy with intraocular gas placement
    c. pars plana vitrectomy with silicone oil placement
    d. intravitreal anti–vascular endothelial growth factor injection

24. An 82-year-old patient who takes warfarin and previously had a central retinal vein occlusion in the left eye presents with an IOP of 39 mm Hg and neovascularization of the iris and angle. The patient has severe eye pain and has had substantially decreased vision for several months. Examination reveals a relative afferent pupillary defect in the left eye and hand motion vision. What is the most appropriate treatment option for the elevated IOP?
    a. selective laser trabeculoplasty
    b. transscleral cyclophotocoagulation
    c. anterior chamber tube shunt implantation
    d. trabeculectomy with mitomycin C

25. A 50-year-old woman presents with an IOP of 27 mm Hg in the right eye and 12 mm Hg in the left eye. On examination, an abnormal corneal endothelium is noted in the right eye; findings in the left eye are normal. Findings from the anterior segment examination are otherwise unremarkable. On gonioscopy, peripheral anterior synechiae anterior to the Schwalbe line are noted in 1 clock-hour. What is the most likely diagnosis?
    a. iridocorneal endothelial syndrome
    b. pseudoexfoliation syndrome
    c. uveitis
    d. Fuchs endothelial corneal dystrophy

26. A patient with primary congenital glaucoma (PCG) asks the ophthalmologist's advice regarding family planning. Notably, she has no relatives with PCG. What is the likelihood of her having a child affected with PCG?
    a. 0%–25%
    b. 25%–50%
    c. 50%–75%
    d. 75%–100%

27. A 2-year-old child is brought in for an eye examination because of persistent tearing. What corneal diameter measurement should trigger concern for glaucoma?
    a. greater than 11.5 mm
    b. greater than 12.0 mm
    c. greater than 12.5 mm
    d. greater than 13.0 mm

28. What finding on examination of a patient with congenital glaucoma can continue to change and indicate progressive glaucoma even though the IOP appears to be controlled?
    a. axial length
    b. corneal thickness
    c. gonioscopic findings
    d. myopia

29. What class of topical ocular hypotensive medication should be discontinued in a patient who also takes an oral monoamine oxidase inhibitor?
    a. prostaglandin analogues
    b. α-adrenergic agonists
    c. β-blockers
    d. carbonic anhydrase inhibitors

30. By what mechanism do Rho kinase inhibitors lower IOP?
    a. increasing uveoscleral outflow
    b. creating an osmotic gradient
    c. decreasing aqueous humor production
    d. increasing conventional (trabecular meshwork) outflow

31. An 84-year-old patient who received multiple-drug therapy for glaucoma returns to the clinic after 1 year and has an IOP of 31 mm Hg, as measured by applanation tonometry, during the follow-up examination. The patient lives alone and has a history of chronic obstructive pulmonary disease, Parkinson disease, and nonadherence. What is the best surgical treatment option for this patient?
    a. laser trabeculoplasty
    b. trabeculectomy
    c. plate-based tube implantation
    d. microinvasive glaucoma surgery

32. A patient with chronic angle-closure glaucoma develops a shallow anterior chamber 3 days after undergoing a trabeculectomy. On examination, the patient has no bleb, no leak, a patent surgical iridectomy, no choroidal effusions, and an IOP of 20 mm Hg. What is the best initial treatment option?
    a. placement of an oversized contact lens
    b. increase in frequency of topical steroid
    c. cycloplegic therapy
    d. injection of viscoelastic into the anterior chamber

Answers

1. **d.** The arterial supply of the anterior optic nerve is derived entirely from branches of the ophthalmic artery via 1–5 posterior ciliary arteries. Typically, between 2 and 4 posterior ciliary arteries course anteriorly before dividing into approximately 10–20 short posterior ciliary arteries, which occurs before these arteries enter the posterior globe. Often, the posterior ciliary arteries separate into a medial and a lateral group before branching into the short posterior ciliary arteries, which penetrate the perineural sclera of the posterior globe to supply the peripapillary choroid, as well as most of the anterior optic nerve. Some short posterior ciliary arteries course, without branching, through the sclera directly into the choroid; others divide within the sclera to provide branches to the choroid and the optic nerve. A discontinuous arterial circle, the circle of Zinn-Haller, is often present within the perineural sclera. The central retinal artery, also a posterior orbital branch of the ophthalmic artery, penetrates the optic nerve approximately 10–15 mm posterior to the globe. The central retinal artery has few, if any, intraneural branches, the exception being an occasional small branch within the retrolaminar region, which may anastomose with the pial system. The central retinal artery courses adjacent to the central retinal vein within the central portion of the optic nerve. The retrolaminar region is supplied by branches of the short posterior ciliary arteries and by branches of the pial arteries coursing adjacent to this region. The pial arteries originate both from the central retinal artery, before it pierces the retrobulbar optic nerve, and from branches of the short posterior ciliary arteries more anteriorly.
2. **b.** The modified Goldmann equation is a mathematical model of the relationship between intraocular pressure (IOP) and the parameters that contribute to its level in the eye at steady state:

   $$P_0 = (F - U)/C + P_V$$

   where P_0 is the IOP in millimeters of mercury (mm Hg), F is the rate of aqueous humor production in microliters per minute (μL/min), U is the rate of aqueous humor drainage through the pressure-insensitive uveoscleral pathway in μL/min, C is the facility of outflow through the pressure-sensitive trabecular meshwork pathway in microliters per minute per millimeter of mercury (μL/min/mm Hg), and P_V is the episcleral venous pressure (EVP) in mm Hg. According to this equation, IOP rises approximately 1 mm Hg for every 1-mm-Hg increase in EVP.

   EVP is often increased in patients with Sturge-Weber syndrome (encephalofacial angiomatosis), carotid-cavernous sinus fistulas, and cavernous sinus thrombosis as a result of obstruction of venous return to the heart or from shunting of blood from the arterial to the venous system. EVP may be partially responsible for the elevated IOP seen in thyroid eye disease. EVP is normally relatively stable, ranging from 6 to 9 mm Hg, as measured with special equipment. Elevated EVP can increase outflow resistance by decreasing the cross-sectional area of the Schlemm canal and may alter uveoscleral outflow.
3. **a.** Like the Goldmann tonometer, the Perkins tonometer is an applanation tonometer and, as such, it is based on the Imbert-Fick principle. The Imbert-Fick principle states that the pressure inside an ideal dry, infinitely thin-walled sphere equals the force required to flatten its surface divided by the area of the flattening. The Goldmann applanation tonometer and the Perkins tonometer use the same measurement tip, which balances the surface tension of the tear film with the rigidity of the cornea to approximate a dry, infinitely flexible,

thin-walled sphere for eyes with central corneal thickness (CCT) of 520 µm. The pneumotonometer, rebound tonometer, and the Schiøtz tonometer do not rely on the Imbert-Fick principle.

4. **d.** Direct measurement of the uveoscleral outflow rate is an invasive process that involves perfusion of a tracer into the anterior segment of the eye, followed by estimation of the tissue distribution of the tracer. Thus, in humans, the uveoscleral outflow rate must be calculated by using the Goldmann equation and the parameters IOP, aqueous humor production rate, outflow facility, and EVP. The rate of aqueous humor production by the ciliary processes cannot be measured noninvasively, but it is assumed to be equal to the aqueous humor outflow rate in an eye at steady state. Aqueous humor outflow can be measured with fluorophotometry; EVP, with venomanometry; and outflow facility, with tonography. All of these procedures are noninvasive.

5. **d.** The Ocular Response Analyzer (Reichert Technologies; see Chapter 2, Fig 2-7C), a type of noncontact tonometer, uses correction algorithms so that its IOP readings more closely match those obtained with applanation techniques, and the effect of corneal biomechanical properties on pressure measurement is reduced. Studies have found that the corneal compensated IOP (IOPcc) has a stronger correlation with glaucoma progression than does IOP measured with Goldmann or rebound tonometry. In addition to measuring IOPcc, the Ocular Response Analyzer calculates indicators of ocular biomechanical properties, including corneal hysteresis, which is the difference between IOP measured during the initial corneal indentation and IOP measured during corneal rebound. Reduced corneal hysteresis has been associated with an increased risk of developing visual field defects in glaucoma suspects and with disease progression in patients with confirmed glaucoma.

   None of the other instruments listed as answer options measure corneal hysteresis. A corneal pachymeter is used to measure CCT. IOP measurement may be affected by a thicker or thinner CCT. The dynamic contour tonometer has a tip that is similar in shape and size to an applanation tonometer tip except that it has a rounded concave surface and a pressure transducer embedded in the center. This allows the device to measure the ocular pulse amplitude in addition to IOP. Evidence suggests that IOP measurements obtained with dynamic contour tonometry may be more independent of corneal biomechanical properties and thickness than those obtained with applanation tonometry. The iCare tonometer is based on a principle of rebound. Rebound tonometry determines IOP by measuring the speed at which a small probe propelled against the cornea decelerates and rebounds after impact (see Chapter 2, Fig 2-7D). IOP readings obtained with rebound tonometry are strongly influenced by CCT.

6. **a.** Obtaining a careful medication history before prescribing new treatments, whether topical or systemic, is essential. Patients with a known allergy to a sulfonamide antibiotic may have an increased risk of a subsequent reaction to multiple classes of medications, including carbonic anhydrase inhibitors (CAIs), although cross reactivity between sulfonamide antibiotics and sulfonamide nonantibiotics such as CAIs may be as low as 10%, as they are different medication classes.

7. **b.** Ultrasound biomicroscopy is the best technique to image the ciliary body and anterior choroid, and it can facilitate diagnosis of plateau iris syndrome, ciliary body cysts, and ciliary tumors. Anterior segment optical coherence tomography does not penetrate deeply enough to adequately image the ciliary body. B-scan ultrasonography is not ideal

for imaging anterior structures. Computed tomography scans do not provide detailed images of anterior segment structures.

8. **d.** Examination of the optic nerve head (ONH) should involve careful comparison with the fellow eye, because cup–disc ratio asymmetry >0.2 between the 2 eyes is unusual in healthy eyes in the absence of ONH size asymmetry (see Chapter 5, Fig 5-1). The vertical cup–disc ratio typically ranges from 0.1 to 0.4, although up to 5% of individuals without glaucoma have cup–disc ratios >0.6 (ie, physiologic cupping). Cup–disc ratio asymmetry values >0.2 occur in fewer than 1% of individuals without glaucoma. This asymmetry may be related to ONH size asymmetry. Increased size of the physiologic cup may be a familial trait, which may be clarified by examination of other family members.
9. **b.** Glaucomatous cups are associated with both generalized and focal ophthalmoscopic signs. Generalized signs include a large optic cup, asymmetry of the optic cup between the eyes, and progressive enlargement of the cup. Focal signs include notching of the neuroretinal rim, vertical elongation of the optic cup, retinal nerve fiber layer hemorrhage, and segmental nerve fiber layer loss. Less specific signs may also be observed, including exposed lamina cribrosa, nasal displacement of rim vessels, baring of circumlinear vessels, and peripapillary atrophy.
10. **d.** In this scenario, before treatment is started, it would be best to obtain at least 1 more visual field test to determine whether the scotoma is reproducible. If the defect has a typical glaucomatous pattern matching the optic nerve appearance, neuroimaging is usually not required. ONH imaging is important in diagnosis and management of glaucoma, but repeating the visual field test would be the most appropriate next step to confirm a defect and obtain a baseline.

    Visual field testing is a subjective examination, and different responses may be obtained each time the test is performed or even during the same test. Such fluctuation can confound the detection of disease progression. To detect true visual field progression, the clinician needs to evaluate whether the observed change exceeds the expected variability for a particular point or area.
11. **d.** A false-positive error occurs when the patient presses the response button even though no stimulus is presented. A false-negative error occurs when the patient does not respond to a stimulus that should have been seen based on prior responses at that location. Fixation losses can be estimated by periodically presenting stimuli within the physiologic blind spot. Patients who see these stimuli are presumed to be looking away from the fixation target. Movement of the eyes from the central fixation point can be detected by modern perimeters, which possess a gaze tracker that monitors pupil location throughout the test.
12. **c.** The Collaborative Normal-Tension Glaucoma Study (CNTGS) was a multicenter randomized controlled clinical trial comparing observation and treatment (30% reduction in IOP) for normal-tension glaucoma. The study found that lowering IOP by at least 30% decreased the 5-year risk of visual field progression from 35% to 12%, after adjusting for the effect of cataract.
13. **b.** Elevated IOP is a significant risk factor for the development of glaucoma, but it is not required for a primary open-angle glaucoma (POAG) diagnosis. Several studies have shown that between 30% and 50% of individuals in the general population with glaucomatous optic neuropathy and/or visual field loss present with an initial IOP measurement below 22 mm Hg. In addition, IOP can vary considerably over a 24-hour period.

14. **b.** The Baltimore Eye Survey found that the prevalence of glaucoma increases considerably with age, particularly among Black individuals. In this group, prevalence exceeded 11% in people 80 years of age and older. Ocular perfusion was not studied in the Baltimore Eye Survey. The Ocular Hypertension Treatment Study found an increased risk of conversion from ocular hypertension to glaucoma with age (per decade). The Collaborative Initial Glaucoma Treatment Study found that visual field defects (ie, glaucoma progression) were 7 times more likely to progress in patients aged 60 years or older than in patients younger than 40 years.
15. **c.** Interlenticular opacification and iris chafing are complications that may occur with implantation of piggyback intraocular lenses within the capsular bag. Iris chafing can result in pigment dispersion syndrome and associated elevated IOP, presumably from obstruction of the trabecular meshwork by pigment granules. On gonioscopy, the trabecular meshwork commonly appears as homogeneous and densely pigmented, with speckled pigment at or anterior to the Schwalbe line, forming a Sampaolesi line. Other findings associated with pigment dispersion syndrome include pigment deposits on the corneal endothelium (Krukenberg spindle); midperipheral iris transillumination defects; and pigment deposits on the zonular fibers, on the anterior hyaloid, and in the equatorial region of the lens capsule (Zentmayer line/ring, or Scheie stripe). The findings listed as other answer choices are not associated with pigment dispersion syndrome.
16. **c.** The most likely diagnosis is phacolytic glaucoma, caused by leakage of high-molecular-weight proteins through microscopic openings in the lens capsule of a mature or hypermature cataract. These proteins obstruct the trabecular meshwork, resulting in elevated IOP. The lack of keratic precipitates helps distinguish phacolytic glaucoma from phacoantigenic glaucoma. Phacoantigenic glaucoma occurs because of sensitization of the eye to native lens protein, causing a granulomatous reaction. Lens particle glaucoma occurs because of retention of lens material after cataract surgery or ocular trauma. Phacomorphic glaucoma is induced by a relatively large lens pushing the iris forward, causing angle closure.
17. **d.** Miotic agents are not recommended in patients with anterior uveitis because they may exacerbate the inflammation and result in the formation of central posterior synechiae. Topical CAIs, α-agonists, and β-blockers are all effective medications in the treatment of uveitic glaucoma.
18. **c.** Corticosteroid-induced glaucoma is an open-angle glaucoma caused by the use of topical, periocular, intravitreous, inhaled, or oral corticosteroids. Approximately 33% of the population without glaucoma demonstrates a mild (6–15-mm-Hg) increase in IOP with corticosteroid use, and 4%–6% of this population has significant IOP elevation of more than 15 mm Hg. In contrast, up to 95% of individuals with POAG develop an ocular hypertensive response to topical corticosteroids. The type and potency of the agent, the route and frequency of its administration, and the susceptibility of the patient all affect the timing and extent of the IOP rise. Risk factors for corticosteroid-induced glaucoma include a history of POAG, a first-degree relative with POAG, very young age (<6 years), or older age.
19. **c.** Although angle closure resulting from rotation of the ciliary body, deposition of tumor cells and inflammatory cells in the trabecular meshwork, direct invasion of the anterior chamber angle, and neovascularization of the angle can all cause glaucoma associated with primary or metastatic tumors of the ciliary body, direct invasion of the anterior chamber angle is the most common cause of glaucoma in this setting. This can be exacerbated by an-

terior segment hemorrhage and inflammation, which further obstruct aqueous outflow. Necrotic tumor and tumor-laden macrophages obstruct the trabecular meshwork and result in a secondary OAG. Tumors causing a secondary glaucoma in adults include uveal melanoma and melanocytoma (see Chapter 8, Figs 8-10 and 8-11), metastatic carcinoma, lymphoma, and leukemia.

20. **d.** This patient has characteristic features of glaucomatocyclitic crisis (also called *Posner-Schlossman syndrome*). Patients with this uncommon form of open-angle inflammatory glaucoma are often mildly or minimally symptomatic despite markedly elevated IOP. On examination, only a few discrete keratic precipitates may be present. Episodes are usually unilateral and recurrent, with normalization of IOP in between attacks. Although attacks are episodic, patients can develop glaucomatous ONH damage and visual field loss. In some cases, filtering surgery is performed to prevent IOP spikes in eyes with advanced optic nerve damage or in those experiencing frequent attacks. Compared with glaucomatocyclitic crisis, herpetic uveitis is generally associated with more inflammation and discomfort. Fuchs uveitis syndrome (formerly, Fuchs heterochromic iridocyclitis) is an insidious and chronic form of uveitis without episodic attacks of elevated IOP. Angle-closure glaucoma is associated with pain and a shallow anterior chamber.
21. **c.** Primary angle-closure glaucoma has been estimated to account for over 90% of blindness due to glaucoma in the Chinese population.
22. **c.** The Zhongshan Angle-Closure Prevention (ZAP) trial identified 889 primary angle-closure suspects. One eye of each subject was randomly assigned to laser peripheral iridotomy (LPI), and the contralateral eye served as a control. The study results showed that very few cases in either group progressed to primary angle-closure glaucoma or an acute attack of angle closure. There was a significantly lower risk of conversion to primary angle closure with treatment. Most cases of conversion to primary angle closure were attributed to formation of peripheral anterior synechiae (PAS) alone.
23. **a.** Scleral buckles (especially the encircling bands) used for retinal detachment repair can produce angle narrowing and frank angle closure, often accompanied by choroidal effusion and anterior rotation of the ciliary body that result in flattening of the peripheral iris with a relatively deep central anterior chamber. With medical therapy (cycloplegics, anti-inflammatory agents, β-adrenergic antagonists, CAIs, and hyperosmotic agents), the anterior chamber usually deepens with opening of the angle over days to weeks. Injection of expansile gas or silicone oil into the eye after pars plana vitrectomy can cause angle closure through forward movement of the lens and/or iris. In general, choroidal effusions are not present in this situation. A surgical iridectomy can be done at the time of the vitrectomy. If a component of pupillary block is present, an LPI may be subsequently performed and beneficial. If performed, the iridotomy or iridectomy should be located inferiorly. Less commonly, the gas or oil may have to be removed. Anti–vascular endothelial growth factor injections can cause elevated IOP, but the mechanism is not due to angle closure.
24. **b.** Neovascular glaucoma (NVG) is a relatively common outcome of central retinal vein occlusion. This patient appears to have an advanced stage of NVG. In this case, given the poor visual prognosis, transscleral cyclophotocoagulation (CPC) may be considered as an alternative to filtering surgery or tube shunt implantation for control of elevated IOP. Complications during filtering surgery or tube shunt implantation often occur in active NVG, so these treatment options are not appropriate for this patient. Lowering the IOP with CPC will likely improve the eye pain. Medical management of the IOP may be instituted at the same

time as treatment of the neovascularization, as a temporizing measure, and/or before surgical treatment. Choosing which class(es) of medication to use will depend on the patient's comorbidities and medical history.

25. **a.** Chandler syndrome, iris nevus syndrome (also called *Cogan-Reese syndrome*), and essential iris atrophy constitute the iridocorneal endothelial (ICE) syndrome. The distinction between the 3 entities is historical and not clearly important for management or prognosis. All are marked by an abnormal corneal endothelium, leading to progressive PAS and elevated IOP. ICE syndrome is unilateral in most cases. In Chandler syndrome, there are minimal anterior segment changes other than high PAS. Iris nevus syndrome is marked by tan pedunculated nodules or diffuse pigmented lesions on the anterior iris surface. Eyes with essential iris atrophy demonstrate heterochromia and corectopia.

    Pseudoexfoliation syndrome typically presents asymmetrically but would not be expected to have the corneal findings described in this scenario. Uveitis can present unilaterally and with PAS but, again, would not be expected to produce the corneal findings noted in this patient. Fuchs endothelial corneal dystrophy causes endothelial changes similar to those observed in ICE syndrome, but these changes typically are bilateral and are not associated with PAS.

26. **a.** This patient has sporadic primary congenital glaucoma (PCG). Without a family history of PCG, an affected patient has a 2% chance of having a child with PCG. The one situation where this calculation would be different is when there is a close familial relationship between parents (consanguinity).

27. **c.** The normal corneal diameter for a newborn is 9.5–10.5 mm. By 2 years of age, the normal corneal diameter is 11–12 mm. A corneal diameter of 11 mm or more in a newborn, greater than 12 mm in a child younger than 1 year, or greater than 13 mm at any age is suggestive of glaucoma.

28. **a.** In children younger than 3 years, the sclera is elastic and will stretch if IOP is not well controlled. This can result in increased axial length despite good IOP during examination under anesthesia. Corneal thickness decreases as corneal edema resolves and, once stable, is often less than the average CCT. The angle can further develop as a child ages, but this does not indicate poor pressure control. Myopia in congenital glaucoma is not necessarily an axial myopia.

29. **b.** Brimonidine is a relatively selective α_2-adrenergic agonist. It lowers IOP by decreasing aqueous production and increasing uveoscleral outflow. Monoamine oxidase inhibitors (MAOIs) (and tricyclic antidepressants) may interfere with the metabolism of apraclonidine and brimonidine, resulting in a toxic effect on the patient. Systemic adverse effects of α_2-selective agonists include xerostomia (dry mouth), lethargy, and headache. Brimonidine should not be used in infants and young children because of the risk of central nervous system (CNS) depression, apnea, bradycardia, and hypotension, due to a combination of the lower volume of distribution and the presumed increased CNS penetration of the drug.

    Latanoprost is a prostaglandin analogue and does not have known interactions with MAOI medications; timolol, a β-blocker, and dorzolamide, a CAI, also are not known to interact with MAOIs.

30. **d.** Rho kinase inhibitors (eg, netarsudil) increase conventional (trabecular meshwork) outflow by increasing phosphorylation and activation of the protein myosin light chain (MLC) phosphatase. Phosphorylated MLC then interacts with actin to affect the physical properties of the cytoskeleton, resulting in relaxation of the cytoskeleton of outflow cells

in the trabecular meshwork and Schlemm canal, allowing increased aqueous outflow. Rho kinase inhibitors also decrease EVP.

Prostaglandin analogues (eg, latanoprost) lower IOP primarily by increasing uveoscleral outflow; they also increase conventional outflow. Topical CAIs (eg, dorzolamide), β-blockers (eg, timolol), and α_2-adrenergic agonists (eg, brimonidine) decrease aqueous humor production. Hyperosmotic agents (eg, mannitol) increase blood osmolality, thus creating an osmotic gradient to draw water from the eye.

31. **c.** A valved plate-based tube implant is the best option for this patient, as the patient has not been seen by an ophthalmologist in the past year and has risk factors that jeopardize the postoperative outcome for a procedure requiring postoperative intervention (as with trabeculectomy). For these reasons, less invasive procedures would also be good; however, because of the disease severity and IOP elevation, this patient likely requires subconjunctival filtering surgery.

    Key considerations when making decisions for the management plan include glaucoma severity, life expectancy, and the presence of any major systemic disease that could affect the outcome. Another key consideration is whether the patient can adhere to medical therapy. For example, a patient who has poor preoperative medication adherence (because of memory loss, poor vision, tremor, or arthritis) is likely to also display poor postoperative adherence to medical therapy. The surgeon should recommend to the patient the procedure that is most likely to successfully reduce IOP with the fewest possible complications. This selection involves considering the patient's ability to return for multiple follow-up visits.

    It is important to minimize risk of surgery in older adult patients through careful preoperative considerations for anesthesia and detailed preoperative evaluation for any potential systemic comorbidities that may affect decisions for the management plan. For this patient, minimizing and simplifying the use of postoperative medications may be important, as well as reducing the frequency of office visits by choosing a procedure that requires the least intensive postoperative management.

32. **c.** When the anterior chamber shallows postoperatively in the absence of overfiltration or choroidal effusions, there should be a high index of suspicion for malignant glaucoma (also known as *aqueous misdirection*). This rare condition is seen most often after trabeculectomy performed for treatment of angle-closure glaucoma. Patients with malignant glaucoma often have elevated IOP; however, the pressure can be "normal."

    Cycloplegic therapy should be initiated in an attempt to normalize the anatomy. Reformation of the anterior chamber is avoided, as the increased posterior pressure will prevent this treatment from being effective. The placement of an oversized contact lens can provide a scaffold for re-epithelialization and may help to stop a bleb leak; with a bleb leak, the IOP invariably will be low in the early postoperative period. Steroids are often increased in the setting of hypotony/choroidal effusions to decrease inflammation.

Index

(*f* = figure; *t* = table)

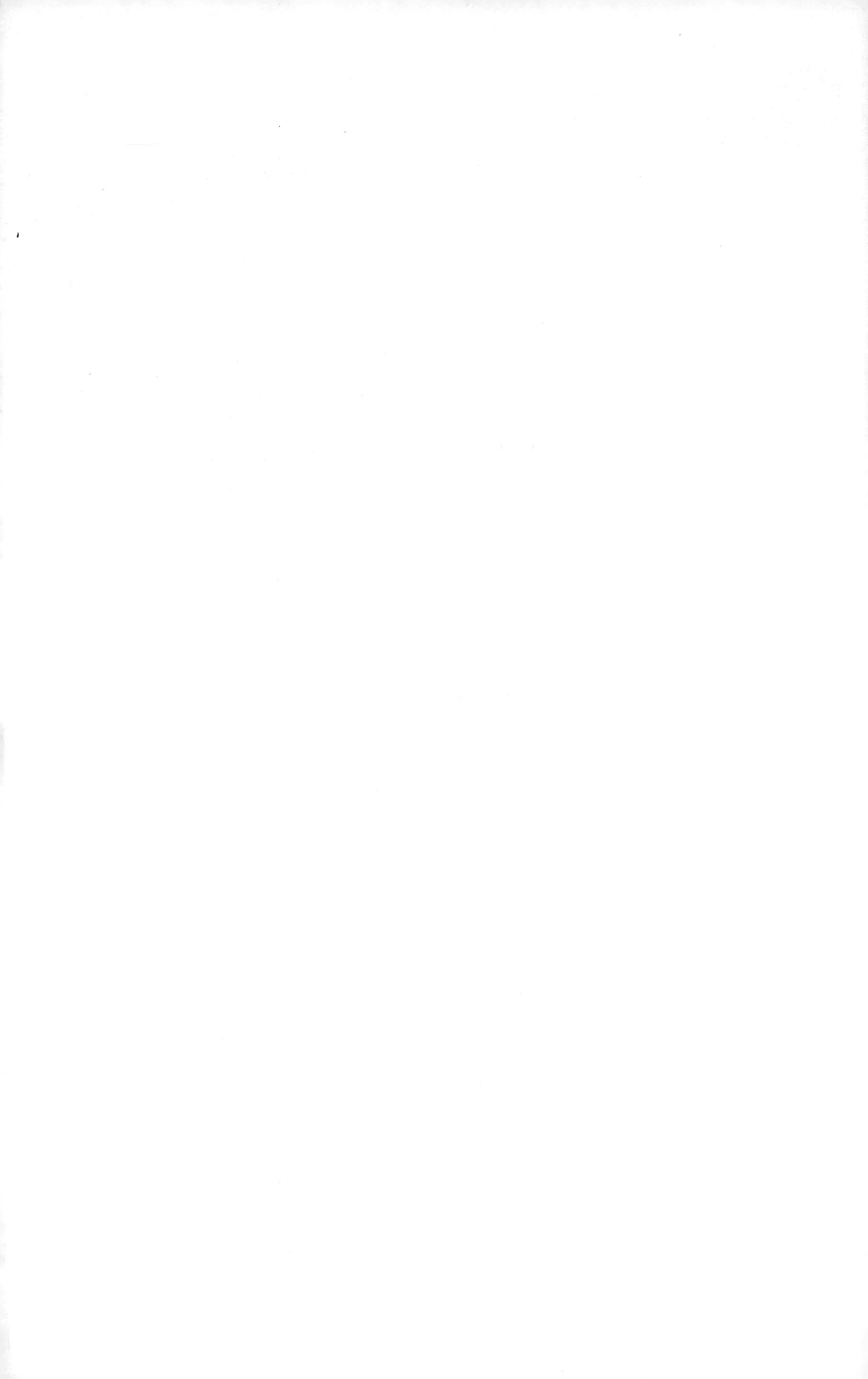